AAOS
Symposium on
Microsurgery
practical use in orthopaedics

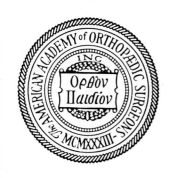

American Academy
of
Orthopaedic Surgeons

Symposium on
Microsurgery

practical use in orthopaedics

Durham, North Carolina
September 1977
May 1979

with 415 *illustrations*

The C. V. Mosby Company

ST. LOUIS · TORONTO · LONDON   1979

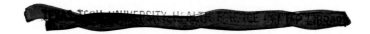

35489

The C. V. Mosby Company
11830 Westline Industrial Drive, St. Louis, Missouri 63141

Library of Congress Cataloging in Publication Data

Symposium on Microsurgery, Durham, N.C., 1977.
  Symposium on Microsurgery.

  Bibliography: p.
  Includes index.
    1. Microsurgery—Congresses.   2. Orthopedic
surgery—Congresses.   I.   American Academy of
Orthopaedic Surgeons.   [DNLM: 1. Microsurgery—
Congresses. 2. Orthopedics—Congresses. WE168
S989s]
RD33.6.S96 1977   617′.05   79-14999
ISBN 0-8016-0066-9

CB/CB/B 9 8 7 6 5 4 3 2 1   01/C/081

Contributors

Donald S. Bright, M.D.

Assistant Professor, Division of Orthopaedic Surgery, Duke University Medical Center, Durham, North Carolina

Richard H. Gelberman, M.D.

Assistant Professor, Division of Orthopaedic Surgery, University Hospital, University of California, San Diego, California

J. Leonard Goldner, M.D.

Professor and Chairman, Division of Orthopaedic Surgery, Duke University Medical Center, Durham, North Carolina

Michael George Hayes, M.B., B.S., F.R.A.C.S.

Former Resident and Microvascular Fellow, Duke University Medical Center, Durham, North Carolina; Visiting Orthopaedic Surgeon, Royal Adelaide Hospital, North Adelaide, South Australia

Hiroo Hiramatsu, M.D.

Department of Orthopaedic Surgery, Hiroshima University School of Medicine, Kasumi, Hiroshima, Japan

Howard W. Klein, M.D.

General Surgery Resident, McGill University, Montreal, Canada

L. Andrew Koman, M.D.

Member of the Orthopaedic Replantation Team, Division of Orthopaedic Surgery, Duke University Medical Center, Durham, North Carolina

Richard S. Kramer, M.D.

Assistant Professor, Division of Neurosurgery, Department of Surgery, Duke University Medical Center, Durham, North Carolina

Joseph E. Kutz, M.D.

Associate Clinical Professor, Department of Surgery, University of Louisville School of Medicine, Louisville, Kentucky

Richard H. Rothman, M.D., Ph.D.

Director of Orthopaedic Surgery, Pennsylvania Hospital, Philadelphia; Professor, Department of Orthopaedic Surgery, University of Pennsylvania School of Medicine, Philadelphia, Pennsylvania

Barry S. Schonwetter, B.S.

University of Florida, College of Medicine, Gainesville, Florida; Former Research Associate, Duke Orthopaedic Microsurgical Laboratory, Duke University Medical Center, Durham, North Carolina

Anthony V. Seaber

Research Associate in Surgery, Division of Orthopaedic Surgery, Duke University Medical Center, Durham, North Carolina

Roni Sehayik, M.D.

Member of Orthopaedic Replantation Team, Division of Orthopaedic Surgery, Duke University Medical Center, Durham, North Carolina

James B. Steichen, M.D.

Assistant Clinical Professor, Department of Orthopaedic Surgery, Indiana University Medical Center, Indianapolis, Indiana

v

Craig R. Stirrat, M.D.

Harvard Combined Orthopaedic Residency Program, Boston, Massachusetts; former Fellow in Orthopaedic Microvascular Surgery, Duke University Medical Center, Durham, North Carolina

Cathy B. Thomson, M.D.

Assistant Professor of Orthopaedics, Department of Orthopaedics and Rehabilitation, University of Miami, Miami, Florida; former Christine Kleinert Hand Surgery Fellow, Department of Surgery, University of Louisville School of Medicine, Louisville, Kentucky

Jack W. Tupper, M.D.

Associate Professor of Orthopaedic Surgery, University of California School of Medicine, Los Angeles, California; Director of Highland Alameda County Hand Clinic, Oakland, California

James R. Urbaniak, M.D.

Professor, Division of Orthopaedic Surgery, Duke University Medical Center, Durham, North Carolina

Fredric H. Warren, M.D.

Member of the Orthopaedic Replantation Team, Division of Orthopaedic Surgery, Duke University Medical Center, Durham, North Carolina

E. F. Shaw Wilgis, M.D.

Assistant Professor of Orthopaedic Surgery and Assistant Professor of Plastic Surgery, The Johns Hopkins Hospital, Baltimore; Attending Hand Surgeon, Union Memorial Hospital, Baltimore, Maryland

Robert H. Wilkins, M.D.

Professor and Chief, Division of Neurosurgery, Duke University Medical Center, Durham, North Carolina

Sydney Wright, O.T.R.

Director, Occupational Therapy Department, Duke Medical Center Rehabilitation Units and Durham Rehabilitation Center, Durham, North Carolina

Preface

The impetus for this Symposium on Microsurgery was provided by two courses on microsurgery sponsored by the Committee on Continuing Medical Education of the American Academy of Orthopaedic Surgeons at the Duke University Medical Center in Durham, North Carolina. The first course, entitled Microsurgery—Practical Use in Orthopaedics, was held on September 15 to 17, 1977, and a second similar course, Microsurgery—Current Status in Orthopaedic Surgery, followed on May 24 to 26, 1979. A faculty of nationally recognized microsurgeons discussed and demonstrated the application of microsurgery in vascular and nerve repair, free tissue transfers, replantation, and spine surgery.

The contents of the 23 chapters of this volume include an updating of many of the formal lectures delivered by members of the Symposium faculty and current pertinent microsurgical topics especially prepared by members of the Duke Orthopaedic Microsurgery Team. In addition, panel discussions conducted by the faculty after the five sections of the first conference were recorded for publication in this text. The readers should find these provocative off-the-cuff discussions to be most informative.

The merits of microsurgery have been proved; no surgical specialty will escape its potential in reconstructive procedures. Although these courses were designed primarily for orthopaedic surgeons, this volume is recommended for imaginative surgeons of all fields of surgery, especially hand surgery, plastic surgery, and neurosurgery. Microsurgery is an extremely demanding discipline that requires patience and perseverance both in the mastering of the skills and in the clinical application. The surgeon may become very frustrated during the early stages of learning the microsurgical techniques; however, once the skills are mastered, the application of the technique is extremely rewarding and satisfying.

We anticipate that microsurgery will become an integral part of the surgical curriculum of most resident education programs. Today microsurgery is a tool for increasing the visualization of an operative field. In the near future, with increased understanding of immunology and physiology of microcirculation, extremity transplantation may become a reality.

We sincerely thank the Symposium faculty and members of the Duke

Orthopaedic Microsurgery Team who donated their valuable time in helping to prepare this text. Special thanks go to Dr. L. Andrew Koman for the initial editing of the audio tapes of the discussions.

James R. Urbaniak
Donald S. Bright

Contents

ix

1. A perspective of microsurgical concepts in orthopaedic surgery

J. Leonard Goldner

This continuing education course sponsored jointly by the American Academy of Orthopaedic Surgeons and the members of the staff of the Division of Orthopaedic Surgery at the Duke University Medical Center indicates the importance of microsurgical concepts as they relate to both research and practice of orthopaedic surgery. The selection of Duke University for this first course related to microsurgical subjects was not done casually by the members of the Academy Committee but with full knowledge that micro-techniques have been practiced at Duke University for many years in the management of musculoskeletal problems and that a replantation team was established as a section of the Orthopaedic Hand Service at Duke University in 1971 although this effort was preceded by less intense attempts at extremity replantation since 1961. We have attempted to maintain an imaginative attitude by planning, teamwork, appropriate laboratory investigation, and rational clinical practice.

Duke Hospital and its outpatient clinics opened in 1930. Dr. W. C. Davison, the first dean, was deeply imbued with the aphorisms of William Osler. The academic and scholastic attitudes prevailed early and continue to this time. Dr. Davison was interested in the "geographic" full-time faculty and stated, "Also, while a medical student at Oxford, I had heard Osler say many times that 'full-time appointments' would subordinate teaching to research."[1]

Deryl Hart was the first professor of Surgery and was instrumental in administering the Surgical Private Diagnostic Clinic, of which we as faculty members in Surgery are members. Lenox Baker was the first medical student admitted to Duke University in 1930 and followed A. I. Shands, Jr., as the second chief of Orthopaedics from 1937 through 1967. I followed Lenox Baker as chief of Orthopaedics, having been appointed to succeed Lenox Baker by David C. Sabiston, Jr., the current chairman of the Department of Surgery. Orthopaedics has expanded during the past 10 years, and the microsurgical aspects of our practice are in keeping with the challenge of solving many complex surgical problems.

1

Although the endowment established by James B. Duke in 1924[1] has been responsible for the development of Duke University, the members of the orthopaedic staff continue to be self-supporting in their role of teachers, clinicians, and clinical and laboratory investigators. Our primary obligation is patient care. We are not protected by the Gothic architecture but do travel out into the state to hold our 12 outlying clinics each month and to provide service and consultation in those outlying clinics for physicians and patients throughout the state.

The Orthopaedic Division includes nine geographic full-time staff, 32 residents at various stages of a 6-year program, two hand fellows, and two microvascular fellows. Five members of the orthopaedic staff are members of the American Society for Surgery of the Hand.

The Orthopaedic Microsurgical Laboratory and the Orthopaedic Research Program are directed by Dr. James R. Urbaniak and myself, and this particular course was organized by Dr. Urbaniak. Dr. Donald S. Bright shares the Microsurgical Clinical and Laboratory Studies with Dr. Urbaniak and other members of the staff, and he has contributed immensely to the development of the Replantation Team at Duke University. Mr. Anthony Seaber is the coordinator of Orthopaedic Research at Duke and has been responsible for most of the organizational details that must be completed in setting up the laboratory for your participation in this practical course.

The reimplantation team at Duke is not mythic but is in constant activity. We have and are treating an average of two reimplantation patients a week and an average of one elective microvascular procedure each week. The team consists of two senior staff, two hand fellows, two microvascular fellows, one physician's associate, four orthopaedic residents, and one combined laboratory and clinical technician, and the usual number of operating room personnel needed for a complex procedure.

Many of you are here today to find out "what it's all about." Others are here to refine their already existing techniques, and others are members of reimplantation teams from elsewhere. Our goal is to present new useful information for each of you at whatever level you are, and, at the same time, place the subject in proper perspective.

The history of microsurgery at Duke in Orthopaedics dates back[2] to 1949 when I organized the Hand Service. Dr. Don Eyler, currently in Nashville, Tennessee, was here as a fellow in Anatomy and was using the dissecting microscope to identify the insertions of the interosseous muscles and to study the microanatomy of the extensor mechanism. I had no difficulty in moving from the Anatomy Laboratory[3] to the operating room by borrowing the Keeler loupes from the ophthalmologists[8] and the magnifying loupes from the otologists.[7] These were used for repairing digital nerves in infants, children, and adults and were also an essential part of the operative procedures on clubfeet.[4] Since the structures of the hand and the foot have the same size, the fear and anxiety of releasing a clubfoot in an infant or in correcting a congenital deformity of the hand before the infant was 6 months of age was eliminated. Tendon repairs of the hand in children, release of contractures associated with clubhand, and early treatment of severe syndactylism were an outgrowth of the availability of magnification equipment.

From 1950 to 1953, nerve grafting was done occasionally and a loupe with 6-power magnification designed for use in industrial work was purchased for actual placement of sutures. The focal distance was short and the circumference of the field was small. I released the transverse retinacular ligament at the wrist of a patient with median nerve compression in 1950 and used magnification to examine the vascular markings of the nerve as the tourniquet was released and to dissect out the motor branch of the median nerve that was compressed by the fascia adjacent to the thenar muscles. Our major problem at that time was not visibility but availability of microinstruments and microsuture.[5] We borrowed the smallest available equipment from the ophthalmologists such as the cataract knife, the spring-lock needle holder, a jewelers' forceps, and 7-0 silk sutures. The needles and suture were too large, and the silk was too reactive to expect an ideal result when 2 mm nerves were sutured.[8] Repair of 1 mm blood vessels was impractical at that time.[9]

In 1960, we secured the Mentor* microscope with a table attachment and oculars of different optics with magnification up to 9 power.[6] During this same period, operating microscopes were being developed for ear and eye surgery, and they were available for hand surgery. Most of the operative procedures on nerves, tendons, or small blood vessels could be done with 3-power magnification supplemented by 6-power loupes at critical times during the procedure and occasionally 9 power with the tabletop microscope.

In 1973, we secured an operating microscope for both laboratory and clinical use. At the same time, the suppliers of operating instruments and suture material made available smaller needles and nylon suture. The progression of the development of BV-3 and BV-6 needles for 8-0 and 10-0 suture resulted in successful repair of vessels with a diameter of 1 mm or less.[9] The development of microinstrumentation complemented the availability of operating-room magnification during this time. As we review many operative procedures in all of Surgery during the past 20 years, we note that the development of surgical procedures marks time while industry and engineers and research grants provide the motivation and the funds for development. The space age, the moon shot, and the centers in the country devoted to development of complex microelectrodes parallel the development of microinstrumentation.

During this same period, we have observed the development of high-density polyethylene, highly polished electrolytically neutral metal, silicone and silicone-Dacron implants, heart valves, Dacron blood vessel grafts, use of

---

*Codman & Shurtleff, Inc., Randolph, Mass. 02368.

the laser beam for detached retinas, and the use of the operating microscope in brain surgery.

There are published accounts of a ruptured intervertebral disc being removed under 40-power magnification, of internal neurolysis of a peripheral nerve at 20-power magnification, and blood vessels of less than 1 mm being sutured by a modification of a Water-Pik forceps and BV-6 needle and 10-0 suture. Other methods of joining vessels are being developed in order to prevent endothelial scarring and to ensure smooth coaptation of blood vessels in order to prevent thrombosis at the suture site.

The field of microsurgery is young, the information explosion continues, and the orthopaedic resident of today must be proficient in the "wonderful world of microsurgery." Harry Buncke, one of the pioneers in the field, uses that description in relating his impression of the improved visibility and likens it to scuba diving.[9] As all of you become familiar with magnifications of 3 to 5 power, you will be impressed by the tissue irritation that occurs during a procedure and will realize the importance of handling tissue gently, performing retraction with minimal force, and protecting soft tissue by appropriate packing and frequent irrigation.

Microsurgical technique as it is used by a surgeon placing a vein graft to make up a defect in a 2 mm blood vessel requires an awareness of the trauma that occurs to the endothelium in completing the anastomosis. The same changes are also apparent and more readily visible on the surface of a high-density polyethylene prosthesis or on the smooth surface of a metal implant. Constant awareness of the small scratches that occur on surfaces of these implants by casual contact, and the microalterations that occur in bone, muscle, tendon, and red cells when these parts of the musculoskeletal system are touched or stressed emphasize the planning and care that must be involved in working with these tissues as well as restoring them to a physiologic level. During this course, we will emphasize the importance of using micro-techniques in decompressing cervical nerve roots, in repairing blood vessels, in managing nerve injuries, and in doing tendon repair. Also, correcting club-foot deformities, working with articular surface irregularities, and identifying small bleeding points to provide a dry field after a big operation are a few of the advantages that occur from recognition of the importance of micro-techniques.

You are here today because you are interested in the subject, you wish to participate in learning these procedures, and you want to take another step in bringing yourself up to date. Microsurgical techniques assist the careful surgeon to be even more careful. The use of certain minimal microtechniques will improve your surgical procedures on a day-to-day basis. Adopting these techniques for suturing small vessels and nerves, however, does take constant practice, good judgment, and high-quality equipment. Replantation is essentially done by the team approach. Physical exhaustion from many hours of work prior to the initiation of the replant, and fatigue during the procedure demand readily available replacements.

Finally, the members of the faculty, both from Duke and from other centers, who have agreed to participate are doing this for many reasons. They are willing to share their past experiences and mistakes, they have a desire to teach and at the same time learn while they are teaching. They have given many hours of their valuable time to prepare their material, they have given up free time to participate in the course, and this time was taken from their family and from their nonmedical activities. Their presence here will benefit you and the public directly. This faculty and other similar groups are yet another panel of unsung heroes of modern medicine who are not well recognized by those who criticize both our present system and the intent of those working in it. I know that you appreciate the selflessness of these faculty members, as do I, and I emphasize to all of you the appreciation that goes to the Academy Committee encouraging those who are willing to take the time to both plan the course and to execute it.

REFERENCES

1. Davison, W. C.: Reminiscences of W. C. Davison, Dean of the Duke University Medical School, 1927-1960, Durham, N.C., 1966, Duke University Press.
2. Eyler, D. L., and Markee, J. E.: The anatomy and function of the intrinsic musculature of the fingers, J. Bone Joint Surg. **36-A**(1):1-9, Jan. 1954.
3. Goldner, J. L., and Wrenn, R.: An experimental study of the effect of cortisone on the healing process and tensile strength of tendons, J. Bone Joint Surg. **36-A**(3): 588-601, June 1954.
4. Goldner, J. L.: Congenital talipes equinovarus, laboratory dissections, observation and techniques, unpublished data, Durham, N.C., 1950-1978.
5. Goldner, J. L.: Repair of peripheral nerves, techniques; presentation, Calgary, Alberta, Canada, 1962.
6. Smith, James: Magnification techniques for repairing peripheral nerves, personal communication, New York, 1962.
7. Arnold, R.: Magnification in otology, personal communication, Durham, N.C., 1956.
8. Anderson, B.: Magnification and instrumentation in ophthalmology, personal communication, Durham, N.C., 1951.
9. Buncke, H.: Suture techniques in repairing 1 mm veins, presentation, Clinical Day, American Society for Surgery of the Hand, 1967.

2. A history of microsurgery

Richard H. Gelberman

In 1917, J. F. Esser, a New Jersey surgeon, first transferred a composite flap based on a single vascular pedicle.[7] Less than 50 years later, in July 1965, in Nara, Japan, after several clinical failures Shigeo Komatsu and Susuma Tamai anastomosed the arteria princeps pollicis and successfully replanted a completely amputated thumb.[13] The notable developments of the intervening 50 years have become the early history of microsurgery.

The development of microsurgery can be conveniently divided into three major stages. The events of the first stage, the early years, were attributable to the efforts of several surgeons in four or five surgical disciplines. Their initial successes in large vessel surgery involved the transfer of tissue from one location to another within the body. This was first accomplished in the early 1900s when composite grafts and transplants were performed by use of macrotechniques for arterial and venous anastomosis. The earliest pedicle tissue transfers are attributed to Carrell and Guthrie as well as Esser.[3,7] It was not until the post–World War II period with advances in renal transplantation, however, that a successful model was established for tissue transplantation with vascular anastomosis. Although Joseph Murray, of Boston, generated much of the new interest in transplantation surgery, it was Sun Lee at the University of Pittsburgh who set up the first transplant laboratory.[8,20] Lee predicted the interest that would ultimately arise in small vessel surgery: "It seems only logical after the resurgence of interest in vascular surgery in the middle of the century, efforts should be exerted towards successful anastomoses of smaller and smaller vessels—both arteries and veins. Induced by the poor results reported after the suturing of vessels less than 4 mm in diameter, pessimism pervaded relative to the feasibility of such vascular surgery by conventional means. Consequently, a variety of techniques and aims have been proposed to improve results."[8]

It was from Lee's laboratory that many of the first clinical microsurgeons emerged. The first stage of development of microsurgery was evolving because of the foresight of Carrell, Guthrie, Murray, and Lee, and the ability to transplant tissues within the body with predictable success had been

6

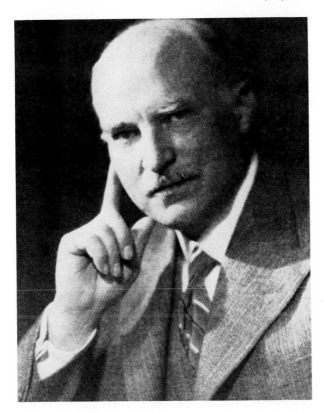

Fig. 2-1. Gunnar Holmgren, Swedish otolaryngologist who originally used the operating microscope in the surgery of otosclerosis in 1921.

achieved. Douglas and Ladanyi individually attempted some early digital reattachments without vascular anastomosis.[6,16] Most of their attempts failed. The need for small vessel anastomosis was appreciated and the concept of tissue revascularization had been established. By 1945, the surgeons' attitude and skill had become unquestionably adequate, but the ability to perform microvascular anastomoses would still be over 20 years away. Composite tissue transfers and elongation of vascular pedicles were being considered with structures of smaller caliber, but the step from stage I to stage II could only be accomplished with the emergence of a completely new surgical discipline, using the most demanding techniques in modern surgery.

Clinical use of the dissecting binocular microscope began in the 1920s when Holmgren first used it in middle ear surgery[11] (Figs. 2-1 and 2-2). It was not until the late 1940s, however, that a realization of a need for higher degrees of magnification for other types of surgery was appreciated, Bernard Seidenberg established an experimental program in New York, involving the anastomosis of arteries varying in diameter from 1.5 to 4 mm. He used magnification

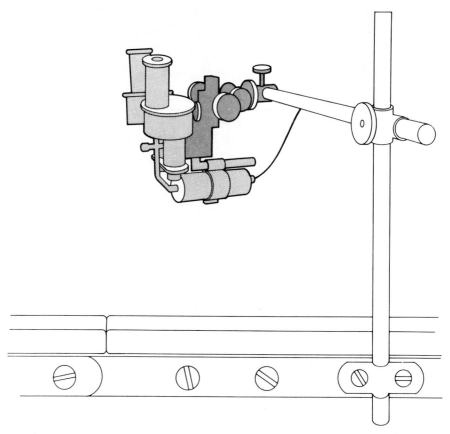

Fig. 2-2. Holmgren-Zeiss operating microscope. One of the early operating microscopes used in 1922.

for successful microvascular anastomoses in dogs in 1950.[23] It was not until 1960, however, that Julius Jacobson, Donald Miller, and Ernesto Suarez of Burlington, Vermont, coined the term "microsurgery."[12] To that time, results of surgery on vessels smaller than 3 to 4 mm had been uniformly poor. They described a new technique for performing anastomoses with the dissecting microscope. It demanded more precision since the anastomosis was performed under 10 to 25 magnifications. For the first time, bits of intima could be trimmed and removed from the suture line. A newer, precise coaptation technique was substituted for previous inversion and eversion macrotechniques. They miniaturized their conventional surgical instruments and achieved a 100% patency rate in 26 dog and rabbit carotids, averaging 2 mm in diameter.

While Jacobson, Miller, and Suarez were introducing the technique for microsurgery, others were developing and refining microscopic instruments. The compound microscope, invented in the 1500s, was not used experimentally until 1921, when Nylen, of Sweden, used it to dissect the inner ear of a rabbit.[21] Nylen is now considered the father of modern operating microscopy. Holmgren introduced the Carl Zeiss binocular operating microscope in 1923.[11] It was used by ear surgeons from that time, but not until 1946 was it adapted clinically by another subspecialty, ophthalmology. Jacobson and Suarez introduced it to coronary artery surgery in 1960,[12] Michon and Masse to peripheral nerve surgery in 1964,[18] Harry Buncke to plastic surgery in 1965,[2] and Donaghy and Yaşargil to neurosurgery in 1967.[5] The microscope had become a sophisticated instrument. Zeiss, Contraves, and Weck had constructed microscopes with motorized focusing units, zoom optics, and single-foot controls to free the hands for uninterrupted surgery. Bernard M. O'Brien made some further modifications to the Zeiss triploscope as it was readied for clinical microvascular surgery and replantation.[22] Acland of Great Britain and Buncke of the United States became interested in finer instrumentation and developed smaller needles and fine metallicized sutures.[1,2] Commercially produced microsuture soon became available in Japan, China, and Australia. With the dissecting microscope and fine suture materials available, the origins of clinical microsurgery were established. The need was apparent. With digital artery lacerations involving inside vessel diameters of 1 mm, would it be possible to perform predictably successful anastomoses? In neurorrhaphy, neurolysis, and nerve grafting under microscopic magnification, would it make a difference?

In its infancy, clinical microsurgery would have as great an impact on hand surgery as any new development of the past 50 years. On May, 23, 1962, Ronald Malt at Massachusetts General Hospital performed the first historical clinical replantation, at the midarm level.[17] In November 1962, Harold Kleinert reanastomosed a digital artery with 9-0 suture and replanted a partially amputated thumb.[14] The first complete digital replant was that of a thumb by Komatsu and Tamai on July 22, 1965.[13] Clinical replantation, transplantation, and free transfers were soon to follow. From isolated pioneer microsurgical work, organized replantation centers appeared in the 1970s. Surgeons like O'Brien, Tamai, Kleinert, Buncke, Urbaniak, and Millesi were to implement the third stage in the development of microsurgery.

In the early 1970s, clinical replant centers were organized in several countries—Kleinert and Kutz in Louisville, Kentucky; O'Brien in Melbourne, Australia; Tamai in Tokyo, Japan; Ikuta in Hiroshima, Japan; Lendvay and Owen in Sydney, Australia; and Urbaniak in Durham, North Carolina. Characteristic of the clinical stage of microsurgery was the emergence of the microsurgical unit. One example of its development was at Duke University Medical Center. In the early 1970s an animal laboratory was organized for the practice of microtechniques and for the exploration of problems with suturing techniques, transplant methods, and vascular spasm.[24-26] In late 1972, the first clinical replant at Duke University, a completely amputated thumb, was performed. The surgical team system had been established, with surgeons and assistants alternating during the procedure. A nursing and microsurgery paramedical team was organized. A transplantation system for the southeast with helicopters and air-flying services was established. With rapid transport, efficient transfer of the patient and digit through the emergency room to the operating room, and cooperating teams of surgeons and assistants, an initial surgical success rate of 76% was achieved. That would improve to almost 90% by 1976.[9] Other centers emerged, and by 1977, clinical replantation was being performed in many metropolitan centers throughout the world. Each of the leaders had done well over 50 replantations by this time, and some had performed more then 100, with success rates of over 80% viability.

The development of microsurgical techniques offered other new possibilities. Microsurgical epineurectomy and internal neurolysis in case of interfascicular fibrosis minimized the risk of damage to the intact fascicles. Hanno Millesi in Vienna, Austria, had introduced the concept of no-tension nerve repair with cable grafting and reported improved techniques with the operating microscope.[19] Thomas Gibson, a plastic surgeon from Glasgow, Scotland, reported a free flap with small vessel anastomosis.[10] Intrafascicular nerve repair, free muscle transfers, toe-to-hand transfers, and free composite flaps were performed with microtechnique in several centers.[15] The development of microsurgery had been a complex one. Surgeons of several disciplines in many countries had made contributions, as they introduced the techniques to their respective fields. The fundamental principles and operative details of successful small vessel anastomosis had been described. It was no longer the experience of surgeons that the percentage of successful results decreased sharply as the vessel size diminished. The dissecting microscope is now being used with increasing frequency for identifying and treating disorders in orthopedic surgery. Filling of defects in long bones by microvascular anastomosis of composite free bone grafts is now being done clinically. Free muscle transfers, intercostal nerve grafts, one-stage toe-to-hand transfers, and arterialized flaps from the foot are being performed with some frequency. The future of microsurgery in the field of orthopedic surgery is growing as the indications for microneural and microangionic repairs increase. The ultimate application of microsurgery at this time continues to be digital replantation. Eventually, this may be just a small part of an entire discipline known as "clinical microsurgery."

REFERENCES

1. Acland, R.: New instruments for microvascular surgery, Br. J. Surg. **59**:181, 1972.
2. Buncke, H. J., and Murray, D. E.: Autogenous arterial interposition graft of less than 1 mm in external diameter, Trans. Fifth Int. Congr. Plast. Reconstr. Surgeons, Melbourne, 1971.
3. Carrell, A., and Guthrie, C. C.: Complete amputation of the thigh with replantation, Am. J. Med. Sci. **131**:297, 1906.

4. Daniller, A. I., and Strauch, B.: Symposium on microsurgery, St. Louis, 1976, The C. V. Mosby Co.
5. Donaghy, R. M. P., and Yaşargil, M. C.: Microvascular surgery. St. Louis, 1967, The C. V. Mosby Co.
6. Douglas, B.: Successful replacement of completely avulsed portions of fingers as composite grafts, Plast. Reconstr. Surg. **23**:213, 1959.
7. Esser, J. S.: Island flaps, N.Y. Med. J. **106**:264, 1917.
8. Fisher, B., and Lee, S.: Microvascular surgical techniques and research surgery, Surgery **58**:904, 1965.
9. Gelberman, R. H., Urbaniak, J. R., Bright, D. S., and Levin, L. S.: Digital sensibility following replantation, J. Hand Surg. **3**:313,1978.
10. Gibson, T.: Modern trends in plastic surgery, London, 1964, Butterworth & Co. (Publishers).
11. Holmgren, G.: Some experience in surgery of otosclerosis, Acta Otolaryngol. (Stockholm) **5**:460, 1923.
12. Jacobson, J. H., and Suarez, E. L.: Microsurgery and anastomosis of small vessels, Surg. Forum **9**:243, 1960.
13. Komatsu, S., and Tamai, S.: Successful replantation of a completely cut off thumb, Plast. Reconstr. Surg. **43**:374, 1968.
14. Kleinert, H. E., Kasten, H. L., and Romero, J. L.: Small blood vessel anastomosis for salvage of severely injured upper extremities, J. Bone Joint Surg. **458**:788, 1963.
15. Kreizek, T. J., Tassboro, T., Desperez, Q. O., and Kiohn, C. L.: Experimental transplantation of composite grafts by microvascular anastomosis, Plast. Reconstr. Surg. **36**:358, 1956.
16. Ladanyi, J.: Trapianto del salante del dito, Minerva Med. **61**:671, 1970.
17. Malt, R. S.: Replantation of severed arms, J.A.M.A. **189**:114, 1964.
18. Michon, J., and Masse, P.: Le moment optimum de la suture nerveuse dans les plaies de membre supérieur, Rev. Chir. Orthop. **50**:205-212, 1964.
19. Millesi, H., and Berger, A.: The interfascicular nerve graft, J. Bone Joint Surg. **54-A**:727, 1972.
20. Murray, J. E.: Correct evaluation of human kidney transplantation, Plast. Reconstr. Surg. **34**:93, 1963.
21. O'Brien, B. M.: Microvascular reconstructive surgery, London, 1977, Churchill Livingstone.
22. O'Brien, B. M., MacLeod, A. M., Miller, T. D. H., Newing, R. K., Hayhurst, J. W., and Morrison, W. A.: Clinical implantation of digits, Plast. Reconstr. Surg. **53**:490, 1973.
23. Seidenberg, B., Hurwitt, E. S., and Carton, C. A.: Techniques of anastomosing small arteries, Surg. Gynecol. Obstet. **106**:743, 1958.
24. Urbaniak, J. R.: Instructional course, American Academy of Orthopedic Surgeons Course on Microsurgery, Durham, North Carolina, September 15-17, 1977.
25. Urbaniak, J. R., and Bright, D. S.: Replantation of amputated hands and digits, presented at the American Orthopedic Association Meeting, Hot Springs, Virginia, 1975.
26. Urbaniak, J. R., Soucacos, P. N., Adelar, R. S., Bright, D. S., and Whitehurst, L. A.: Experimental evaluation of microsurgical techniques and small vessel anastomoses, Orthop. Clin. North Am. **8**(2):249-273, April 1977.

3. The microsurgery laboratory

Craig R. Stirrat
Anthony V. Seaber

The microsurgery laboratory serves three major functions. First, it introduces the novice surgeon to the basic techniques of microsurgery. Second, it allows the experienced microvascular surgeon an opportunity to refine his ability and experiment with innovative techniques. Third, it provides a facility for research and development.

The distinction between the first two functions is an important one. Microvascular technique is a surgical skill of increasing importance in clinical surgery. As a surgical skill, it is unique compared to other skills acquired within the operating room because it can be learned in a small-scale laboratory. This aspect is particularly important for the beginning surgeon who may not have the opportunity to participate in the surgery within the operating room, but can perform the same procedures on vessels and nerves in the laboratory.

For the experienced surgeon, the laboratory offers an opportunity for practice and improvement in dexterity. Such dexterity may take years to develop in clinical work, whereas in the microvascular laboratory there are models that can improve dexterity and refine surgical judgment in short periods of time.

Laboratory setting

Because of the high level of concentration required to perform microsurgery, the area chosen for the laboratory should be a self-contained room. Distractions from noise and vibrations should be kept at a minimum. All planning for the laboratory area should acknowledge that the slightest distraction while the microscope is in use will hamper the student performing microsurgery.

Electrical fittings should be adequate so that many pieces of equipment can work simultaneously. When it is possible to design the laboratory from the beginning, it is important to have the location of the operating microscope and major pieces of equipment on the plans. Then all electrical outlets can be placed to avoid overhead wires or cords crossing the room.

12

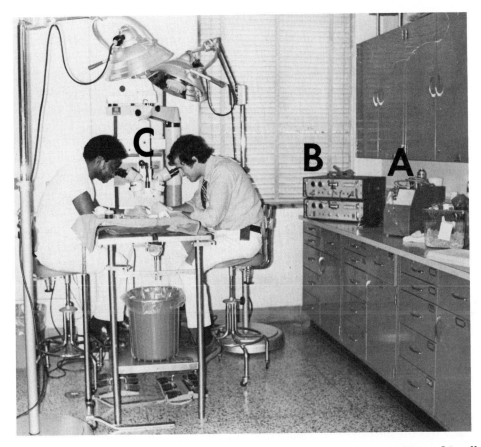

Fig. 3-1. An orthopaedic microsurgery laboratory at Duke University. **A,** Harvard Small Animal Respirator (Harvard Apparatus, 150 Dover Road, Millis, Mass. 02054). **B,** Two Micron Magnetic Flowmeters (Micron Instruments, Inc., 1519 Pontius Ave, Los Angeles, Cal. 90025). **C,** Weck Microscope, Model no. 10122. Although a Weck Microscope is pictured, other companies manufacture microscopes that can be used in the laboratory.

Microscope

Knowing that the laboratory is the training ground for clinical work, ideally the same or similar instrumentation should be used in the laboratory as in the operating room. The most expensive piece of equipment in the laboratory is the operating microscope (Fig. 3-1). The cost of a microscope is related to the quality of its optics and to built-in or added-on features. In microsurgical procedures the microscope adds a magnification interface between the surgeon and the operative site. Depending on the sophistication of the microscope purchased, the intrusion of this interface can be minimized.

In the initial stages of acquiring microsurgical skills, a single-person binocular microscope with a magnification capability of 10× to 15× is quite functional. Such a microscope allows the beginning surgeon to practice on microsurgical models and develop dexterity in using the microscope.

As one's skill increases, the appeal of a more sophisticated microscope will become apparent. Features that are desirable include the ease of changing powers of magnification and the ease of focusing. Foot-controlled focusing and magnification changes can greatly lessen the fatigue and distraction of adjusting the microscope. Depth of focus, field of view, and strength of illumination are also important considerations in lessening fatigue when the microscope is used.

A microscope that allows two surgeons to view the field can be important in the laboratory when more difficult procedures are performed. The success of many microsurgical procedures will depend on a team effort, which is enhanced by two surgeons seeing the operative field with equal facility. Whether this is achieved with split-beam imaging or separate binocular units depends on personal preference and comfort.

Despite the appeal of an elaborate laboratory microscope, the cost can be prohibitive. With the expanded interest in microsurgery, the competitiveness of microscope suppliers is increasing. Lender microscopes are frequently available for trial periods. If one is available, perform a microsurgical procedure with it in the lab. Experience the depth of focus, field size, ease of focusing, range of magnification, and ease of changing magnification. Check the brightness of illumination at higher powers of magnification. Find out what features can be added, such as another binocular head or photographic equipment. Try to work with a basic microscope that will allow additions to it as a more sophisticated microscope is required.

Surgical instruments

The laboratory should have separate instrument sets for gross dissection and microsurgical work.

The following will be needed for gross dissection:
> Scalpel for cutting skin
> Tenotomy scissors for dissecting
> Ring-handled scissors for heavier cutting
> Self-retaining skin retractor
> Needle holder
> Adson forceps
> Anesthetic (sodium pentobarbital) and syringe
> Skin sutures for retraction and closure
> Animal board

Microsurgery instruments needed include the following (Fig. 3-2):
> Needle holder, Barraquer type (curved) without lock
> Forceps with tying platform
> Forceps, jewelers', nos. 3, 4, and 5

Microscissors, spring loaded (curved or straight)
Fine ring-handled iris scissors (straight)
Vessel dilator—lacrymal dilator of hockey-stick shape
Vessel dilator—pencil tip shape
Irrigating cannula with 27-gauge or filed-down 27-gauge needle
Weck-Cels or Q-Tips
Sponges, 2×2s
Plastic beaker with foam liner
Normal saline for irrigation
Heparin
Syringe for irrigation and lidocaine (Xylocaine)
Lidocaine (Xylocaine) 1%
Suture
Bipolar cautery and forceps or battery-powered cautery

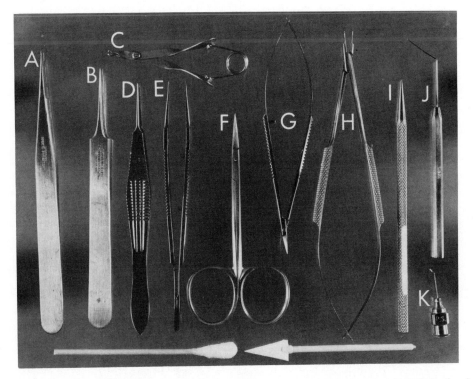

Fig. 3-2. Basic set of microsurgery instruments. **A,** Jewelers' forceps no. 3. **B,** Jewelers' forceps no. 5. **C,** Microvascular clamp–applying forceps. **D** and **E,** Forceps with tying platforms. **F,** Straight, fine ring-handled iris scissors. **G,** Spring-handled microscissors with straight blades and pointed tips. **H,** Curved Barraquer type of needle holder without lock. **I,** Vessel dilator, pencil-tip shape. **J,** Vessel dilator, hockey-stick shape. **K,** No. 27-gauge irrigating cannula. *Bottom of picture,* Weck-Cel and Q-Tip for sponging.

Fig. 3-2 represents an example of a set of microvascular instruments. *A* and *B* are two types of jewelers' forceps that can be modified to either very fine points for grasping tissue or rounded points for holding the suture. Jewelers' forceps (5*B*) are the most delicate and represent an inexpensive, versatile forceps for microsurgery use. Forceps *D* and *E* represent ones with tying platforms to allow better grasping of the suture. The fine ring-handled iris scissors, *F*, is used only for cutting the vessel in preparation for the anastomosis. The microscissors, *G*, which in this case have straight blades, are spring loaded and allow for fine dissection. Other pairs are available with curved blades or rounded points. The needle holder, *H*, is the curved Barraquer type without a lock. It is important to have instruments without locks because the jarring action of the lock release will be increased by the microscope's magnification and disrupt the fine control of the needle. The dilators, *I* and *J*, are used for opening the vessel ends prior to repair. The pencil-tipped dilator, *I*, works well on millimeter-sized vessels. Additionally there is a hockey stick–shaped dilator that will work well on vessels smaller than a millimeter. A 27-gauge irrigation cannula, *K*, can be modified from existing needles or purchased separately. At the bottom of the figure are examples of a Weck-Cel* and Q-Tip, either of which can be used for sponging the field during repair. *C* is a microvascular clamp applicator used with the clamps in Fig. 3-3.

Fig. 3-3 represents five types of microvascular clamps. There are two mi-

———

*Edward Weck & Co., Inc., Long Island City, N.Y. 11101.

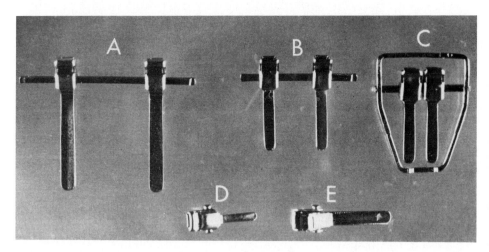

Fig. 3-3. Different types and sizes of microvascular clamps and anastomotic approximators. **A,** Microvascular clamp approximator useful for repairs on larger vessels and interposing vein grafts. **B,** Microvascular clamp approximator for anastomosis of vessels of 1 mm diameter. **C,** Microvascular clamp approximator with outrigger. **D** and **E,** Single microclamps of different sizes.

crovascular clamp approximators of different sizes, *A* and *B*. The larger size, *A*, functions well for interposing vein grafts in segmented defects. Additionally there is a microvascular clamp with an outrigger, *C*, to support the stay sutures. This type of clamp is of great assistance to the beginning microvascular surgeon who is learning the procedures without assistance. There are also two single clips, *D* and *E*, that are useful in various microvascular models to be discussed later in this chapter.

Care and maintenance of instruments. In surgical endeavors, surgeons are instrument-dependent artisans. Malfunctioning of instruments from either mistreatment or neglect can disrupt the concentration of the surgeon and contribute to a less desirable result. Because microvascular instruments are designed for work under magnification, imperfections of the slightest nature can become evident and disrupt the function of the instrument. For this reason, microsurgery instruments require careful handling throughout the surgical procedure and during their cleaning and storage. For storage, a rubber-lined metal case can give protection to the entire set of instruments. Such a case is represented in Fig. 3-4. This case has the benefits of being compact and autoclavable. It is opened on the surgical table only when the microvascular portion of the operation begins. This restriction on availability of the instruments prevents their use in gross dissection, which is a frequent cause of damage.

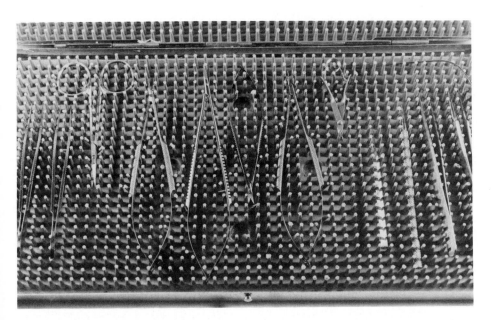

Fig. 3-4. Rubber-lined, autoclavable metal case for microsurgery instruments. Storz Microinstrument Case Model E7212.

Another frequent cause of damage to instruments occurs as the surgeon replaces the used instrument on the metal tray or into a stainless steel bowl. As seen in Fig. 3-5, *A*, this damage was done to a pair of microforceps that were roughly placed into a stainless steel bowl. To eliminate such damage, a successful method has been to line a disposable plastic beaker with packing foam rather than using steel bowls (Fig. 3-6).

Fig. 3-7 demonstrates a standard tool cart that can be converted into a laboratory workbench. The cart is fully portable and can store all instruments and suture. In this instance the cart has been fitted with a jewelers' wheel and magnification light for modification and repair of instruments. Laboratory personnel can repair or modify most instruments with the use of the jewelers' wheel and magnification light or microscope. Fig. 3-5, *B*, demonstrates the damaged forceps of Fig. 3-5, *A*, after repair in the laboratory.

After their use, all instrument joints should be irrigated free of particles and dried blood. This is particularly important for the microclamps, which can

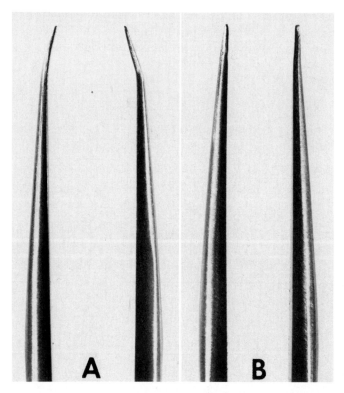

Fig. 3-5. A, The tip of this jewelers' forceps was damaged as it was replaced onto the tray during a training session. The impact rendered the instrument useless for additional microsurgery. **B,** Same forceps is shown after it has been repaired in the laboratory by laboratory personnel using the instrument cart and jewelers' wheel.

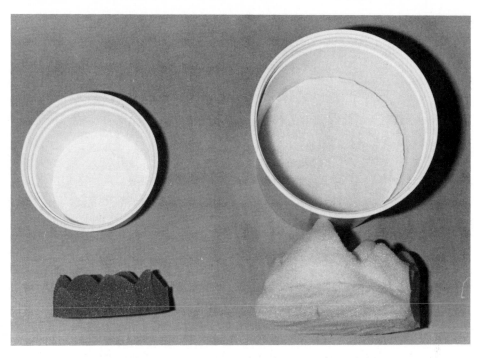

Fig. 3-6. By using packing foam cut to the dimensions of the plastic specimen container, the laboratory has virtually eliminated such damage as is seen in the microsurgery forceps in Fig. 3-5, A.

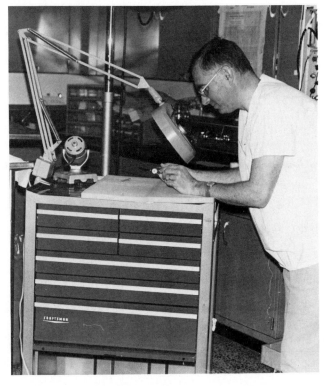

Fig. 3-7. The instrument cart shown above houses all of the spare microinstruments together with the operating microscope accessories. Using this cart, laboratory personnel can repair and modify instruments.

malfunction if dried blood is retained in their spring mechanism. Once irrigated, the instruments should be placed in an antimicrobial water-soluble lubricant.* Never use mineral oil, silicone oil, or machine oil for lubrication as steam cannot penetrate these oils and therefore microorganisms, especially spores, on the instrument surface may not be destroyed by sterilization.

Bipolar cautery

One important addition to the basic microvascular laboratory is the bipolar cautery. This form of cautery allows precise control of the coagulating current. With the use of bipolar forceps, which act as the electrical terminals, the coagulating function is limited to the tissue between the forceps tips. This allows hemostasis of small branch vessels without damage to the main vessel. Many units available allow for the adaptation of microforceps to become coagulating forceps.

The advantage of bipolar cautery in the laboratory is the preparation of vessels for microvascular procedures. Frequently on animal models it is necessary to free the main vessel from branch vessels. If this is done poorly, then bleeding, subadvential hematoma, spasm, or wall damage in the main vessel may result. Fig. 3-8, *A*, demonstrates the precision with which the bipolar cautery can coagulate branch vessels. In this instance the main vessel is 1 mm in diameter and the branch vessel is 0.2 mm in diameter. Fig. 3-8, *B*, shows the result after coagulation without evidence of central vessel damage. The branch can then be safely severed through the area of coagulation. Coagulation is best effected in a wet field as this minimizes tissue shrinkage and adhesion of tissue to the forceps.

A less expensive method of coagulation is the battery-powered cautery. This unit creates an intense heat source, which can coagulate tissue. If touched directly to a vessel, it will frequently burn a hole in the wall without coagulating it. To avoid creation of a hole, one must bring the tip into proximity with the vessel but not touch it and then move the cautery tip back and forth along the vessel until coagulation has occurred.

Microsutures

Inexpensive microsutures† exist for use in the laboratory. These sutures are provided in nonsterile multiple-strand packages with the choice of several needle sizes. The 130- and 143-micron needles are suitable for initial knot-

---

*Codman & Shurtleff, Inc., Randolph, Mass. 02368.
†Davis & Geck, Pearl River, N.Y. 10965:
10-0 Dermalon TE-143 (143 micron needle): product no. 1820-38 (nonsterile)
Ethicon, Inc., Sommerville, New Jersey 08876:
10-0 Ethilon BV-5(130 micron needle): product no. 2887 (nonsterile)
10-0 Ethilon BV-7(75 micron needle): product no. 2888 (nonsterile)

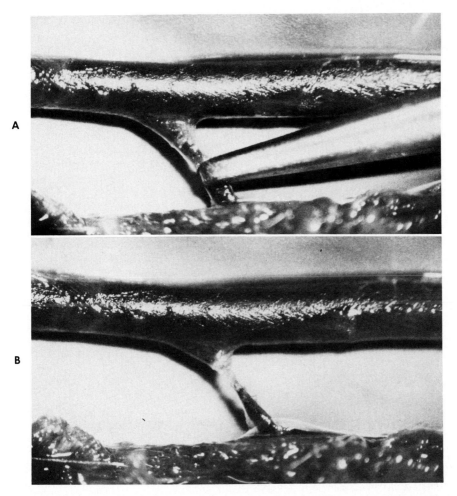

Fig. 3-8. A, An example of a branch vessel measuring 0.2 mm in diameter being coagulated with the bipolar cautery forceps. The central vessel is 1 mm in diameter. **B,** The result after coagulation with no evidence of transmitted damage to the central vessel.

board practice or suturing of a thick-walled vessel such as the aorta of a hamster. As skill increases, the 75-micron needle is used for practice on vessels with diameters of 1 mm. The nonsterile sutures may be used directly from the package or be gas sterilized with the microsurgical set.

BASIC PRINCIPLES IN MICROSURGERY

Before beginning at the microscope, it is important that you adjust the microscope exactly to your individual needs. Make sure the seat and forearm support are at a comfortable height and that there is no strain on the neck or back or shoulders. Adjust the eyepieces for interpupillary distance to allow for

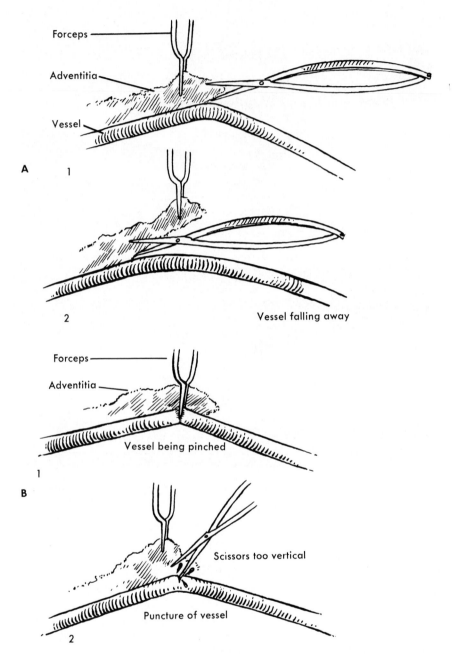

Fig. 3-9. *A,* Right way to dissect—scissors parallel to vessel and forceps holding only adventitia. *B, 1,* Wrong way to dissect—forceps grasping vessel instead of adventitia; *2,* scissors too vertical so that vessel wall risks being cut during dissection.

a single visual field. Adjust each eyepiece individually to ensure that both eyes are in focus, since doing so will maximize the depth of field.

Figs. 3-9 to 3-12 demonstrate the basic principles for dissecting the vessel and performing a microvascular anastomosis. In dissecting vessels, it is important to use the surrounding tissue to protect the vessel wall. The vessel should only be handled by its surrounding tissue. When possible, all dissection should be performed in planes parallel to the vessel as demonstrated in Fig. 3-9. This minimizes the possibility of puncturing the vessel wall as frequently occurs with veins where the thin wall is tented up during the dissection.

Fig. 3-10 shows the cleaning off of the adventitia in preparation for suturing. Two pairs of forceps are sometimes useful in teasing the adventitia so that it can be cut.

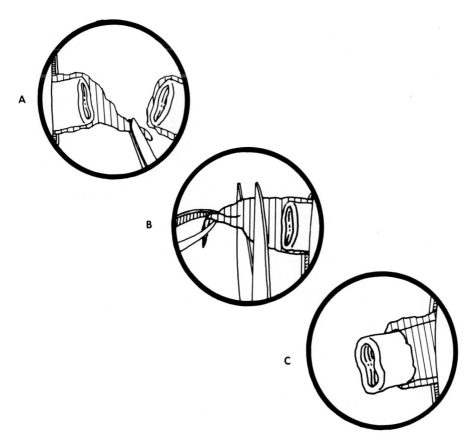

Fig. 3-10. Cleaning off the adventitia. **A,** Adventitia is picked up by a pair of microforceps and advanced well over the end of the vessel. This is in preparation for cutting the adventitia. **B,** Adventitia is cut with a straight pair of microscissors. When the vessel is fully prepared for anastomosis, the end should be cleaned of all adventitia, as shown in **C.**

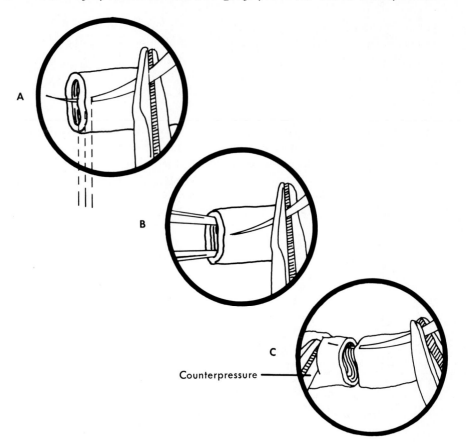

Counterpressure

Fig. 3-11. A, When entering, the needle for *arterial anastomosis* is placed the same distance from the end of the artery as the thickness of the arterial wall. When a *vein anastomosis* is performed, the distance of the entrance of the needle should be more than twice the wall thickness. **B,** Microforceps (tying or jewelers' forceps) or a small blunt probe is inserted into the lumen for the initial needle passing. This protects the back wall while giving counterpressure to the front wall. **C,** Use of microforceps on the receiving vessel during the exit of the needle acts as a counterpressure for better control of placement of the needle.

Irrigation with heparinized saline to wash out retained blood and gentle dilatation with a forceps or dilator will prepare the vessel end for suturing. Figs. 3-11 and 3-12 show the suturing technique, which is termed the "triangulation method." Here the first two sutures are placed from 120° to 160° apart, depending on the vessel size. If an outrigger clamp is available, it can greatly facilitate the repair for the unassisted surgeon by stabilizing these stay sutures. Once the stay sutures are placed, the in-between sutures are placed,

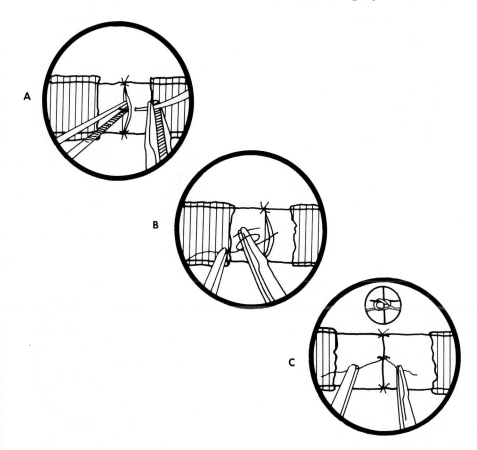

Fig. 3-12. A, In placement of a secondary suture the back wall can be protected by use of a blunt microforceps to receive the needle. Also, frequent irrigation with heparinized Ringer's lactate solution helps to float the vessel walls apart. *At NO stage of the anastomosis is the intima grasped by the forceps.* **B,** Microsurgical square knot is demonstrated. Since the stay sutures may be inserted under some tension at the anastomosis site, a surgeon's knot (double loop) should be placed in these initial two sutures. Subsequent knots do not require a surgeon's knot. Three knots in a square fashion are sufficient for each suture placement. **C,** Loop of the knot should be visible so as not to cause the vessel walls to overlap.

with care taken to avoid the back wall. When the front wall is sutured, the vessel is flipped over and the back wall carefully completed without engagement of the front wall. As illustrated in Fig. 3-12, A, a pair of forceps or the needle can be used to gently lift the wall away from the other side.

Once the anastomosis is completed and the clamp removed, small leaks will generally seal off. At this stage the patency test or "flow test," as shown in Fig. 3-13, can be performed.

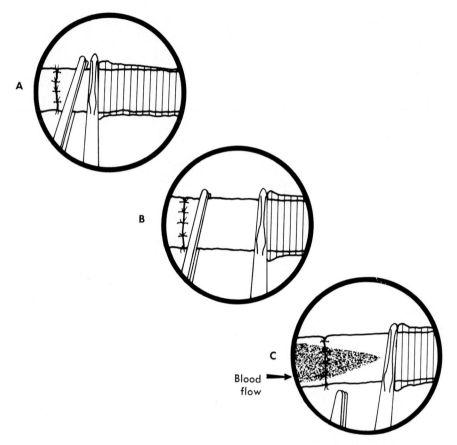

Fig. 3-13. After anastomosis is achieved, the procedure from **A** to **C** is usually performed, commonly known as the "patency test." When accomplished, this test will help to determine the patency of the lumen and the amount of blood flow across the anastomosis. Tying forceps are best used so as not to damage the vessel wall. The vessels must be gently stroked.

MODELS FOR TEACHING MICROSURGERY IN THE LABORATORY

Once the instrumentation of the microvascular laboratory is established, there are various models that will teach the techniques of microsurgery to the surgeon and also provide a continuing challenge to his skills.

The four models discussed here require skills from simple to complex.

Model 1: knot board

This model is composed of a knot board to familiarize the surgeon with the operating microscope, the microvascular instruments, and the microvascular suture and needle. The purpose of this exercise is to improve one's dexterity in controlling the needle tip and suture. As seen in Fig. 3-14, A, a latex glove

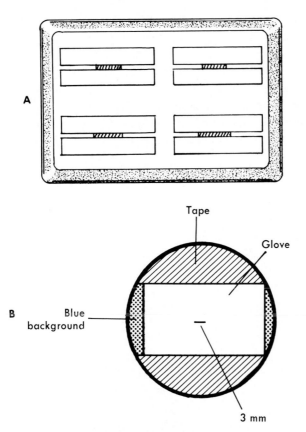

Fig. 3-14. A, Used food tray measuring 12 × 9 inches has areas where the student can learn the first stages in microsurgery. **B,** Practice area is made from a small piece of surgical rubber glove and placed over a blue piece of plastic. It is secured with white tape, and a 3 mm incision is made in the glove for practice in passing the suture and knot tying.

and a disposable food tray measuring 12 by 9 inches are used for the knot board. The board is constructed to have four areas where the student can practice passing the needle and knot tying. As shown in Fig. 3-14, *B*, a 3 mm incision is made in the glove prior to starting with the suture. If desired a very narrow strip of latex glove may be removed from the incision to add resistance to the knot tying. Initially the 140-micron needle should be used in an attempt to gain perfect needle control. The surgeon should be able to repeatedly poise his needle point next to the lip of the incision and then puncture the wall, pass the needle through one or both walls, and tie a knot.

Model 2: hamster aorta

This model depends on the use of the hamster aorta and vena cava for the microvascular procedure. In hamsters weighing 100 gm, the central abdominal vessels are approximately 1 to 1.5 mm in external diameter. For the beginning surgeon, the aorta is appealing because of its thick wall, which provides a cut surface easily seen by the surgeon as the vessel ends are approximated. Additionally, preparation of the aorta offers good dissection practice, and the aorta resists vasospasm more than do the peripheral vessels.

Preparation of hamster. The hamster, weighing about 100 gm, is anesthetized with intraperitoneal sodium pentobarbital (Nembutal), 3.5 mg per 100 gm of body weight. The hamster's abdomen is shaved and the animal placed

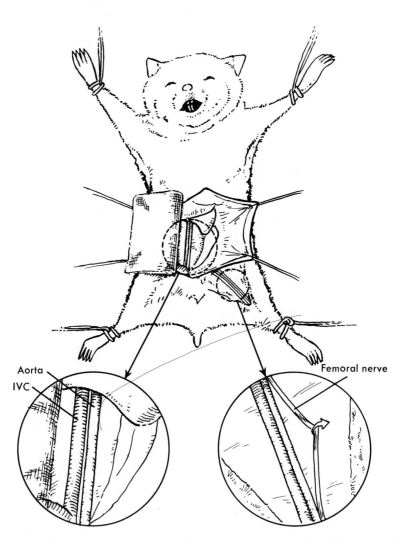

Fig. 3-15. Hamster weighing approximately 100 grams prepared for microsurgery. *Inset on right,* Incision necessary to expose the femoral nerve. *Inset on left,* Dissection necessary to expose the aorta and the inferior vena cava.

on an animal board with its limbs secured by rubber binders and tape (Fig. 3-15). A midline abdominal incision is made from the xiphoid cartilage to the pubis. Scissors can be used to open up the peritoneum.

The intestines are wrapped in a moistened sponge and pulled to the right side of the animal as the mesentery is mobilized and the retroperitoneal space opened. Stay sutures may be necessary to stabilize the intestines and mesentery out of the operative field.

The animal is now ready for dissection of the central vessels with the microscope. If the hamster requires additional anesthetic during the case, several drops of sodium pentobarbital can be applied to the liver surface. It is usually necessary to coagulate one renal vein in mobilizing the central vessels. Once the aorta is free for about 2 cm above the bifurcation, a colored background (yellow, blue, or green latex from a balloon) is placed beneath the vessel and the microvascular approximating clamp is applied. It is important to apply the approximator with the clamps widely separated, since after the vessel is cut, the clamps may be pushed together. This can be achieved by the use of an Adson forceps to allow tensionless approximation of the vessel ends. For severing the vessel when in the microclamp, use a straight, sharp scissors like the straight iris scissors seen in Fig. 3-2, *F*. This scissors is used only for this part of the procedure because it gives a straight cut leaving a clean vessel edge for repair.

The surgeon is now ready to proceed as described in Figs. 3-10 to 3-12. It is important to place sutures evenly to prevent outpouching of the vessel wall and subsequent leaks. With evenly spaced sutures the vessel will dilate and seal its edges when the clamp is removed.

Anastomosis of the hamster vena cava can be attempted after the aorta is completed. Although the vein size is larger, its thin wall makes it a more difficult task. Vein repairs will usually require an assistant to hold the stay sutures or a microclamp with an outrigger. The hamster's femoral nerve is also available for repair.

Model 3: rat femoral vessels

This model depends on the use of the rat's femoral vessels for microvascular repair. The major advantage of this model is the flexibility of surgical procedures that can be done with the anatomy in this area. Only the straightforward repair of the vessels will be described here, and the reader is referred to the references that describe other procedures that can be performed on this model.[1-4]

Preparation of rat. A white rat weighing 350 to 400 gm is anesthetized with intraperitoneal sodium pentobarbital, 5 mg/100 gm of body weight. When asleep, the animal is placed on the animal board in the usual fashion. The inguinal region is shaved. A perpendicular incision is made to the inguinal ligament of the medial surface of the thigh. The femoral artery, vein, and nerve are exposed. With the femoral vessels exposed, the branches can be coagulated to allow better mobilization of the artery. It is important to maintain the femoral vessels dilated with topically applied lidocaine (Xylocaine) 1%. Once adequate vessel length is exposed, the microvascular clamp may be applied and the repair performed as described previously. The common femoral artery at the level of the inguinal ligament is appreciably larger than the superficial femoral but exposure is more difficult. The femoral nerve allows practice repair of its fascicles.

Model 4: replantation of rabbit ear

Replantation of the rabbit's ear as first described by Buncke in 1966, represents a challenging microvascular model for the laboratory.[3] This model provides both an excellent procedure for replantation practice and a setting in which the variables for the success of the replant can be manipulated for research purposes.[5-7]

In the rabbit ear, the vessels are easily accessible and approximate 1 mm in diameter. The ear is supplied by a central set of blood vessels and can withstand amputation and replantation of those vessels alone without causing undue stress on the animal. Rabbit ears have been removed for as long as 28 hours for cold (4° C) ischemic time and still survived replantation. In the Orthopaedic Microvascular Research Laboratory at Duke University Medical Center, the rabbit ear model has served as an excellent one for both practice and research purposes. Within the laboratory, a greater than 90% success rate has been achieved by using 2 to 3 kg rabbits with central ear vessel size of 1 mm in diameter.

Preparation of rabbit and method of replantation of ear. New Zealand white rabbits weighing from 2.5 to 3 kg are anesthetized with intraperitoneal sodium pentobarbital, 40 mg/kg body weight. The ear to be replanted is shaved and washed with PhisoHex. The rabbit is secured in a lateral position with tape and the operative ear is placed superiorly. Once the rabbit is adequately anesthetized by the sodium pentobarbital, it will tolerate the lateral position without difficulty. Two milliliters of 1% lidocaine are injected subcutaneously around the central vessel at the base of the ear for additional anesthesia. A cruciate incision (Fig. 3-16) is made at the base of the ear, and the central vessels and nerve are dissected free for approximately 2 cm. Retraction sutures are used to maintain the ear in a suitable position while dissection is carried out. When the central vessels are free of all soft tissue, they may be measured with a millimeter rule after being maximally dilated with 1% lidocaine. The incision is then extended across the entire posterior surface of the ear with extra lidocaine anesthesia as needed. Additional vessels are cauterized with a bipolar cautery. Along both edges of the ear are located large veins, which may be saved at the operator's discretion for additional venous anastomoses. Once all soft tissue bleeding is controlled, the cartilage is stripped on the posterior

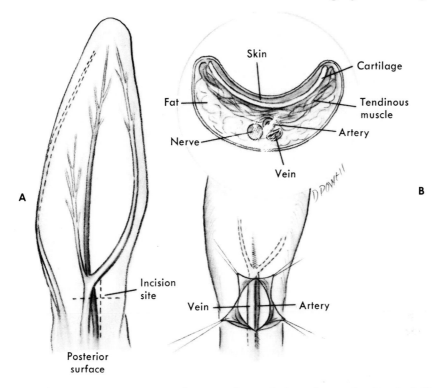

Fig. 3-16. A, Cruciate incision over the central vessels is made proximal to the bifurcation of the vein. **B,** Skin-retraction sutures stabilize the soft tissue while the central structures are dissected free for approximately 2 cm.

surface of the ear at the level of amputation. A 6-0 silk tie is placed around the artery at the level of the amputation, and the vessel severed distal to it (Fig. 3-17). The vein and nerve are then severed at the same level. Ligation of the central vein is unnecessary as it usually will not bleed.

When the ear is removed, it may be immersed in chilled Ringer's lactate solution at a temperature of 4° C to minimize the effects of warm ischemia. The ear should be milked of all residual blood. While immersion is maintained, the skin of the inside proximal edge of the amputated ear is stripped away from the cartilage for approximately 1 cm (Fig. 3-18).

While the amputated ear is being prepared, the proximal stump of the ear is inspected and any additional bleeding vessels are cauterized.

Replantation of the ear can begin within several minutes of amputation. If longer periods of ischemic time are desired, the chilled ear may be left in the Ringer's lactate solution and placed in the refrigerator. If prolonged ischemic time is planned, one can close the proximal ear stump by pulling the dorsal soft tissue over the exposed cartilage and central vessels.

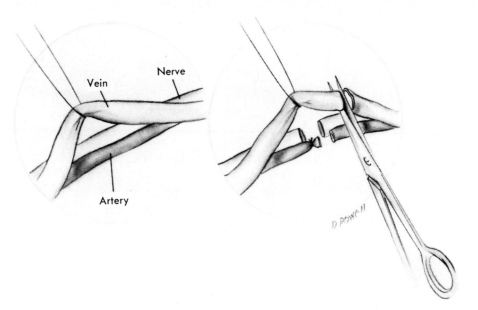

Fig. 3-17. This shows the orientation of the central structures with the artery beneath the vein and nerve. (See the cross section in Fig. 3-16.) Only the artery is ligated with a tie before severance of the structures. The central vein will usually not back-bleed.

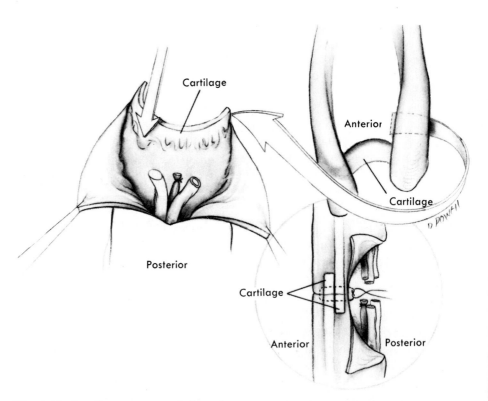

Fig. 3-18. Cartilage is stripped clean for approximately 1 cm on the posterior surface of the ear stump and the anterior surface of the amputated part. This allows cartilage-to-cartilage approximation, which is secured with multiple mattress sutures. Once secured, the reattached ear will remain upright.

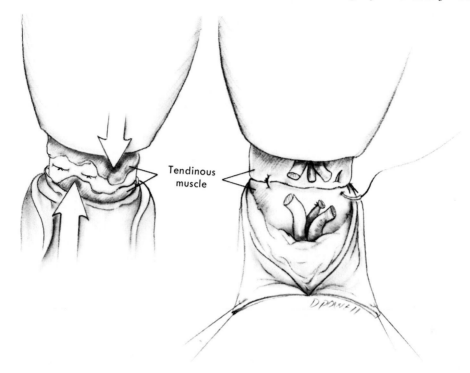

Fig. 3-19. The musculotendinous layer is repaired beneath the central vessels and thus pulls the central vessels into tensionless approximation.

Once replantation is started, the cartilage is overlapped 1 cm with interrupted 5.0 nylon mattress sutures (Fig. 3-18). The musculotendinous layer that lay beneath the vessels is reapproximated with 5-0 absorbable sutures (Fig. 3-19).

At this point, the central vessels may be repaired in either order. If the artery is repaired first, the vein may be repaired either bleeding or with the arterial clamp remaining on. No attempt should be made to perform the venous anastomosis with the clamp on the distal vein while the artery is patent. This will lead to extreme venous congestion within the ear.

If the vein is done first, the surgeon needs to dilate the vein ends with irrigation solution to decide how much redundancy exists in the vein. It may be necessary to excise a short segment of the vein to compensate for the shortening of the ear. This will pervent kinking of the repaired vein.

In repairing the artery, it is important to bathe the proximal portion with 1% lidocaine during the early stages of replantation to maintain it in a dilated state. When it is time for the artery to be repaired, the artery is sharply transected just proximal to the tie. This allows the artery to bleed profusely and wash out any proximal clots. A single microclamp as shown in Fig. 3-3 is applied approximately 1 cm from the proximal end. Care is taken not to stretch the artery while the clamp is applied because observations have indicated that when the artery is stretched, the segment that is clamped develops significantly more residual spasm after clamp removal. The distal end of the artery does not need to be placed in a clamp approximator for alignment of the vessel ends. The arterial repair is then performed in the appropriate fashion.

When the arterial clamp is removed, the presence of arterial flow can be recognized from dilatation of the distal artery segment and filling of the venous anastomosis. Inspection of the ear surface shows dilatation of the central artery throughout the ear's length and filling of the peripheral veins.

The central nerve may be repaired at this time with either epineurial or fascicular sutures.

Closure is performed in layers with running absorbable sutures. The layers closed are on the posterior surface of the ear and include the musculotendinous layer, the subcutaneous fat, and the skin. The skin on the inside portion of the ear is not closed. The entire incision is sprayed with an antimicrobial sealant. Additionally, the rabbit may be given 0.5 ml of Combiotic* intramuscularly each day for 3 days. No special postoperative care is necessary, and the rabbit is allowed to be active in his cage throughout the postoperative period.

In monitoring the success of the replanted ear postoperatively, it is possible to see the filling of the central artery on the dorsum of the ear. Frequently, the ear will swell and droop slightly. If the ear assumes a leathery appearance, arterial thrombosis has occurred. If the ear becomes grossly swollen and blue, venous thrombosis is likely. Both of these problems will manifest themselves within the first 24 to 48 hours postoperatively.

Frequently, by the end of the first postoperative week, a successful replantation will appear as an upright ear with minimal to no swelling. By 2 weeks after the procedure, the ear should be normal in all appearances.

ACKNOWLEDGMENT

Work in this chapter was partly supported by NIH Grant no. 1 RO1 GM25666.

REFERENCES

1. Acland, R. D.: Practice manual for trainees, Louisville Microsurgery Laboratory, Louisville, Ky., 1975.
2. Buncke, H. J., Chater, M. L., and Szabo, Z.: The manual of microvascular surgery, Pearl River, N.Y., 1975, Davis & Geck Co.
3. Buncke, H. J., and Schulz, W. T.: Total ear replantation in the rabbit utilizing microminiature anastomosis, Br. J. Plast. Surg. **19:**15, 1966.
4. Gordon, L., and Buncke, H. J.: Models and techniques for microsurgery research, Orthop. Clin. North Am. **8:**273, 1977.
5. Shearn, J. C., Serafin, D., and Georgiade, N. G.: Microvascular anastomosis: an experimental model utilizing the rabbit ear, Plast. Reconstr. Surg. **58:**451, 1976.

*Combiotic is penicillin and dihydrostreptomycin in aqueous suspension, from Pfizer Agricultural Division, New York, N.Y. 10017.

6. Tsai, Tse-Ming: Experimental and clinical application of microvascular surgery, Ann. Surg. **181:**169, 1975.
7. Urbaniak, J. R., Seaber, A. V., and Bright, D. S.: Orthopaedic microsurgery: laboratory manual, Durham, North Carolina, 1977.

ADDITIONAL READINGS
Microinstruments

Acland, R. D.: Microvascular anastomosis: a device for holding stay sutures and a new vascular clamp, Surgery **75:**185, 1974.

Acland, R. D.: New instruments for microvascular surgery, Br. J. Surg. **59:**181, 1972.

Assimacopoulos, C. A., and Salmon, P. A.: A modified pneumatic needle holder suitable for fine suture techniques, Surg. Gynecol. Obstet. **119:**356-358, 1964.

Berci, G., and Nyhus, L. M.: A new vessel clamp for microsurgery, Med. Pharmacol. Exp. **16:**45, 1967.

Broggi, R. J.: A combined tissue and tying forceps for microsurgery, Am. J. Ophthalmol. **77**(5):763-764, 1974.

Castroviejo, R.: A new needle holder, Trans. Am. Ophthalmol. Soc. **48:**331, 1950.

Castroviejo, R.: Improved needle holders, Trans. Am. Acad. Ophthalmol. Otolaryngol. **56:**929, 1952.

Cobbett, J. R.: Microvascular surgery, Surg. Clin. North Am. **47:**521, 1967.

Dujovny, M., Vas, R., and Osgood, C.: Bipolar jeweler's forceps with automatic irrigation, for coagulation in microsurgery, Plast. Reconstr. Surg. **56**(5):585-587, 1975.

Greenwood, J.: Two point coagulation. A new principle and instrument for applying coagulation current in neurosurgery, Am. J. Surg. **50:**267, 1940.

Greenwood, J.: Two-point or interpolar coagulation, review after a twelve-year period with notes on addition of a sucker tip, J. Neurosurg. **12:**196, 1965.

Healey, J. E., Moore, E. V., Brooks, B. F., et al.: A vascular clamp for circumferential repair of blood vessels, Surgery **51:**452, 1962.

Henderson, P. N., O'Brien, B. M., and Parel, J. M.: An adjustable double microvascular clamp, Med. J. Aust. **1:**715, 1970.

Henderson, P. N., Peričic, L., and O'Brien, B. M.: Mobile arm rests, Med. J. Aust. **1:**720, 1970.

Hickman, G. A., and Mortenson, J. D.: A comparative evaluation of vascular clamps, J. Thorac. Cardiovasc. Surg. **44:**561, 1962.

Hiebert, C. A.: An instrument to facilitate construction of miniature vascular suture lines, Ann. Thorac. Surg. **18**(6):640-641, 1974.

Ikuta, Y.: Microvascular surgery, Hiroshima, 1975, Lens Press.

Jacobsen, J. H.: Microsurgical technique. In Cooper, P., editor: Craft of surgery, ed. 2, Boston, 1971, Little, Brown & Co.

Kleinert, H. E., Serafin, D., and Daniel, R. K.: The place of microsurgery in hand surgery, Orthop. Clin. North Am. **4:**929, 1973.

Malis, L. L.: Bipolar coagulation in microsurgery. In Donaghy, R. M. P., and Yaşargil, M. G., editors: Microvascular surgery, Stuttgart, 1967, Georg Thieme Verlag.

Maroon, J. C., Roberts, E., Numoto, M., et al.: Microvascular surgery: simplified instrumentation, technical note, J. Neurosurg. **38**(1):119-126, 1973.

Mayfield, T. N.: Cited in McFadden, J. T.: The origin and evolutionary principles of spring forceps, Surg. Gynecol. Obstet. **130:**356, 1970.

McFadden, J. T.: Metallurgical principles in neurosurgery, J. Neurosurg. **31:**383, 1969.

McFadden, J. T.: Modifications of crossed-action intracranial clips, J. Neurosurg. **32:**116, 1970.

McFadden, J. T.: The origin and evolutionary principles of spring forceps, Surg. Gynecol. Obstet. **130**:356, 1970.

McLean, D. H., and Buncke, H. J.: Use of the Saran Wrap cuff in microsurgical arterial repairs, Plast. Reconstr. Surg. **51**:624, 1973.

Moller-Christensen, V.: The history of the forceps, Copenhagen, 1938, Levin & Munksgaard.

Nakayama, K.: A new device for small vessel anastomosing instruments, J. Jap. Pract. Surg. Soc. **22**:14, 1961.

O'Brien, B. M., and Hayhurst, J. W.: Metallized microsutures and a new microneedle holder, Plast. Reconstr. Surg. **52**:673, 1973.

Parel, J., Crock, G. M., O'Brien, P., et al.: Prototypal electro-microsurgical instruments, Med. J. Aust. **1**:709, 1970.

Rigg, B. M.: A microirrigator, Plast. Reconstr. Surg. **56**(3):349, 1975.

Salmon, P. A., and Assimacopoulos, S. W.: A pneumatic needle holder suitable for microsurgical procedures, Surgery **55**:466, 1964.

Scarff, T.: Bipolar suction cautery forceps for microneurosurgical use, Surg. Neurol. **2**:213, 1974.

Scoville, W. B.: Miniature torsion bar spring clip, J. Neurosurg. **25**:97, 1966.

Smith, J. W.: Microsurgery: review of the literature and discussion of microtechniques, Plast. Reconstr. Surg. **37**:227, 1966.

Terzis, J., Faibisoff, B., and Williams, H. B.: Use of polyethylene bag background in microsurgical repair of peripheral nerves, Plast. Reconstr. Surg. **53**:596, 1974.

Terzis, J., Faibisoff, B., and Williams, H. G.: A diamond knife for microsurgical repair of peripheral nerves, Plast. Reconstr. Surg. **54**(1):102-103, 1974.

Vogelfanger, I. J., and Beattie, W. G.: A concept of automation in vascular surgery; a preliminary report on a mechanical instrument for arterial anastomosis, Can. J. Surg. **1**:262, 1958.

Williams, C. L., and Takaro, T.: The Russian stapler in small artery anastomoses and grafts, Angiology **14**:470, 1963.

Zirkle, T. J., and Seidenstricker, K. L.: An adjustable double clamp for use in microvascular surgery, Plast. Reconstr. Surg. **51**(3):340-341, 1973.

Microinstrument companies

Codman & Shurtleff, Inc.,
Pacella Drive
Randolph, Mass. 02368

Edward Weck & Co., Inc.,
49-33 31st Place,
Long Island City, N.Y. 11101

Medsonics, Inc.,
790 Hemmeter Lane,
P. O. Box M,
Mountain View, Cal. 94042

Mizuto-Ika-Kogyo Co.,
3-29-10 Hongo, Bunkyo-ku,
Tokyo, Japan

Muranaka Medical Instrument Co.,
33, 2-Chome, Funakoshi-Cho,
Higashi-Ku,
Osaka 540, Japan

S & T Chirurgische Nadeln,
7893 Jestetten/FRG,
West Germany

Sparta Instrument Corp.,
305 Fairfield Ave.,
Fairfield, N.J. 07006

Storz Instrument Co.,
3365 Tree Court Industrial Blvd.,
St. Louis, Mo. 63122

Microsutures

Acland, R.: A new needle for microvascular surgery, Surgery **71**:130, 1972.

Acland, R.: Note on the handling of ultrafine suture material, Surgery **77**:507, 1975.

Bernhard, W. F., Cummin, A. S., Vawter, G. F., and Carr, J. G.: Closure of vascular incisions utilizing a new flexible adhesive, Surg. Forum **13:**231, 1962.

Buncke, H. J., and McLean, D. H.: The advantage of a straight needle in microsurgery, Plast. Reconstr. Surg. **47:**602, 1971.

Carton, C. A., Kessler, L. A., Seidenberg, B., and Hurwitt, E. S.: Experimental studies in the surgery of small blood vessels. IV. Nonsuture anastomosis of arteries and veins, using flanged ring prostheses and plastic adhesive, Surg. Forum **11:**238, 1960.

Chase, M. D., and Schwartz, S. I.: Consistent patency of 1.5 millimeter arterial anastomoses, Surg. Forum **13:**220, 1962.

Cobbett, J.: Small vessel anastomosis: a comparison of suture techniques, Br. J. Plast. Surg. **22:**16, 1967.

Hafner, C. D., Fogarty, T. J., and Cranley, J. J.: Nonsuture anastomosis of small arteries using a tissue adhesive, Surg. Forum **11:**417, 1963.

Inokuchi, K.: A new type of vessel-suturing apparatus, A.M.A. Arch. Surg. **82:**337, 1958.

Jacobson, J. H., Moody, R. A., Kusserow, B. K., Reich, T., and Wang, M. C. H.: The tissue response to a plastic adhesive used in combination with microsurgical technique in reconstruction of small arteries, Surgery **60:**370, 1966.

Mannax, W. G., Bloch, J. H., Longerbeam, J. K., and Lillehei, R.: Plastic adhesive as an adjunct in suture anastomosis of small blood vessels, Surgery **54:**663, 1963.

McCulloch, C.: Needle with wire loop for drawing sutures through tissue, Am. J. Ophthalmol. **72**(5):1012-1013, 1971.

Nakayama, K., Yamamoto, K., and Makino, H.: A new vascular anastomosing instrument and its clinical applications, Clin. Orthop. **29:**123, 1963.

O'Brien, B. M., and Hayhurst, J. W.: Metallized microsutures and a new microneedle holder, Plast. Reconstr. Surg. **52:**673, 1973.

O'Brien, B. M., Henderson, P. N., and Crock, G. W.: Metallized microsutures, Med. J. Aust. **1:**717, 1970.

Padula, R. T., and Ballinger, W. F.: A new clamp for rapid vascular anastomosis, Surgery **57:**819, 1965.

Phelan, J. T., Young, W. P., and Gale, J. W.: The effect of suture material on small artery anastomoses, Surg. Gynecol. Obstet. **107:**79, 1958.

Polack, F. M., Sanchez, J., and Eve, F. R.: Microsurgical sutures. I. Evaluation of various types of needles and sutures for anterior segment surgery, Can. J. Ophthalmol. **9:**42, 1974.

Sanchez, J., Polack, F. M., Eve, F. R., and Troutman, R. C.: Microsurgical sutures. II. Corneal endothelial healing and posterior wound closure after "through and through" suturing, Can. J. Ophthalmol. **9:**48, 1974.

Shuhmacker, H. B., and Lowenberg, R. I: Experimental studies in vascular repair. I. Comparison of reliability of various methods of end-to-end arterial sutures, Surgery **24:**79, 1948.

Sigel, B., and Acevedo, F. J.: Vein anastomosis by electrocoaptive union, Surg. Forum **13:**233, 1962.

Sigel, B., and Acevedo, F. J.: Electrocoaptive union of blood vessels. A preliminary experimental study, J. Surg. Res. **3:**90, 1963.

Sigel, B., and Dunn, M. R.: The mechanism of blood vessel closure by high frequency electrocoagulation, Surg. Gynecol. Obstet. **121:**823, 1965.

Winfrey, E. W., and Foster, J. H.: Prevention of arterial thrombosis with a negatively charged wire suture, Surg. Forum **13:**229, 1962.

Zingg, W., and Khodadadeh, M.: Vascular anastomosis—sutures, staples or glue? Can. Med. Assoc. J. **91:**791, 1964.

Microsuture companies

Davis & Geck,
Middletown Road,
Pearl River, N.Y. 10965.

Ethicon Inc.,
3640 Allendale Drive
Sommerville, N.J. 08876.

MicroFine,
Medical Applications Pty. Ltd.,
Buffalo Road,
Gladesville, N.S.W.,
Australia 2111.

S & T Chirurgische Nadeln,
7893 Jestetten/GRD,
Postfach 93,
West Germany.

Microscopes

Barraquer, J. I., Barraquer, J., and Littman, H.: A new operating microscope for ocular surgery, Am. J. Ophthalmol. **63**:90, 1967.

Becker, S. C.: A miniature head mounted surgical microscope, Arch. Ophthal. **82**:216, 1969.

Brambring, D. F.: Chair-tripped for the operating microscope—a new micro-surgical operating unit, Klin. Monatsbl. Augenheilkd. **162**(3):412-413, 1973.

Dohlman, G. F.: Carl Olof Nylen and the birth of the otomicroscope and microsurgery, Arch. Otolaryngol. **90**:161, 1969.

Guis, J. A.: Surgical explorations in the area between the macroscopic and the microscopic: the "metascopic" zone, Am. J. Surg. **104**:296, 1962.

Harmes, H., and Mackensen, G.: Ocular surgery under the microscope, Chicago, 1966, Year Book Medical Publishers.

Heerman, J.: Ringplate on the Zeiss surgical microscope objective for the attachment of the sterile cover, Z. Laryngol. Otol. **51**(10):690-692, 1972.

Horenz, P.: The design of the surgical microscope, parts I and II, Ophthalmic Surg. **4**:40, 89, 1973.

Jacobson, J. H.: Microsurgery, Curr. Probl. Surg. February 1971.

Jacobson, J. H.: Microsurgical technique. In Cooper, P., editor: The craft of surgery, ed. 2, Boston, 1971, Little, Brown & Co.

Littman, G., and Wittekind, R.: Operation microscope with new camera attachment and new observation tube for a second observer, Zeiss Information **58**:149, 1965.

Littman, G., Reidel, H., and Jakubowski, H.: Assistant's viewing tube and cine (television) adapter for Zeiss operating microscope, Zeiss Information **75**:5, 1970.

Littman, H.: The Zeiss diploscope—a new aid in microsurgery, Zeiss information **43**:24, 1962.

Littman, H.: Two new motorized operating microscopes with physiologically adapted magnification control, Klin. Monatsbl. Augenheilkd. **157**:61, 1970.

Nylen, C. O.: The microscope in aural surgery, its first use and later development, Acta Otolaryngol. **116**:226, 1954.

O'Brien, B. M.: The triploscope—a triple operating microscope, Plast. Reconstr. Surg. **45**:279, 1970.

O'Brien, B. M.: A modified triploscope, Br. J. Plast. Surg. **26**:301, 1973.

Owen, E. R.: Practical microsurgery: a choice of optical aids for fine work, Med. J. Aust. **1**:224, 1971.

Rand, R. W.: Microneurosurgery, ed, 2, St. Louis, 1978, The C. V. Mosby Co.

Thomson, J. R.: Operating under magnification, Aust. N.Z. J. Surg. **41**:160, 1971.

Troutman, R. C.: Microsurgery of the anterior segment of the eye; vol. I, Introduction and basic techniques, St. Louis, 1974, The C. V. Mosby Co.

Yaşargil, M. G.: Microsurgery: as applied to neurosurgery, Stuttgart, 1969, Georg Thieme Verlag.

Microscope companies

Applied Fiberoptics,
46 River Street,
Southbridge, Mass. 01550.

Carl Zeiss,
444 Fifth Ave.,
New York, N.Y. 10018.

Codman & Shurtleff, Inc.,
Pacella Drive
Randolph, Mass. 02368.

Edward Weck & Co., Inc.,
49-33 31st Place,
Long Island City,
New York, N.Y. 11101.

Sparta Instrument Corp.,
305 Fairfield Avenue,
Fairfield, N.J. 07006.

Microsurgery technique

Acland, R. D.: Signs of patency in small vessel anastomosis, Surgery **72:**744, 1972.

Acland, R. D.: Thrombus formation in microvascular surgery: an experimental study of the effects of surgical trauma, Surgery **73:**766, 1973.

Baxter, T. J., O'Brien, B. M., Henderson, P. N., and Bennett, R. C.: The histopathology of small vessels following microvascular repair, Br. J. Surg. **59:**617, 1972.

Derman, G. H., and Schenck, R. R.: Microsurgical technique—fundamentals of the microsurgical laboratory, Orthop. Clin. North Am. **8:**229, 1977.

Hayhurst, J. W., and O'Brien, B. M.: An experimental study of microvascular technique, patency rates, and related factors, Br. J. Plast. Surg. **28:**128, 1975.

O'Brien, B. M., Henderson, P. N., Bennett, R. C., and Crocke, G. W.: Microvascular surgical technique, Med. J. Aust. **1:**722, 1970.

Urbaniak, J. R., Soucacos, P. N., Adelaar, R. S., Bright, D. S., and Whitehurst, L. A.: Experimental evaluation of microsurgical techniques in small artery anastomoses, Orthop. Clin. North Am. **8:**249, 1977.

4. Techniques of microsurgery

Donald S. Bright

BACKGROUND AND GENERAL USES

The ability of the microsurgeon to anastomose small vessels has stimulated interest in the field of microvascular surgery.[8] With the development of more precise instrumentation, advanced techniques, more appropriate microscopes, and smaller suture material and needles, the microsurgeon can predictably obtain the patent anastomosis in vessels less than 1 ml in diameter.

The several areas currently recognized in microsurgery[11] include replantation and revascularization,[16,18] nerve repairs and grafting,[10] free groin flaps,[5,9] and composite tissue transfers.[1,7]

Several factors determine the success of microsurgery: (1) the experience of the surgeons and assistants in working together during lengthy procedures and in sufficient numbers to relieve each other periodically, (2) the surgeon's knowledge of the physiology of the microcirculation, (3) the use of proper microscopes, instrumentation, and suture material maintained to close tolerances, and (4) extensive laboratory practice for all team members.

This chapter presents the instrumentation, the microscopes, the procedure for laboratory practice, and our methods of clinical microvascular surgery developed over 5 years in 600 clinical anastomoses.

MAGNIFICATION, INSTRUMENTATION, AND ACCESSORY EQUIPMENT
Microscopes

The magnifying device usually used is the surgical telescope (Fig. 4-1). These can be individually fitted to the surgeon with prescriptions ground into them when necessary. The working distance varies from 14 to 19 inches and a depth of field of several centimeters is possible. The most useful magnification is 3.5 to 4.5.

More complex surgery demands operating microscopes (Fig. 4-2). Available models include the Zeiss (OMPI pH 7), the Weck, and Applied Fiberoptics. Operating microscopes should not be moved, even from one room to another. Several essential features of the microscope are necessary for com-

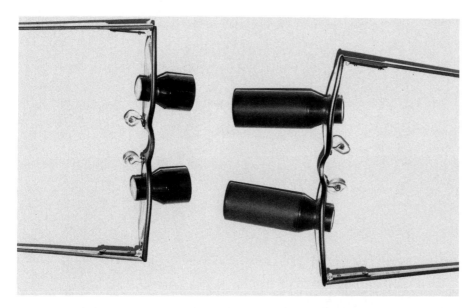

Fig. 4-1. Surgical telescopes with individually fitted interpupillary distance and predetermined working distance. *Left*, 3.5 power with 17-inch working distance. *Right*, 6 power with 16-inch working distance.

plex microsurgery: (1) a double head to permit the surgeon and his first assistant to view the same fields, (2) an easily controlled zoom allowing magnification from 7.5 to at least 30 power, (3) a convenient focusing method, usually electrically controlled, (4) a fiberoptic light source to adequately illuminate the vessel under high magnification. Several other features are desirable: (5) a power XY control movement, (6) a third head with a separate zoom for another assistant, (7) a camera and a color video system for documentation.

Microscopes easily lose adjustment; so trained service people must be available. Because of the different technical requirements and the undesirability of moving microscopes to different operating rooms, no more than one service should use a microscope.

Instrumentation

Many commercial designs of special instrumentation are available (Figs. 4-3 and 4-4). They should have fine tips that approximate accurately; fairly large, comfortable handles with a light spring mechanism to prevent fatigue of the intrinsics of the hand; and a nonglare surface. They can be damaged or ruined by slight mishandling and should be kept separate from other instruments and handled only by those involved in microsurgery.

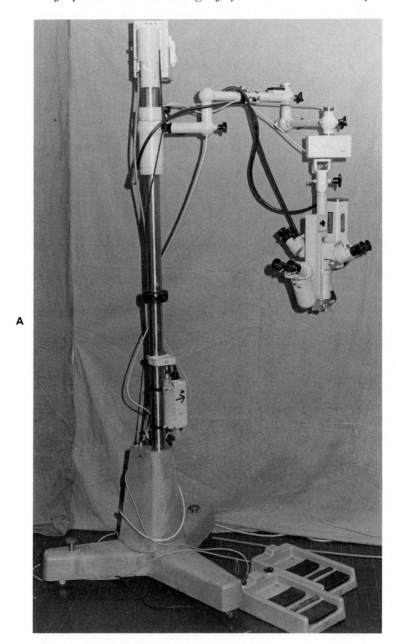

Fig. 4-2. Microscopes. **A,** Zeiss OPMI pH 7 with the following features: foot-control electrical focus, foot-control zoom from 7.5- to 35-power magnification, power foot XY control movement, a third head with a separate zoom for another assistant, and a color video camera for documentation. Features of the OPMI pH 7 that are desirable include the fact that the operator and first assistant see the same field and have the power focusing. The base shown is generally inadequate and unable to handle all the accessory equipment and a newer electrically controlled base should be used if many accessories are planned.

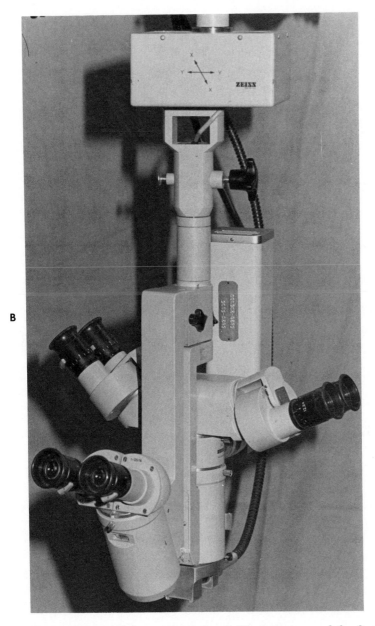

Fig 4-2, cont'd. B, Close-up of the operating head. The operator and the first assistant see the same field while the third head attachment allows the third assistant to individually control zoom. The XY control unit is very helpful when the surgeon works at 10× and above. House Urban video camera is mounted on the beam splitter and is most useful for teaching purposes.

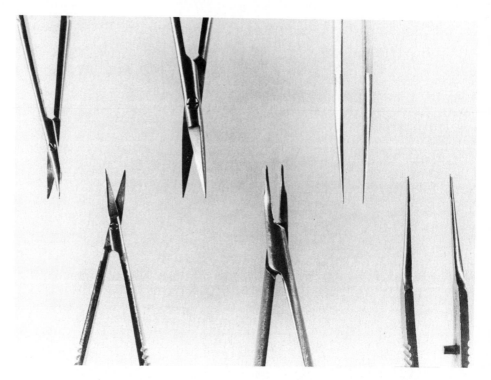

Fig. 4-3. Microinstrumentation. The instruments needed are few but must be precisely machined and maintained. *Top row from left to right,* Curved spring-loaded microdissection scissors, straight sharp scissors for transecting nerves and arteries, no. 5 jewelers' forceps. *Bottom row from left to right,* Straight spring-loaded dissecting scissors, spring-loaded needle driver, tying forceps for handling the adventitia of vessels and tying sutures. The tying forceps have a flatter, less damageable tip.

Forceps (Fig. 4-3). Tying forceps are blunt nosed and are used for handling vessels and tying sutures. Several pairs are necessary in various sizes. Jewelers' forceps (nos. 5 and 6) are sharp tipped and are used for nerves and for gripping the adventitia of vessels. It is essential for the points to come together precisely at the tip. The fine tips lose their points quickly and must frequently be replaced. Fortunately, they are not expensive. Toothed forceps are used to dissect larger structures.

Scissors (Fig. 4-3). Spring-loaded microscissors must be available for sharp and blunt dissection. Curved blunt-tipped scissors are used for most dissection around vessels and their branches. Sharp straight scissors are used for cutting vessels and for sharp dissection around the nerves. Several extra pair should be available since these are easily damaged.

Needle drivers (Fig. 4-3). Frequently used needles have 30-, 50-, and 65-micron diameters. Fine-tipped spring-loaded needle drivers are important.

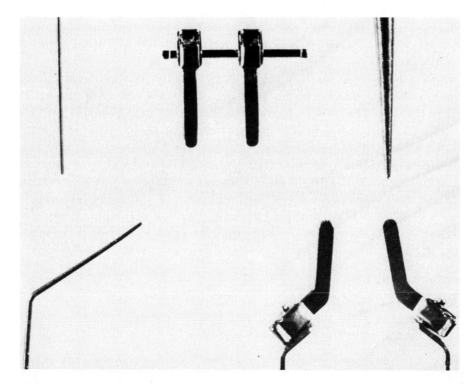

Fig. 4-4. Microinstrumentation dilators and vascular clamps. *Top row from left to right,* Irrigation tip made from spinal needle for irrigating the lumens of the vessels. Bar-loaded microclips with opening pressures of 30 gm for holding smaller arteries. Graduated dilator for dilating the tips of vessels. *Bottom row from left to right,* Angle dilator for gentle probing of smaller vessels and tips of Kleinert clamps for larger vessels.

These should have a slight curve at the end with the locking mechanism either absent or disengaged. The force necessary to lock or unlock the mechanism will often tear small vessels.

Vascular clamps (Fig. 4-4). Vascular clamps are used for occluding vessels during anastomosis. For smaller vessels, they should have less than 30 grams of opening pressure. The most convenient is a dual clamp mounted on a frame or bar with or without a mechanism for sliding the clamps together. Larger clamps (Klinert) have a higher closing pressure, making them unsuitable for smaller vessels, but they can be satisfactory for larger 2 to 3 mm vessels. Clamps are not recommended for many vessels, including veins and smaller arteries, since they produce some damage and, in some cases, can cause a decrease in flow through the vessel.

Dilators (Fig. 4-4). Several sizes of dilators are necessary for dilating the ends of vessels to relieve spasm. The small, constant-gauge type is used for initial probing and for small vessels. The larger size is used for enlarging the end of the vessels. Lacrimal dilators are used occasionally for spasm along the length of the vessels.

Fogarty catheters. Smaller size Fogarty catheters can be used for larger vessels within the hand or wrist. They are of no use distal to the mid palm.

Irrigation tips (Fig. 4-4). Vessels require frequent irrigation. The irrigation tips should be angled with a blunt tip and can be easily made from cut-off spinal needles with the ends smoothed by a burnishing wheel.

Suture material (Fig. 4-5). Nonreactive monofilament should be used with a noncutting needle (Fig. 4-4). The commonly used suture for small vessels is a 30-, 50-, or 65-micron needle on a 20 micron or less suture (10-0 or 11-0 on a BV-6 or BV-8 needle). Either moderately curved or a straight needle is satisfactory. Larger sizes are available for the tagging of vessels or the anastomosis of larger vessels or nerves.

Accessory equipment

Essential additional equipment includes the following:
1. Warmed heparinized Ringer's lactate solution, which is used for irrigation of the vessel

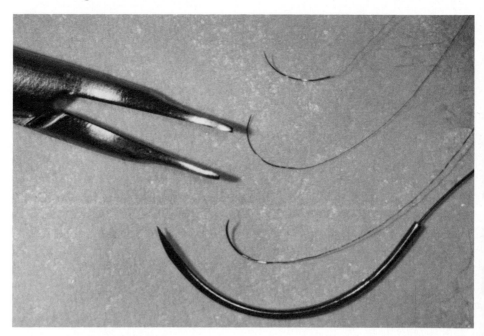

Fig. 4-5. Microsuture. Sutures shown are compared in size to the microneedle drivers. *From top to bottom,* 11-0 suture on a BV-8 needle (18-micron suture on 50-micron needle); 10-0 on a BV-6 needle (65-micron needle and 18-micron suture); 8-0 nylon with a BV-2 needle for tagging vessels and repairing nerves; bottom suture is a 6-0 nylon on a cutting needle for comparison.

2. Bipolar electrocautery with microtips, to avoid damage to the surrounding vessels
3. Fiberoptic headlight, used with surgical telescopes
4. Small sponges, cotton applicators, or cellulose sponges on holders
5. Instrumentation for postoperative and intraoperative monitoring

The small size of vessels and the frequent difficulty in determining patency, both before and after surgery, requires that special instrumentation be used for monitoring the patency of small vessels (Fig. 4-10). These instruments and our method of postoperative management are discussed in the following chapter. We have found, however, that the digital plethysmograph and the ultrasonic Doppler scanner are useful in preoperative management of arterial injuries. In the emergency ward or in the operating theater application of the Doppler scanner or the digital plethysmograph can determine whether or not there is patent arterial flow. This can help in planning whether to use microsurgical techniques and whether to plan for microvascular anastomosis.

Documentation

Photographs. Cameras should be fitted to the microscope to document the microvascular surgery. Most microscopes have a beam splitter that divides the light coming from the object for the use of photographic equipment (Fig. 4-2). The microscopic lens serves as the camera lens. One can focus the camera by focusing the microscope on a vessel at the highest magnification. Without changing the focus, the zoom or magnification is changed to the desired viewing field. A flash attachment is then used to illuminate the field while the photograph is taken. With the Zeiss microscope and a 180 mm objective lens, the *f* stop is set at *f* 14 and a flash with a guide number of 25 is placed 200 mm from the field. This gives good slides with slow, ASA 64 film.

Video tape (Fig. 4-2). There are several commercially available color video systems for use with operating microscopes. One focuses at a higher power and then zooms down to the desired power without changing the focus and adjusting the eyepieces. After this is done, the video tape will be in focus when the image of the surgeon is in focus. A color television is brought into the operating room to help the operating technicians and assistants. Video recordings can be made of surgical procedures, which are useful for teaching purposes.

Movie cameras. These are also available for use with the beam splitter. They are usually used only when a permanent recording is to be made. They require more editing and more light than normally available in the operating room.

LABORATORY PREPARATION AND PRACTICE

To attain and maintain efficiency in microsurgery, laboratory preparation and practice are essential.[17] The laboratory can be small, since only smaller animals are used. It should be separated from other laboratories and have a calm and quiet atmosphere. It should contain only the basic laboratory microscope and instrumentation, plus monitoring equipment.

Greater proficiency is gained if each participant has a specified project with an attainable goal. This will enable each person to obtain efficiency in microvascular surgery and to contribute to the knowledge of the group. The basics of microvascular surgery can be learned by having two to three sessions a week over several months. Each session should last several hours.

Laboratory training begins when one learns to use the microscope. This should include focusing, adjustment of interpupillary distance, and focusing with an assistant using the high- and low-power zoom.

After the participant is familiar with the microscope, he should learn to handle the instruments and to tie the suture with an instrument tie by using a section of a thin rubber glove with a slit. Then he can use a laboratory animal to learn the techniques of dissection and basic anastomosis of arteries and veins.

When each participant is proficient with the microscope and the instrumentation and suture techniques, simple revascularization and nerve repairs can be done in the operating room. Progression to more difficult procedures follows naturally.

We have used several animal models for microvascular repair. These are listed below with instructions for preparation.

Hamster, rat, or mouse. Rodents weighing 100 to 200 grams have several sites that are satisfactory for microvascular and microneural practice. The animals are inexpensive, easy to maintain, and can be disposed of after the dissection. The aorta and vena cava below the renal artery and above the bifurcation, the femoral artery and femoral vein, and the carotid are all areas readily accessible for anastomosis. The animal is anesthetized with 0.1 ml of sodium pentobarbital (Nembutal) intraperitoneally and fixed supine on a board. A midline abdominal incision is made, and the abdominal contents are gently lifted outside the peritoneum to expose the aorta and vena cava. By use of bipolar cautery, the branches of the aorta and vena cava are cauterized and divided. The vessel to be anastomosed is placed in a clamp apparatus and divided, and the anastomosis is carried out. The carotid artery is also available and is large enough for a good anastomosis.

Rabbit ear. The ear in 3- to 5-pound rabbits can be used as a model for amputation and replantation. A box is necessary to hold the rabbit and to administer anesthesia. Anesthesia can be either ether or thiopental (Pentothal). A clean amputation of the ear is made, and the artery and central vein are dissected proximally and distally. The ear cartilage is overlapped 0.5 cm, and interrupted sutures are applied for fixation. The anastomosis begins with the artery and proceeds to the vein. The skin is closed loosely. A light dressing is applied postoperatively, and the animal should be kept in a protective cage. Some animals will damage the replanted ear, but a success rate of 80% or more can be expected with practice.

Cat. The femoral and brachial arteries of the cat are larger than the rodent, easier to anastomose, and can serve as a model for investigation.

The cat is anesthetized with intraperitoneal phenobarbital at 1 ml per 5 pounds. An incision is made over the femoral or brachial artery, and the branches are cauterized and divided for the desired length. This model can be used for simple anastomosis, vein-to-artery grafts, vein-to-vein grafts, and artery-to-vein grafts.

The tail can be used as a model for study. It contains a volar artery and two dorsal veins. The tail can be completely or partially amputated and an intramedullary wire used in the vertebra for fixation. Anastomosis can be carried out and patency expected. Survival rates will be low when the tail is used because of its rich sympathetic supply. This model is more appropriate for the study of the sympathetic nervous system.

CLINICAL MICROSURGERY
Anesthesia and preparation

The safest and most rapid anesthesia for microvascular surgery is brachial block. In over 200 replantation patients, we have had no major complications. The failure rate is low with experienced personnel and high with inexperienced personnel. In an adult, 20 ml of 1% lidocaine and 20 ml of 0.5% bupivacaine HCl (Marcaine) are used. The solution is placed in the axillary sheath by a 22-gauge needle without penetration of the artery; the solution is then administered slowly. Anesthesia occurs within 20 minutes and lasts 6 to 16 hours. Blood flow to the extremity is increased because of the sympathetic blockade. General anesthesia is necessary in young children after the block wears off.

A tourniquet can be inflated and deflated as needed, usually painlessly. Occasionally, after an hour and a half of tourniquet time, there will be some discomfort.

The patient should be placed on an extrathick, soft mattress to avoid back fatigue during a long operation. The hand is fixed firmly to the hand table to prevent motion. Arm rests for the surgeon and assistant should provide support from the elbow to the fingertips. This prevents fatigue and permits control of fine motor movements of the hand. The surgeon's chair should be adjustable in height and comfortably padded.

Detriments to fine motor movements for the surgeon include heavy exercise and the use of coffee, alcohol, and cigarettes.

Before beginning to use the microscope, the surgeon and his assistant focus both at low and high power on a well-defined object so that they will be in focus throughout the range of powers available in the microscope.

Arterial anastomosis

After performing over 600 clinical anastomoses during the last 4 years, with a patency rate of over 85% even in the most traumatized vessels (see Chapter 5), we have evolved the following technique.

First, the proximal vessel is dissected until the surrounding tissue is normal. Under tourniquet control, routine midlateral incisions are made and carried down to the artery. Incisions must be planned so that proximal and distal dissection can take place if damage to the artery extends further than expected. We follow four major principles in our anastomosis. The artery is

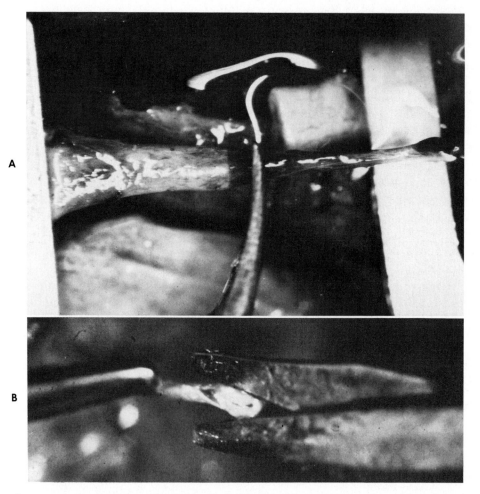

Fig. 4-6. A and **B,** Preparation of the vessel ends is most important. Here the adventitia is pulled out and trimmed to prevent occlusion of the vessel lumen, and the vessel is trimmed sharply with straight, sharp microscissors.

dissected sharply on either side of the anastomotic site. Branches are cauterized with bipolar cautery, with minimal handling of the artery.

Second, both vessel ends are resected so that normal intima is observed under the highest power available on the microscope. Under high power the artery is cut back to good intima (Fig. 4-6, *A* and *B*) with straight sharp scissors and inspected (Fig. 4-6, *C*). Overhanging adventitia is cleared off and the vessel is dilated gently. The tourniquet is released to ascertain flow. The blood should spurt freely 6 inches or more. If flow is impaired, the vessel is dilated gently more proximally to ascertain whether further damage has occurred proximally or distally at a point where the vessel branches. Locally acting dilating agents (such as papaverine) mixed 1:3 with normal saline can be placed on the vessel or gently irrigated into the lumen.[3] After good flow is obtained, the patient is given a loading dose of heparin, and the tourniquet is reinflated.

Third, absolutely no tension is permitted on the anastomosis site. When both vessels have been cut back to good intima, the ends should come together without any tension (Fig. 4-7). If there is tension, a graft is used. Clamps are not usually used during the anastomosis of veins and small arteries, especially

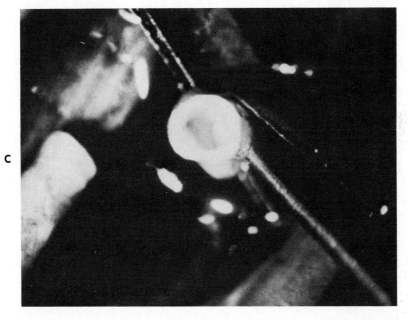

C

Fig. 4-6, cont'd. C, After resection of the vessel and trimming of the adventitia, the intima is noted to be clean with no imperfections. The wall should be of normal thickness and the vessel healthy-appearing both externally and internally. Figs. 4-6 to 4-9 show steps in a microvascular anastomosis and are shown on an artery less than 1 mm in diameter as seen through the operating microscope.

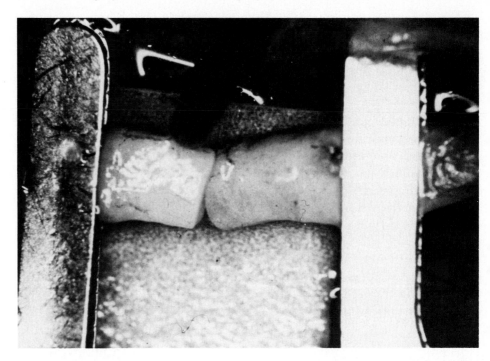

Fig. 4-7. Vessels should approximate without any tension whatsoever. Often no clamps are used and the first 10-0 suture should easily bring the vessel together.

in children.[2] Clamps may be used in larger arteries, but they should have an opening pressure of only 30 gm.

Fourth, there must be excellent technique in the vessel anastomosis. Care must be taken to adjust the length of the vessel after anastomosis. It should not be too long, or kinking will occur. If clamps are not used, the first suture placed should easily approximate the vessels without tension. Sutures should be placed without the intima being touched by the forceps. On most vessels 10-0 or 11-0 monofilament is used (Fig. 4-8). It is wedged on a BV-6 or a BV-8 needle (50 to 70 microns). Either jewelers' or tying forceps are used.

Corner sutures are first placed 120 to 180 degrees apart (Fig. 4-8, A). The width of the suture bite should equal one to two times the thickness of the wall on most arteries and veins. The suture is tied with an instrument tie with the help of the assistant and with three knots squarely laid down. The corner sutures are left long.

One should grasp the corner sutures by lifting the anterior from the posterior wall while exposing the arterial lumen. From one to three sutures are placed in the front wall so that there are no visible gaps. The first knot should be a surgeon's knot so that it will not slip during the tying of the other knots.

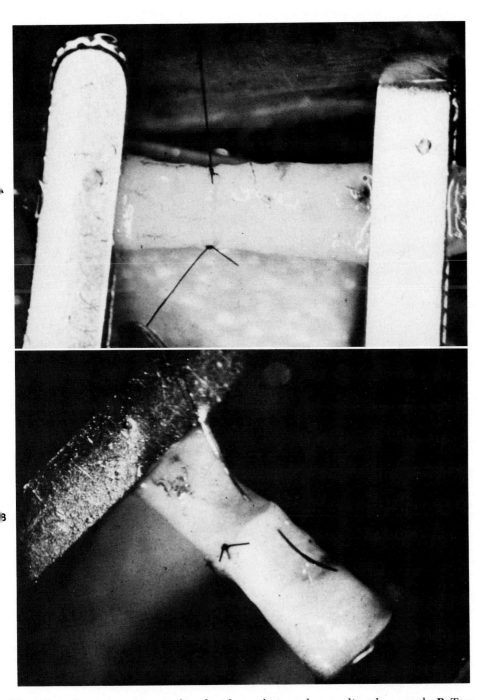

Fig. 4-8. A, Corner sutures are placed with care being taken to align the vessels. **B,** Two or three sutures are placed between these corner sutures so that there are no gaps.

The vessel ends should be drawn together gently until they come together, and then very slight tension is placed on them while the knots are being completed. The vessel is turned 180 degrees by the use of corner sutures or by turning of the clamps.

After each suture, the vessels should be irrigated with warm heparinized Ringer's lactate solution.

When the back side is exposed, a right-angle dilator is gently placed in each lumen. This ensures that the back wall has not been caught in one of the front wall sutures. The back wall is completed and the second inspection is made to see that no additional sutures are needed.

The tourniquet or clamps are released, and the initial flow observed under the microscope. Blood should come through the anastomosis quickly and freely with only a slight ooze at the anastomosis site (Fig. 4-9). Any large spurt should be repaired with an additional suture.

Usually the repaired digit or hand will immediately regain its normal color, but when there has been a long time from amputation to replantation, or when there has been an avulsion injury, this may take up to 15 or 20 minutes. There should be no manipulation of the artery during this time, and local vasodilating agents can be used. This is often an appropriate time to anastomose a nerve while waiting to reevaluate the vessel.

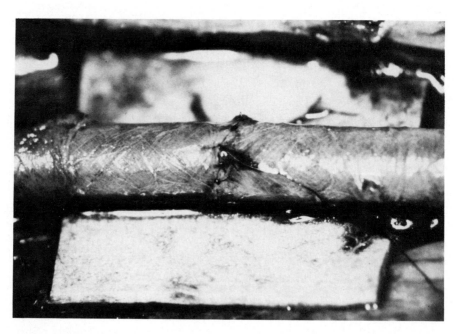

Fig. 4-9. Completed anastomosis with rapid flow proximally and distally. Major leaks should be repaired and no tension should be present. Our studies have shown that after anastomosis, the vessel should have 70% or greater flow through the anastomotic site.

It is important to decide when reanastomosis of a vessel is necessary. Reanastomosis should be considered in the following circumstances:

1. There is too much tension. The vessel should be redone with an interposition graft or a reversed vein graft.[14]
2. The repaired vessel fails the patency test. With two smooth-tying forceps, the vessel is occluded just distal to the anastomosis, and the second clamp is used to extract the blood distally for a distance of 1 cm. The proximal forceps is then released, and the blood should flow rapidly and freely.
3. There is an obvious clot or technical problem at the anastomosis site.
4. There is no back bleeding.

We have found that the digital plethysmograph or pulse volume recorder is a relatively objective indication of flow to the digit (Fig. 4-10). Twenty to 30 minutes after anastomosis, the recorder can be placed on the digit. Pulsations should be greater than 50% of the opposite control digit. If there is good pulsation on the plethysmograph, the chances for continued patency are excellent. (See Chapter 6.)

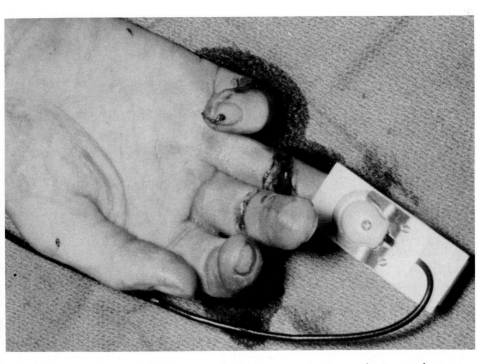

Fig. 4-10. Transducer of plethysmograph used in preoperative evaluation to determine flow characteristics of partial amputation of ring finger. The ring finger had absence of pulsatile flow and laceration of both digital arteries, which were repaired. The long finger, on the other hand, had only one artery lacerated and had good pulsatile flow, but no arterial anastomosis was needed.

Venous anastomosis and vein grafts

We do venous anastomosis after arterial anastomosis in replantation or composite tissue transfers. Only veins that are patent and flowing will be done initially. This allows accumulated toxins in the digit or especially the arm to be washed out to avoid their potentially dangerous effects.

Prior to doing venous anastomosis, all veins to be sutured should be identified, tagged with 8-0 nylon or clips, and dissected the necessary amount so they can be approximated without tension. This prevents retraction on an already anastomosed vein.

Most veins are lateral to the midline, and horizontal communication is usually present between veins. One can identify veins on the digit by finding one large vein and dissecting it out. Its branches will lead to other veins. These branches can be divided and used to add length to a venous anastomosis if necessary.

Proximal veins can easily be identified by the bleeding. The tourniquet can then be elevated so that they can be dissected free. They should be dissected sharply, with any tension on the vein being avoided.

After all veins have been identified, the anastomosis is carried out sequentially from one side of the digit to the other, placing a skin suture over each anastomosis after it is completed.

Veins have a thinner wall than arteries, and more sutures must be placed to help maintain dilatation by the blood. Sutures must be placed slightly farther back in relation to the thickness of the wall than in arteries. Often communicating branches prevent turning of the vein 180 degrees. The back sutures must be taken with the vein held at an angle by the corner sutures. Clamps should be avoided whenever possible. Often the anastomosis can be carried out without the use of either the tourniquet or clamps.

The adventitia is carefully trimmed so that it cannot occlude the lumen. The corner sutures are taken 120 to 180 degrees apart, and the front wall is completed. The back wall is then completed; flow is assessed by the patency test. The skin is then closed loosely over the veins for protection.

Often because of damaged intima and segmental losses, anastomosis cannot be carried out without undue tension. This is probably the greatest deterrent to successful microvascular anastomosis in replantation surgery. If tension is noted on either the venous or arterial side, a graft should be done without hesitation.

There are always ample veins available. The first choice would be the dorsum of the affected extremity. Digital veins can be chosen from the dorsum of an adjacent digit, or veins on the dorsum of the hand can be easily identified by application of a venous tourniquet and cutting down directly over the vein. The dorsal veins of the foot are also available but are somewhat larger. The brachial vein can be used for larger arteries. It is constant, and a 10 cm graft can be obtained with use of this vein.

After the vein has been located, the branches are cauterized with bipolar cautery or are ligated. An identification suture is placed on the proximal end, and this fact should be written down to ensure reversal of the vein in an arterial graft and no reversal in a venous graft. Even in the smallest veins, valves are present. When doing an arterial anastomosis, the vein must be reversed, and in a venous anastomosis, it should not be reversed. Doing the first anastomosis in the direction of flow ensures that blood is flowing through the vein graft toward the second anastomosis.

After ligation, the vein is immediately taken to the vein graft site and the anastomosis completed in the direction of flow. The tourniquet or clamp is then released. Patency is evaluated through the first anastomosis. The correct length of vein graft is determined and the vein divided appropriately. The second anastomosis is then carried out.

Ideally, the diameter of the vein graft should be no more than 20% different from the diameter of the recipient artery or vein. End-to-end anastomosis should be carried out in lieu of end-to-side whenever possible, since the flow characteristics are better.

Difficult vascular repairs

During microvascular surgery, problems on both the arterial and venous sides can occur. Below are listed some of the problems commonly encountered in replantation and composite tissue transfers and the solutions we have used successfully.

Arterial flow from the proximal vessel is poor. This is commonly encountered in an avulsion injury. Often after the part is amputated, the artery is stretched, and proximal to the amputation site there will be constriction where a branch leaves the artery. The artery should be dissected back proximally for several centimeters for identification of intimal tears and sites of constriction. Dilators can be used to dilate up to 10 to 12.5 cm proximally.

Local lidocaine will relax smooth muscle a small amount, although papaverine, in a 1:3 dilution, placed on the artery and injected into the proximal vessel, is much more effective.[3]

The last measure to increase arterial flow is to dissect the artery to the arch. Then the arch is divided, with part of the arch brought up for the anastomosis. Likewise, an adjacent digital vessel can be dissected from a normal finger and brought across for the anastomosis.

The princeps pollicis can be dissected back to the anatomic snuff box with an additional several centimeters of length made up (Figs. 4-11 and 4-12).

There is tension on the suture line. This is probably the most common deterrent to successful anastomosis. The vessel ends should come together easily with the first suture.

There is often insufficient length in segmental defects because the vessel ends have to be cut back to reach normal intima. Some length can be made up

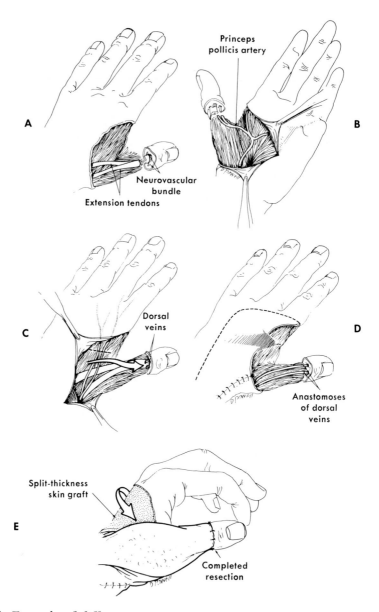

Fig. 4-11. Example of different anastomoses. Patient had an injury to thumb with segmental loss of skin and veins. **A,** Showing segmental loss of dorsum skin and veins. **B,** Incision made in palm and princeps pollicis dissected to gain length and anastomosis carried out. Good flow following. **C,** Incision on the dorsum of the hand and veins draining the index finger swung over and anastomosed to veins draining the replanted thumb. **D,** Closure of incision and outline of flap. **E,** Flap from the dorsum of the hand covers the venous anastomosis with split-thickness graft over the donor area.

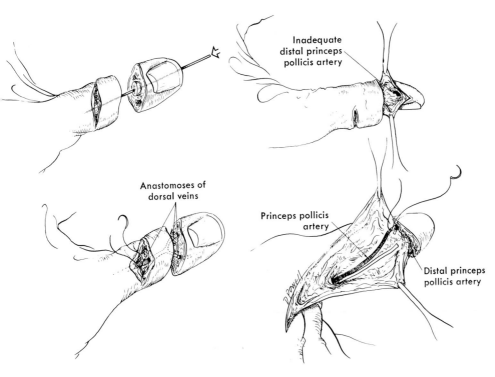

Fig. 4-12. Another example of vascular problems and thumb amputation with seg-mental venous interruption on the dorsum. **A,** Intramedullary fixation. **B,** Segmental loss of princeps pollicis. **C,** Dissection proximally to regain length with anastomosis and good flow in princeps pollicis artery. **D,** Dorsal veins anastomosed at two levels with successful replantation.

by proximal and distal dissection with cautery and dividing of the branches (Fig. 4-12).

The bone can be shortened or a tension suture can be taken on the skin to relieve tension on the anastomosis; however, a graft is preferable.

It is preferable to use a segment of artery for grafting material when avail-able. However, there are usually sufficient veins on the dorsum of the hand to use for a venous graft of sufficient length.

There are defects in the veins to be anastomosed. In some instances with segmental defects, flexion of the digit, or intimal damage, there is insufficient length of the veins for anastomosis.

Several steps can be taken. First, the vein should be dissected back, and the branches cut and cauterized to give 5 mm or so. Second, if the venous plexus is dissected, there are many horizontal connecting veins that can be cut in appropriate places and swung up to make up the defect. Third, a venous interposition graft can be done successfully. Finally, in several instances, a full-thickness flap, including its venous supply, can be swung from the dorsum of the arm or the hand (Fig. 4-11). In this way, not only will skin coverage be sufficient, but proximal veins will be present for any number of venous anastomoses. The defect from which the flap was taken can be covered with a split-thickness graft.

Skin coverage and anticoagulation

A routine midlateral incision should be used on the digit. Vertical incisions should not generally be sutured because of the expected postoperative edema. This avoids constriction. Horizontal incisions can be sutured for coverage over the vessels.

Split skin is poor coverage over exposed vessels. When local skin is not available, a flap can be used on both the volar and dorsal sides to cover the anastomosis. Dressings should be loosely applied and plaster placed only on one side of the extremity.

Postoperative monitoring and maintenance of flow

Vessels are small and have a relatively low flow, properties that make them susceptible to postoperative clotting. This is not apparent in many patients until the digit begins to necrose, making reversal of the thrombosis impossible.[4] Because of this, we have found continuous intraoperative and postoperative monitoring essential. Doing so allows the surgeon to alter hemodynamics or return the patient to the operating room to salvage the vascular anastomosis.

Intraoperatively, monitoring can be done with the digital plethysmograph. The height of the wave is roughly proportional to the amount of flow entering the digit. The flow should be at least 50% of the control digit or extremity.

Postoperatively, several methods to monitor flow are available[12] and are discussed in Chapter 6.

Nerve repair

In severe tissue injury and replantation, nerve injury is often severe, extending several centimeters or more along the trunk of the nerve. Repairs are difficult, but return of sensory and motor function is essential for function of the extremity.

Nerve trunks are made up of an epineurial sheath that continues to the center of the nerve and contains connective tissues and blood vessels derived from mesenchymal tissues. Its collagen is relatively coarse. This epineurial tissue makes up from one-fourth to three-fourths of the cross-sectional area of peripheral nerves depending on its location. Within the epineurium are the fascicles (funiculi), which are surrounded by perineurium. It is responsible for the strength of the peripheral nerves, provide a diffusion barrier, and maintain an interfascicular pressure gradient. Within the fascicles or funiculi is the endoneurium of neuroectodermal origin with a finer collagen. The endoneurium forms tubules within which the axons lie surrounded by Schwann cells and myelin.

Fascicles vary in size from about one twentieth of a millimeter to several millimeters. Several fascicles will often join together to form bundles.

There is a great deal of anatomic variation within a given nerve trunk throughout its length. These variations often make repair difficult:

1. The percentage of epineurial tissue compared to funicular tissue varies from about 25% to 75% throughout the nerve.
2. The cross-sectional fascicular pattern varies, because of interconnections between fascicles. Axons will travel from one fascicle to another as they move distally along the nerve.
3. There is also a difference in the composition of any fascicle throughout the length of the nerve. More distally the fascicles are divided into those that contain primarily sensory and those that contain primarily motor axons. More proximally, however, each fascicle will contain a significant number of motor and sensory fascicles.

When a nerve is injured through trauma, the axons distal to the site of division will degenerate. Proximally, the nerve will die back several millimeters through one or more nodes of Ranvier. A certain number of central cell bodies will undergo degeneration. Thus a certain number of axons will be forever lost to the nerve.

In regeneration, the axons grow from the proximal cut end of the nerve in an effort to find endoneurial tubes. Each axon can produce many sprouts and those sprouts entering endoneurial tubes will hypertrophy and start the nerve regeneration. For useful regeneration, the axons must find *functionally* related endoneurial tubes. For instance, motor axons going down endoneurial tubes that have sensory endings will be of little use to the patient.

Axons are able to cross significant gaps. However, they are impeded by scar formation from the epineurium, or by the use in the reparative process of a section of the nerve that has been damaged during the original trauma. Our preferred method of nerve repair has evolved from these facts and it is based on several principles.

First, the nerve must be cut back to healthy tissue. Healthy tissue often cannot be ascertained early in severe injury; thus late repairs are made necessary. Proper magnification will help in determining where the nerve injury ends and healthy fascicles begin.

Second, the fascicular pattern must be identified, both proximally and distally. The fascicular pattern can be identified in clean lacerations. This pattern and external markers, such as branches of arteries or veins within the epineurium, enable proper orientation to be achieved for the repair.

Where the fascicular pattern differs because of segmental loss of the nerve, one should be familiar with the anatomy of the trunk well described by Sunderland.[13] In segmental losses, knowledge of the funicular anatomy throughout the nerve trunk can help in correct repair of the nerves so that functionally related fascicles are opposed.

Third, the nerve must be approximated without tension. This occasionally requires dissection proximally and distally and, when large gaps are present, requires a sural-nerve cable graft. When there is a high proportion of connective tissue compared to fascicular tissue within the nerve, or when there is a variation in fascicular pattern from the proximal cut end to the distal cut end, a bundle or fascicular suture may be more appropriate.[10]

However, when there is (1) a higher proportion of nerve tissue compared to connective tissue, or (2) a similar funicular pattern, or (3) a proximal lesion in which each funiculus contains a significant amount of sensory and motor axons, then epineurial repair may be preferable. In most instances, epineurial repair without grafting is most appropriate.[6,15]

When the repair is performed, magnification and fine suture material (8-0 or less) prevent intraneural damage. Proper orientation is stressed, and the nerve must be handled as gently as possible to prevent further damage to proximal axons and cell bodies.

In later repairs, especially in lacerations in the distal portion of the nerve, correct orientation can be obtained by use of the procedure under local anesthesia. When the skin and subcutaneous tissue are infiltrated, the proximal cut end can be identified and the fascicular localization of primarily sensory and motor fascicles can be done. When the nerve is dissected distal to the previous area, the motor and sensory branches can be identified. When both the proximal and distal fascicles that contain primarily motor and sensory branches are identified, correct fascicular orientation can be accomplished with either epineurial or fascicular repair.

When early repairs are done, especially in clean cuts, the distal cut end of the nerve can be stimulated to determine which fascicles contain motor axons. When the proximal cut end of the nerve is stimulated under local anesthesia, the patient can identify which nerves contain primarily sensory axons. Therefore, fascicular orientation can be accomplished by either fascicular or epineurial repair.

After the repair the nerve must be protected for at least 3 weeks. The extremity can then be mobilized gradually.

ACKNOWLEDGMENT

Work in this chapter was partially supported by NIH Grant no. 1 RO1 GM25666.

REFERENCES

1. Adelaar, R. S., Soucacos, P. N., and Urbaniak, J. R.: Autologous cortical grafts with microsurgical anastomosis of periosteal vessels, Surg. Forum **25:**1974.
2. Bright, D. S., Schonwetter, B., and Urbaniak, J. R.: Effects of microclips on blood flow in the microcirculation, Department of Surgery, Division of Orthopaedic Surgery, Durham, N.C. In preparation.

3. Bright, D. S., Urbaniak, J. R., Schonwetter, B., and Seaber, A. V.: Effects of vaso-active agents on microvascular spasm, Department of Surgery, Division of Ortho-paedic Surgery, Duke University Medical Center, Durham, N.C. In preparation.
4. Bright, D. S., and Urbaniak, J. R.: The physiology of the microcirculation after amputations and replantation, J. Hand Surg. **1**:80, July 1976.
5. Daniel, R. K., and Taylor, G. I.: Distant transfer of an island flap by microvascular anastomoses, Plast. Reconstr. Surg. **52**:111, 1973.
6. Goldner, J. L.: Biological principles of repair and regeneration of nerve and ten-don, South. Med. J. **64**:121-122, Jan. 1971.
7. Ikuta, Y., Kubo, T., and Tsuge, K.: Free muscle transplantation by microsurgical technique to treat severe Volkmann's contracture, Plast. Reconstr. Surg. **58**:407, 1976.
8. Jacobson, J. H., and Suarez, E. L.: Microsurgery and anastomosis of the small vessels, Surg. Forum **11**:243, 1960.
9. McCraw, J. B., and Furlow, L. T., Jr.: The dorsalis pedis arterialized flap: a clinical study, Plast. Reconstr. Surg. **55**:177, 1975.
10. Millesi, H.: Interfascicular grafts for repair of peripheral nerves of the upper ex-tremity, Orthop. Clin. North Am. **8**:387, April 1977.
11. O'Brien, B. M.: Microvascular reconstructive surgery, New York, 1977, Churchill Livingstone.
12. Stirrat, C. N., Seaber, A. V., Urbaniak, J. R., and Bright, D. S.: Temperature mon-itoring in digital replantation, J. Hand Surg. **3**:342, 1978.
13. Sunderland, S.: Nerves and nerve injuries, Baltimore, 1968, The Williams & Wilkins Co.
14. Tupper, J. W.: Vascular defects and salvage of failed vascular repairs. Presented at the American Academy of Orthopaedic Surgeons, Course on microsurgery: prac-tical use in orthopaedic surgery, Durham, N.C., Sept. 16, 1977.
15. Urbaniak, J. R., Bright, D. S., and Gelberman, R.: Sensory recovery in replanted digits. Presented at the Combined Meeting of the Australian and American So-cieties, Vienna, Austria, May 23, 1977.
16. Urbaniak, J. R., and Bright, D. S.: Replantation of amputated digits and hands in children, Interclinic Information Bull. **14**:1, 1975.
17. Urbaniak, J. R., Soucacos, P. N., Adelaar, R. S., Bright, D. S., and Whitehurst, L. A.: Experimental evaluation of microsurgical techniques in small artery anastomoses, Orthop. Clin. North Am. **8**:248, 1977.
18. Weiland, A. J., Villarreal-Rios, A., Kleinert, H. E., Kutz, J., Atasoy, E., and Lister, G.: Replantation of digits and hands: analysis of surgical techniques and functional result in 71 patients with 86 replantations, J. Hand Surg. **2**:1, 1977.

5. Replantation of amputated parts— technique, results, and indications

James R. Urbaniak

In 1962, Malt in Boston first successfully replanted a completely amputated arm of a 12-year-old boy.[12] The groundwork had been developed over 50 years earlier on animal limb replantation by Hopfner[5] of Europe and Carrel and Guthrie[3] of this country. However they were able to achieve viability in their dog-limb replantations for only about 3 weeks. There was a half century void in replantation interest until Lapchinsky of Russia and Snyder of Salt Lake City succeeded in obtaining long-term results in dog-limb reattachment in the early 1960s.[10,16]

Developments in the field of microsurgery have resulted in successful replantation of completely amputated hands and digits, which is becoming rather commonplace. Although the use of the operating microscope had been routine in the surgical specialties of otolaryngology and ophthalmology for more than 25 years, inexplicably its use was not applied to the reconstruction of small blood vessels until the work of Jacobson and Suarez[7] in 1960. Distally amputated fingers have been frequently reported as surviving as composite grafts; however most replantations of digits without vascular anastomoses have failed to survive. Proficiency in obtaining patent anastomoses of vessels 1.5 mm or less is necessary to accomplish viability of replanted hands and digits.

In 1963 Kleinert and Kasdan emphasized the importance of revascularization of severely damaged digits by repair of the small digital vessels.[8] Buncke's pioneer investigations in the successful replantation of partial hand amputations in monkeys proved that complete digital and hand amputations could be replanted successfully by use of microvascular techniques to anastomose vessels of 1 ml or less in diameter.[2] The first successful replantation of a human thumb by microvascular anastomosis was accomplished by Komatsu and Tamai[9] in Japan in 1965. A year later the Chinese reported a successful replantation of a completely amputated finger.[14] Over the next decade several microsurgery centers around the world have reported impressive series of successful replantations, with current viability rates approaching 85%.[6,11,13,15,17,19,20,22]

THE REPLANTATION TEAM

Surgeons engaged in the replantation of amputated parts should realistically be able to achieve a survival rate of 80%. A recent survey by the Microsurgery Committee of the American Society for Surgery of the Hand revealed that centers that perform 20 or more replantations per year are obtaining 80% or greater viability. The concept of a well-organized team is essential if a continually good success rate of survival is to be obtained. A microvascular surgeon functioning alone will find it extremely difficult to obtain and maintain consistency of quality because of the great demands placed on him. Everyday the replantation team must be readily available around the clock if a replantation service is to be provided. Since the replantation of multiple digits on an individual patient may require up to 16 hours, surgery can be very demanding. Even the replantation of a completely amputated single digit requires a minimum of 3 to 4 hours by an experienced microsurgeon or a team of microsurgeons. Since the patient with his amputated part usually arrives at inconvenient times, these emergency procedures can be extremely disrupting to the routine clinical day of a physician. Around the clock availability of an adequate number of accomplished microsurgeons enables relatively fresh surgeons to operate in a platoon system and thus eliminates the fatigue factor in these extremely tedious procedures. Proficiency in the anastomosis of microvessels (vessels of 1 mm diameter or less) must be developed by a team of microsurgeons in the animal laboratory. By practicing on vessels approximately 1 mm in diameter (the size of adult digital vessels) on femoral vessels of rats, brachial and femoral vessels of cats, or ear vessels of the rabbit, the prospective microsurgeon should be able to achieve a patency rate of 90%. This success rate of anastomosis is necessary if the replantation surgeon expects to accomplish an acceptable clinical survival rate of 80%. Microvascular techniques in the laboratory and in a clinical situation, as well as the instrumentation have been thoroughly described in earlier chapters of this text and will not be repeated in this chapter. Personnel other than skilled microsurgeons are vital to a successful replantation team. The operating microscope and microinstruments are delicate and easily damaged. This equipment must be kept in absolute functional condition for optimal performance. Our center has found it essential to have one person (technician, research fellow, nurse, or physician associate) responsible for the orderly arrangement and maintenance of the equipment. It is extremely frustrating for the microsurgeon to be compelled to use malfunctioning microinstruments or operating microscopes during a stressful and fatiguing microsurgical procedure at an inconvenient hour. A harmonious team concept is paramount in the operating room. It is extremely disturbing to be assisted in the operating room by an operating nurse who is unfamiliar with microsurgical instruments, microtechnique, and surgical sequence. Because the surgery is precise and fatiguing, and frequently the surgeon's field is confined to the view through the microscope, the operator's emotional and physical performance is improved by a knowledgeable accomplished scrub nurse.

In addition personnel well versed in the postoperative management of patients who have had replantations of amputated parts play an extremely important role in maintaining a high survival rate. Our 5 years of experience with more than 200 replantations has demonstrated that many replantations have been successful because of a careful postoperative program. Personnel well-trained in postsurgical management can diminish the labors of the surgeons as well as increase survival rates. The detailed postoperative management will be described in a later section.

INDICATIONS FOR REPLANTATION

Almost any amputated part can be successfully replanted by an experienced microsurgery team. However, success and survival must not be misconstrued with success in useful function of the replanted extremity. Our current criteria for indications for replantations are based on our follow-up evaluations of replantations in more than 200 patients. Even with this knowledge, the decision is still frequently difficult. Many factors, such as type, level, hand dominance, ischemic time of amputation, sex, age, health, occupation, and the economic and social situations, influence the surgeon's decision.

Guillotine type of amputations certainly are ideal; however in our experience this type of amputation is uncommon. Most amputations are ragged, avulsed, or crushed, conditions that complicate the surgical repair and diminish the success rate.

Good candidates for replantation are amputations of the following:
1. Thumb
2. Multiple digits
3. Amputation through the palm
4. Child (almost any part)
5. Wrist or forearm
6. Above elbow—only if sharp or moderately ragged or avulsed
7. Individual digit distal to the flexor superficialis insertion

This list is not necessarily a rigid order of priority. However, attempts at replantation in the first six should be performed if other factors are favorable. Certainly the prime considerations for digit replantations are thumbs and multiple-digit amputations (Fig. 5-1). A projection of the overall function of the hand always outweighs the cosmetic result. In some instances of multiple digital amputations, the surgeon may wisely choose to replant only some of the digits by transferring the least damaged digits to the least damaged or most useful stumps. The shifting of digits can result in a very functional hand with a good grip.

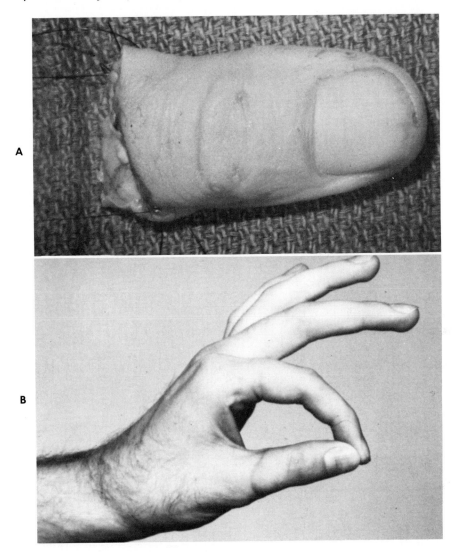

Fig. 5-1. Sharply amputated thumb in a teen-age boy was successfully replanted. The patient obtained 6 mm of two-point discrimination, independent metacarpal and interphalangeal motion, and tolerance to cold.

Replantations of amputations at the palm or metacarpal level, wrist, or forearm, if they survive, will result in a better functioning extremity than can be achieved by any type of prosthetic device (Fig. 5-2). Most amputations above the elbow are of the severe avulsion type, which makes successful replantation difficult and the rehabilitation period extremely long. Therefore, the surgeon must be very selective at this level. Our criteria for selection are less rigid in a child, because if the replantation remains viable, useful function

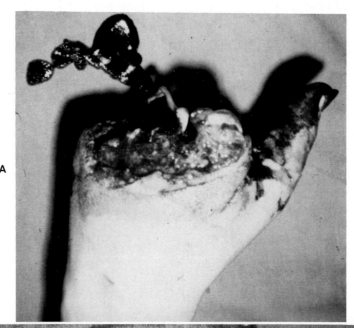

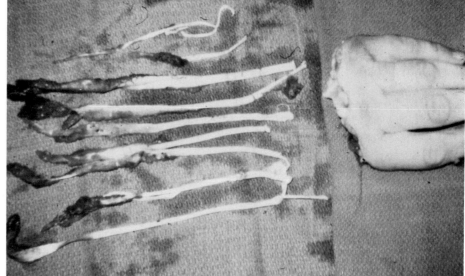

Fig. 5-2. **A** and **B,** This hand of a 30-year-old woman was avulsed by a horse rope. **C,** The four fingers were successfully replanted, and 9 months later two-point discrimination was 10 mm or less. Useful flexion and extension was obtained by delayed tendon grafting.

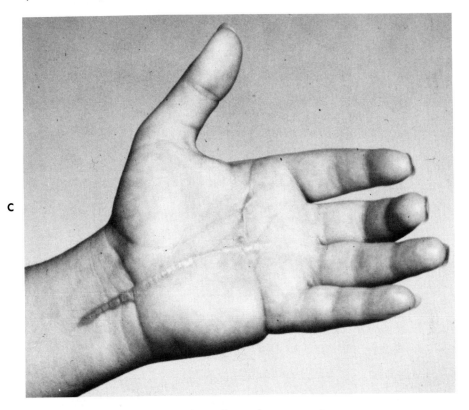

C

Fig. 5-2, cont'd. For legend see opposite page.

can be expected (Fig. 5-3). Even the lower extremities in a child, if cleanly amputated, deserve serious consideration for replantation.

Amputations of single or multiple digits that are distal to the flexor superficialis insertion are excellent candidates for replantation because the functional as well as cosmetic results are excellent and the operative time is relatively short (less than 4 hours) (Fig. 5-4).

Poor candidates for replantations are amputations as follows:
1. Severely crushed or mangled parts
2. Amputations at multiple levels
3. Amputations in patients who have had previous serious injuries to the amputated extremity
4. Amputations in patients with serious injuries or diseases
5. Amputations in which the vessels are arteriosclerotic
6. Amputations in mentally unstable patients
7. Individual digit with the amputation proximal to the superficialis insertion (in adults)

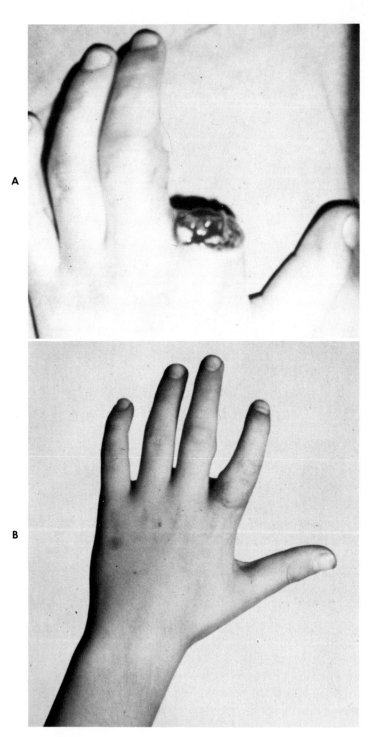

Fig. 5-3. Index finger of a 6-year-old male was cleanly amputated, **A.** Successful replantation resulted in a total active range of motion of 160 degrees of the digital joints and 3 mm of two-point discrimination, **B.**

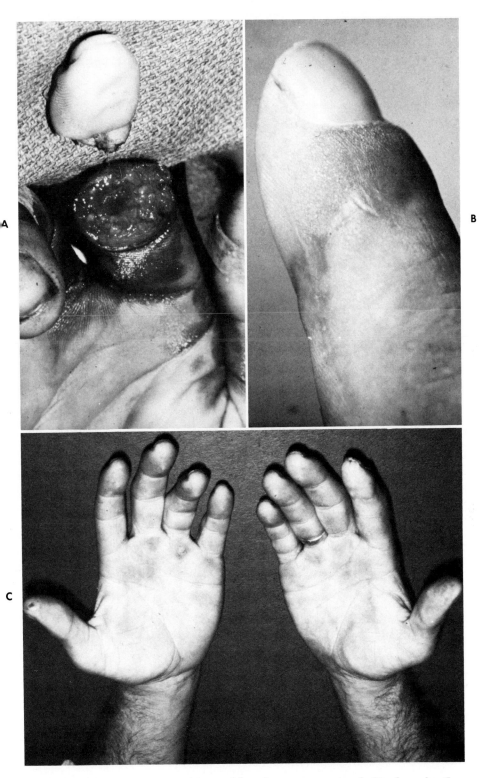

Fig. 5-4. A, Index finger of a 28-year-old male was amputated distal to the flexor superficialis insertion. **B,** Sensibility of 7 mm of two-point discrimination returned. The carpenter uses this digit on his dominant hand, as **C** indicates, since all fingertips are equally soiled from his labor.

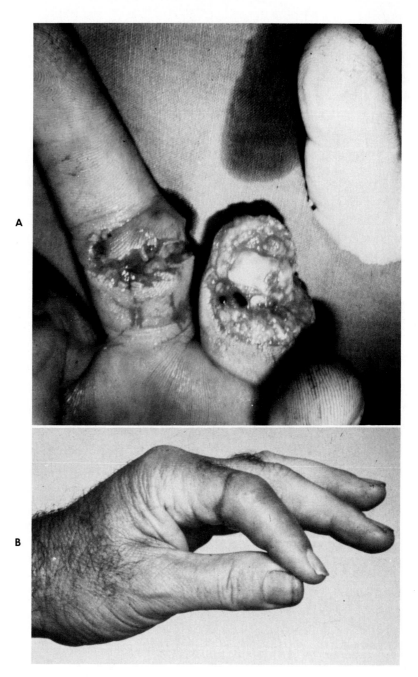

Fig. 5-5. Index finger of a 53-year-old contractor was amputated proximally to the proximal interphalangeal joint, **A.** The replantation was successful, but the patient avoided use of the digit in his daily work, **B.**

If the mechanism of the amputation has produced severe damage to the main vessels, then successful replantation is not possible. Although we frequently use vein grafts to replace injured vessels in the ragged or avulsed type of injuries, there is no method of replacing the most distal vessels in the amputated part. In older patients, the arteries should be examined for arteriosclerosis, for this precludes successful reanastomosis of small vessels. We have experienced failures in patients on whom we have tried to reattach arteries with definite arteriosclerotic plaques in the region of the anastomosis.

Careful appraisal of the patient's mental status is somewhat difficult in the immediate preoperative period because of the recent injury to the extremity. However, it has been the experience of the replantation surgeons that patients who have their upper extremity severed are not uncommonly emotionally unstable; in fact, this may play a role in the mechanism of their injury. Therefore, the emotional state of the patient is an important part of the initial history-taking on admission.

An isolated finger amputation proximal to the superficial tendon insertion generally should not be replanted in the adult. Even the index finger that has been completely amputated is not a good selection for replantation as the patient will usually bypass this digit on prehension (Fig. 5-5). Special considerations, for example, a musician who plays a stringed instrument, or even a young woman, may influence the decision.

We have attempted replantations for those patients 10 weeks to 60 years of age, and age is therefore not necessarily a limitation. An amputated thumb or hand, even in a patient 60 years or older, should be replanted, unless there are negating factors such as general health, economics, or the patient's opposing decision. We have found that on occasions the decision cannot be made until the vessels of the amputated part are examined under the operating microscope. In severe avulsions, particularly involving an important part such as the thumb, the decision may be delayed until the arterial anastomosis has been completed. If no venous backflow can be achieved, the replantation attempt is aborted. Family influence should not sway the surgeon to make an ill-advised decision in replanting an amputated part, for the family usually always wants the amputated part reattached, but they are not aware of the difficulty of the surgery, length of hospitalization, and functional outcome. Sometimes certain replantations are unwise in laborers, because of predicted loss of work time and functional result. However, our experience has revealed that a loss of work time in a successful replantation is frequently no longer than if the amputation is revised. Certainly the rehabilitation of a replanted digit, partial hand, or complete hand is easier and shorter and results are better than in many cases of mangled, crushed, or burned injuries to the hand.

PRESERVATION OF AMPUTATED PART

Proper primary care of the amputated part is critical. The referring physician must be given clear and brief instructions in the preparation of both the amputated part and the injured patient. The preparatory instructions for the primary care physician are as follows:

1. The amputated part or parts are placed in a bag containing Ringer's lactate or saline solution.
2. The plastic bag is placed in ice.
3. Direct contact of the amputated part with ice is avoided to prevent freezing of tissues.
4. The stump is wrapped in a sterile compressive dressing.
5. A tourniquet should not be used.
6. The vessels should not be ligated or perfused in any solution, such as heparin, for fear of producing intimal damage.

If the amputated part is not cooled, tissue will survive for approximately 6 hours before undergoing necrosis from lack of oxygen supply from arterial blood flow. However, an amputated digit will survive longer since there is no muscle tissue in a digit. An amputated part that has been cooled may survive for as long as 12 hours, or even longer if it is a digit. Although the transportation should be as rapid as possible, the referring physician is cautioned that there is no need for panic since successful replantation has been achieved as late as 20 hours after amputation.

INITIAL MANAGEMENT

When a patient with an amputated part arrives in the emergency room, the microsurgery team that has been alerted divides into two subteams. If replantation surgery is elected, one team cares for the amputated part and immediately transports it to the operating room where it is cleansed with pHisoHex and sterile Ringer's lactate solution. The amputated part is placed on a bed of ice covered with a sterile plastic drape. If there are multiple digits, they are preserved by keeping them under ice packets until they are required for reattachment. With the aid of operating loupes or an operating microscope (depending on the size of the amputated part), the amputated part is debrided and the nerves and vessels are located and tagged with 8-0 nylon suture. Preliminary shortening of the bone is performed at this stage and an intermedullary Kirschner wire is inserted in a retrograde fashion for immediate bone stabilization.

Simultaneously the other team assesses the patient with a routine physical examination, roentgenograms of the injured extremity and chest, electrocardiogram, blood chemistries, complete blood count, urinalysis, blood type and cross-matching, and an activated partial thromboplastin time. Intravenous fluids are instituted, and the patient is given intravenous antibiotics and tetanus prophylaxis if indicated.

An axillary block using a combination of 20 ml of 0.5% bupivacaine HCl (Marcaine) and 20 ml of 1% lidocaine is given in the emergency room prior to the patient's transfer to the operating theater. Usually general anesthesia is required in children under 12 years of age, although if the child is cooperative, we have used axillary block even in children as young as 9 years of age.

With the aid of tourniquet ischemia and magnification, one team debrides the stump and identifies the nerves and vessels and tags them with 8-0 nylon sutures. Identification of the veins on the stump and amputated part is particularly difficult, and the surgeon learns to identify them more rapidly with experience. Their identification requires meticulous tissue dissection and patience, since successful replantation depends on careful anastomosis of an adequate number of veins (a minimum of three venous anastomoses is usually attempted in all types of replantation). Replantation of amputated hands or digits must be performed by the surgeon experienced in hand surgery as well as microsurgery. The team members involved in these important preparatory phases must be thoroughly knowledgeable of the anatomy of the hand and experienced in the techniques of hand surgery. Any additional damage to or mishandling of the already traumatized vessels will jeopardize the success of revascularization. The location and labeling of vital structures are critical time-saving steps of replantation and are particularly important in the patient with multiple amputations. Neglecting to label these important structures can induce extreme frustration in the microsurgeon in later stages of replantation where the fatigue factor influences the surgeon's proficiency.

SEQUENCE OF SURGERY

The operative sequence of replantation varies slightly with the type of injury, that is, a clean-cut injury or an avulsing type, and the location of the injury, that is, digit and hand versus areas proximal to the wrist. Since digital and hand to partial hand, and hand replantations are much more common than proximal replantations, the sequence of the surgery will be described for digital and hand replantations first and then variations in the technique will be mentioned later.

The sequence for digital replantation is as follows:
1. Bone shortening and fixation
2. Extensor tendon repair
3. Flexor tendon repair (optional)
4. Arterial anastomosis
5. Nerve repair
6. Venous anastomosis
7. Skin coverage

The technique of each of these surgical steps will be described in detail.

Bone shortening and fixation

Bone shortening and fixation is a crucial step in replantation surgery.[19] To insure the approximation of normal intima in the vascular anastomoses, adequate bone must be resected. The connection of arteries, veins, and nerves must never be performed under tension. Therefore the bone ends must be adequately shortened to achieve ease in approximation of the vital structures. A greater amount of bone must be resected in the crushing or avulsion type of injuries to allow ease of coaptation of undamaged vessels. In the digit it is usually necessary to resect 0.5 to 1 cm of bone, and in amputations proximal to the hand or wrist level, it is frequently necessary to resect 2 to 3 cm of bone. Even more resection may be indicated in the avulsing type of injury. Tupper has emphasized that bone shortening is rarely necessary and prefers vein grafting when there is considerable intimal damage.[18] However, it is our impression that bone shortening should generally be favored over vein grafting because one anastomotic site is more favorable than two. In addition, in a situation where vessels require grafting because of extensive damage, there is frequently concomitant damage to the nerves and other soft-tissue structures, which likewise need to be shortened. Also, the shortened replanted digit, which frequently has a restricted range of motion, is generally less obvious and less likely to "get in the way." We hasten to add, however, that we do not hesitate to perform vein grafts when we believe they are indicated. Certainly it is easier, quicker, and less frustrating to perform a vein graft rather than to redo a difficult anastomosis several times. Also, any difficult anastomosis when performed under tension is unlikely to remain a patent vessel.

In amputations of the thumb, it is of extreme importance that the major portion of the bone shortening in the replantation of the thumb be on the severed distal end, so that a maximal amount of bone is preserved proximally (on the stump) to ensure good bone stock should the replantation fail. Our preference for digital bone fixation is a single intramedullary Kirschner wire inserted by a motorized, cordless drill. The reasons for this selection are (1) simplicity and speed of technique, (2) less bone exposure required, (3) less skeletal mass needed for fixation, (4) rotation of the replanted digit possible if needed to realign the vessels, and (5) ease of reshortening after fixation if further shortening is indicated during the vascular repair.

A second longitudinal intramedullary pin may be used for better stability, although this has usually not been necessary. We have been reluctant to insert cross pins for better stabilization at the end of the procedure, for fear of damaging a repaired neurovascular bundle by tethering of the vessel or its supporting structures by the pin. However, on occasions we have used cross Kirschner wire fixation, and this has been a preferred choice when fusion is elected at a joint level.

We have also used circular wire, inserted through drill holes in a longitudinal axis of the bone, or perpendicular to the fracture site. We sometimes insert two circular wires at right angles to each other. This method does eliminate the interference of the Kirschner wires with the soft-tissue structures and may make earlier motion easier if good stability is obtained. However, we have not always found this a reliable method of obtaining good stability and it does require more exposure of bone and frequently more surgical time.

Amputations at the wrist level have been stabilized by cross Steinmann pins, and amputations more proximal have been stabilized usually by large intramedullary pins such as Rush rods with the addition of a wire through drill holes to prevent distraction. If the time factor is not critical, that is, a need for immediate arterial inflow, then plates and screws are used. Most of our bone fixation has been obtained by a single longitudinal intramedullary pin. Nonunion has not been a serious problem in our experience of over 200 replants. We have not found it necessary to perform a secondary procedure because of nonunion. Angulation or malunion has occurred in less than 5% of patients. Superficial infections secondary to the pins, which are usually immediately beneath the skin, have occurred in 5% of the patients but have always responded rapidly to removal of the pins.

Extensor tendon repair

After bone shortening and fixation, the extensor tendon is repaired with two 4-0 polyester sutures placed in a horizontal mattress fashion. Extensor tendon repair further stabilizes the bone junction by diminishing rotational instability, particularly if intramedullary pin fixation is used. In amputations in the proximal phalangeal area it is extremely important to repair the lateral bands of the extensor tendon if optimal extension of the distal interphalangeal joint and proximal interphalangeal joint is to be expected. In the earlier years of our replantation experience, we repaired only the central portion of the extensor mechanism, and inadequate or incomplete extension of the two distal joints of the digit was apparent. During the past 2 to 3 years, we have noted an improvement in distal joint extension after reestablishment of the lateral bands when it has been possible.

In some instances of a severe avulsing injury there is no extensor available either on the amputated part or the proximal stump. In these situations, interphalangeal joint fusion or extensor tendon grafting as secondary procedures are necessary.

Flexor tendon repair

Primary flexor tendon repair should be attempted in clean-cut amputations. In the ragged or avulsion type of injuries, we do not advocate extensive dissection or lengthy incisions to retrieve or reconstruct avulsed tendon. In such a situation we prefer to do secondary flexor tendon repair, often using two-stage silicone-rod grafting for flexor tendon reconstruction. If the flexor tendon transection occurs in the proximal portion of the digit that is being replanted, it may be expeditious to insert the sutures into the free flexor tendon ends but not coapt the tendon ends until after the vascular and nerve anastomoses have been completed on the flexor surface. The advantage of this method is that the digit may be held in full extension for better exposure for the vascular and nerve repairs on the flexor surface of the hand.

There is no urgency in performing primary flexor tendon repair as secondary tendon reconstruction may be safely performed as early as 3 months after replantation. In amputations through the palm or wrist we prefer to repair all flexor and extensor tendons primarily because of the difficulty of reentering this scarred area. However, in avulsion injuries, as mentioned, this may not be possible or advisable. Delayed two-stage silicone-rod flexor tendon grafting is frequently used successfully in our replanted digits. Delayed Z-lengthening of the flexor pollicis longus at the wrist and advancement distally has been successfully used in seven of our thumb replantations.[21]

Arterial and venous microsurgery repair

The microvascular techniques have been thoroughly described in the previous chapter by Bright, and only a few points will be emphasized in this section. Table 1 provides suggestions for needle and suture size at the various levels. Monofilament nylon or polypropylene (Prolene) is used in all vascular repairs distal to the wrist. The needle size may be as large as 150 microns at the wrist and as small as 50 microns at the distal digit particularly for the veins. Suture size is usually 9-0 nylon for the wrist vessels and as small as 11-0 nylon for distal digital vessels.

After fixation, extensor tendon repair, and possibly flexor tendon repair, the arteries are anastomosed. In a digit, we always attempt to repair both digital arteries, and in a partial hand or wrist amputation, we repair all arteries that can possibly be salvaged. The artery must be resected until normal intima is visualized under high-power magnification; *only normal intima is reconnected.* If this is not possible, the bone must be further shortened or a vein graft used.

The two most important determining factors in achieving successful microvascular anastomosis are (1) skill and expertise of the microsurgeon and (2) easy coaptation of normal intima. Clinical revascularization in replantation procedures is not the setting for training of microvascular techniques. These skills must be developed and perfected in the animal laboratory, and only the

Table 1. Appropriate needle and suture size for microvascular repairs in the hand

Location	Needle size in microns	Suture size
Wrist	150	9-0
Palm	100	10-0
Proximal digit	75-50	10-0
Distal digit	50	11-0

most experienced microvascular surgeon should perform the vascular repairs in replantation surgery. We never deviate from this rule.

We have found it more advantageous to use a pneumatic tourniquet with frequent inflation and deflation during the replantation procedure. This enables us to repair the arteries first and then control bleeding. We have found tourniquet use has no effect on clotting across the anastomosis site. Since all available microclips do produce some amount of intimal changes, we attempt to use them as little as possible and certainly their application time should be less than 30 minutes.[1] The use of the tourniquet does diminish the need for microclips; however we use them when the exposure is difficult, but generally we refrain from using them on veins, particularly small fragile veins. Immediately after the anastomosis has been accomplished, there should be flow through the repaired artery, and pinking of the distal skin should occur within a few minutes if not instantly. A long delay from amputation to revascularization, combined with cooling, may result in a prolonged latency period from reanastomosis to apparent perfusion of the distal portion of the digit. Venous backflow must occur if the part is to survive.

Prior to the completion of the arterial anastomosis, intravenous heparin (3000 to 5000 units) is administered. Subsequently 1000 units of intravenous heparin are given hourly during the operation. This dosage is adjusted for children. We attempt to anastomose two veins for each artery, and if necessary the veins are mobilized or "harvested" to obtain anastomoses without tension. Vein grafts may be necessary to obtain a ratio of two veins per artery, and every attempt is made to anastomose at least three veins per amputated part.

Many recognized replantation surgeons repair veins prior to the arteries to decrease the blood loss and maintain a bloodless field for better vision. However, by judicious use of the tourniquet, we have been able to repair the artery first, maintain a dry field, and have the advantages of early revascularization of the amputated part and easier location of the most functional veins detected by their spurting backflow. In addition, if the veins are repaired first, particularly in a severe avulsion injury, and subsequent arterial anastomosis fails to show adequate arterial inflow, then the surgeon will have wasted valuable time on a nonsalvageable part.

Since small veins are considerably more fragile than arteries, the microclips should be avoided when possible. Proper use of the tourniquet usually obviates the necessity for using microclips on veins.

Nerve repair

Because the bone has usually been shortened in replantations, nerve repair is generally not difficult, since it is easy to approximate the severed ends with no tension at the suture line. With the aid of the microscope, careful fascicular alignment can be achieved in the freshly injured nerve. However, in some instances where there has been avulsion, it is difficult to tell how much nerve to resect in the acutely injured nerve. However, it has been our principle to repair the peripheral nerves primarily in all replantations, except those in which there has been severe avulsion, making primary repair impossible.

We use 8-0 or 9-0 monofilament nylon or polypropylene (Prolene) for repair of the peripheral nerves. An epineurial suture is repaired after the fascicles are properly aligned. Nylon 8-0 or 9-0 is of sufficient strength, since the nerves are repaired with no tension. In the digital nerves, only two or three sutures are usually necessary, and as the repair of nerves moves more proximally in the upper extremity, more interrupted sutures are indicated.

We have not used nerve grafts to make up large defects as a primary procedure. However, sural nerve grafts have been used in secondary repair. Approximately 5% of our primary repairs have had to have further resection and end-to-end repair or nerve grafting at a later date because of evidence of poor sensory recovery.

Skin coverage and dressing

Meticulous hemostasis using a bipolar coagulator is obtained after all the structures have been repaired and revascularization of the amputated part has been assured. The skin is loosely approximated with interrupted nylon sutures. All damaged skin that may become necrotic is carefully excised and no tension should be placed on the skin during the closure. The vessels should be covered without compression or constriction from the overlying skin or sutures. If doing so is not possible, a local flap or split-thickness skin is used. Fasciotomies are indicated if there is the slightest indication of distal or proximal compression. The wounds are covered with small strips of gauze impregnated with petrolatum. Care is taken in the placement of these petrolatum strips so that they are not continuous or circumferential in the digits.

The upper extremity is immobilized in a bulky compression hand dressing that extends above the elbow to prevent slippage. Extreme care is taken to prevent circumferential pressure.

Plaster splints should be placed only on the volar aspect of the dressing to permit ease of exposure of the dorsum of the digits if this is necessary in the postoperative course.

The postoperative management will be discussed in a subsequent chapter.

RESULTS

From 1973 to 1978 the Duke Orthopaedic Replantation Team has attempted revascularization on 187 complete or incomplete amputations (Table 2).

Seventy-five of 80 incomplete amputations have been successfully revascularized. Eighty-eight of 107 complete amputations have been successfully replanted for a viability of 82%.

Table 2. Revascularizations—187 total

	Number	Type	Viability
	107	Complete	88 (82%)
	80	Incomplete	75 (94%)

Sensory recovery in replanted digits is nearly as good as that seen in isolated peripheral nerve repairs.[4] Of the patients studied, 90% have recovered protective sensibility, two thirds have two-point discrimination of 15 mm or less, and 50% of the patients have a sensibility rating of 10 mm of two-point discrimination or less. Most patients do experience some degree of cold intolerance, but this usually improves with time and requires about 1 year before there is a significant decrease in the intolerance and it completely or nearly completely subsides about 2 years after surgery in most of the patients.

Replanted thumbs offer the best functional results for excellent sensation (frequently two-point discrimination of 6 mm or less), and adequate joint motion and pinch strength can be expected. Likewise replantations of fingers amputated distal to the superficialis insertion restore good distal sensation (two-point discrimination of 10 mm or less), pulp, turgor, and cosmesis while maintaining good range of motion of the proximal joints. Replantations of multiple digits, partial hands (through the palm), or complete hands provide good sensation and gross grasp, but usually poor prehension and dexterity. In adults, isolated finger amputations proximal to the superficialis insertion usually result in digits that "get in the way." Only two patients have stated that they felt the replanted digit was not worthwhile in follow-up interviews. The time out from work has averaged about 4 months in all replantations; however patients with isolated digits are frequently able to return to work in about a month. In industrial or compensation injuries, the total cost for the insurance carrier for a patient with a replantation compares favorably with the cost of compensating the patient who does not have his parts replanted. One of the best advantages of the replanted digit is that painful neuromas do not occur as they frequently do in finger stumps from amputations.

CONCLUSION

Successful replantations proximal to the elbow consistently restore useful function that is superior to any type of prosthetic device. Our 5-year follow-up of over 200 replantations has shown that although the technical procedures are long and involved, the results are generally satisfactory with good functioning digits and hands. A well-organized and proficient microsurgical team should statistically be able to achieve an 80% viability in the replantation of amputated hands and digits.

REFERENCES

1. Bright, D. S., Schonwetter, B., and Urbaniak, J. R.: Effects of microclips on blood flow in one millimeter vessels—experimental analysis with microflow probes. Unpublished study.
2. Buncke, H. J., Buncke, C. M., and Schulz, W. B.: Experimental digital amputation and reimplantation, Plast. Reconstr. Surg. **36**:62-70, 1965.
3. Carrel, A., and Guthrie, C. C.: Results of a replantation of the thigh, Science **23**:393, 1906.
4. Gelberman, R. H., Urbaniak, J. R., Bright, D. S., and Levin, L. S.: Digital sensibility following replantation, J. Hand Surg. **3**:313-321, 1978.
5. Hopfner, E.: Über Gefässnaht, Gefässtransplantation und Reimplantation von amputierten Extremitäten, Arch. Klin. Chir. **70**:417, 1903.
6. Ikuta, Y.: Microvascular surgery, Hiroshima, 1975, Lens Press, p. 42.
7. Jacobson, J. H., and Suarez, E. L.: Microsurgery and anastomosis of the small vessels, Surg. Forum **11**:243, 1960.
8. Kleinert, H. E., and Kasdan, M. L.: Anastomosis of digital vessels, J. Kentucky Med. Assoc. **63**:106, 1963.
9. Komatsu, S., and Tamai, S.: Successful replantation of a completely cut-off thumb: case report, Plast. Reconstr. Surg. **42**:374, 1968.
10. Lapchinsky, C. A.: Recent results of experimental transplantation of preserved limbs and kidneys and possible use of this technique in clinical practice, Ann. N.Y. Acad. Sci. **64**:539, 1960.
11. Lendvay, P. G.: Replacement of the amputated digit, Br. J. Plast. Surg. **26**:398-405, 1973.
12. Malt, R. A., and McKhann, C.: Replantation of severed arms, J.A.M.A. **189**:716-722, 1964.
13. O'Brien, B. M.: Microvascular reconstructive surgery, London, 1977, Churchill Livingstone.
14. Sixth People's Hospital, Shanghai: Reattachment of traumatic amputations. A summing up of experience, Chinese Med. J. **1**:392, 1967.
15. Sixth People's Hospital, Shanghai: Replantation of severed fingers: clinical experiences in 162 cases involving 270 severed fingers, pamphlet, July 1963.
16. Snyder, C. C., and Knowles, R. P.: Autotransplantation of extremities, Clin. Orthop. **29**:113, 1963.
17. Tsai, T. M.: Experimental and clinical applications of microvascular surgery, Ann. Surg. **181**:169, 1975.
18. Tupper, J. W.: Vascular defects and salvage of failed vascular repairs. Presented at the AAOS Course. Microsurgery—practical use in orthopaedic surgery, Durham, N.C., Sept. 16, 1977.
19. Urbaniak, J. R., Hayes, M. G., and Bright, D. S.: Management of bone in digital replantation: free vascularized and composite bone grafts, Clin. Orthop. **133**:184, 1978.
20. Urbaniak, J. R.: Replantation of amputated digits and hands. Instructional Course Lectures—AAOS **27**:15, 1978.
21. Urbaniak, J. R., and Goldner, J. L.: Laceration of the flexor pollicis longus tendon, delayed repair by advancement, free graft or direct suture. A clinical and experimental study, J. Bone Joint Surg. **55-A**:1123-1148, 1973.
22. Weiland, A. J., Villarreal-Rios, A., Kleinert, H. E., Kutz, J., Atasoy, E., and Lister, G.: Replantation of digits and hands: analysis of surgical techniques and functional result in 71 patients with 86 replantations, J. Hand Surg. **2**:1-12, 1977.

6. Postoperative management in replantation

Donald S. Bright
Sydney Wright

Postoperative care in replantation begins in the operating room and continues for 3 weeks. For the last 5 years, we have concentrated on postoperative management in the belief that this will increase not only the survival rate in amputations, but also the final functioning of the replanted hand or digit. We believe that the final functional result relates proportionally to the flow and that proper postoperative management will help to ensure that maximum flow is achieved.

INSTRUMENTATION

The small size of vessels and the frequent difficulty in determining patency both prior to and after surgery require that special instrumentation be used in monitoring patency.

The *ultrasonic Doppler scanner* is the most readily available. It gives a qualitative estimate of flow through arteries, but is difficult to use in small venous anastomoses. It has been used by others with a chart recorder to give a semiquantitative value of flow, but this can be inconsistent. The Doppler scanner is difficult to apply to a digit if the hand is in a dressing. Although we have used it in the postoperative period in major extremity replantations, its use in digital replantations is limited because of the presence of the dressing.

The *digital plethysmograph* or *pulse volume flowmeter* (Figs. 6-1 to 6-3) has been found useful for preoperative, intraoperative, and postoperative monitoring. The recording can be demonstrated on a chart recorder or oscilloscope and is generally proportional to flow through the vessel. It can be used for estimating the flow through an anastomosed artery intraoperatively and can also be used periodically throughout the postoperative period to determine the extent of flow. It is of limited value in determining venous patency.

We have found the *temperature gauge* to be the most convenient tool in determining patency in digital replantation (Figs. 6-4 to 6-7). Three temperature gauges are necessary: one on the replanted digit or hand, the second on

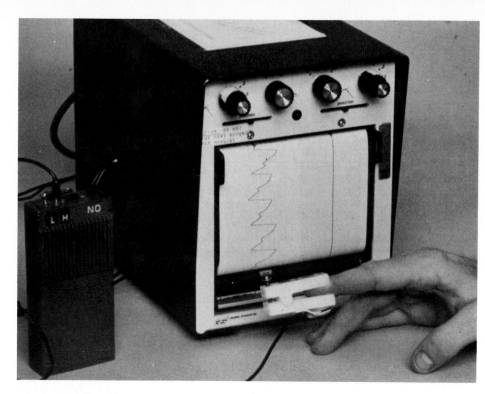

Fig. 6-1. Pulse volume flowmeter or digital plethysmograph. A piezoelectric crystal records the change in pulp volume with increased arterial flow. The recording on the strip chart is roughly proportional to the flow in the digit when compared to the height of the wave on the opposite or adjacent digit. This is a semiquantitative measurement of flow and is useful both in determining the state of flow and in assessing measures that increase or decrease flow.

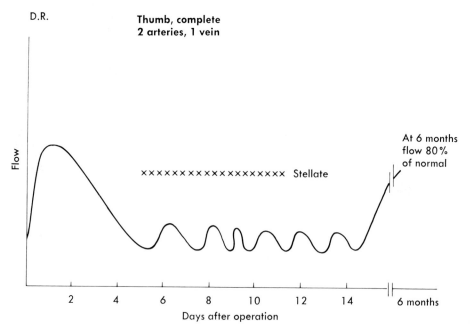

Fig. 6-2. Patient with complete amputation of thumb with replantation. On the sixth postoperative day there was a decrease in flow, but the flow was increased with periodic stellate blocks. When measured 6 months later, the flow had increased to 80% of the opposite normal digit, and color, tissue turgor, and recovery were all good.

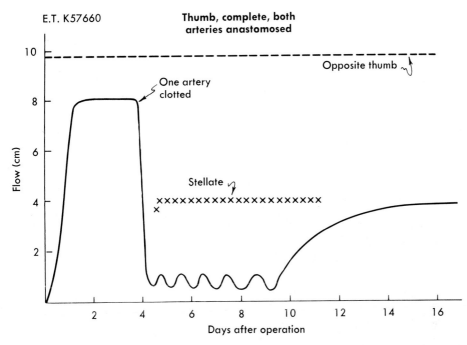

Fig. 6-3. Patient with complete amputation and replantation of thumb. At day 4 the ulnar digital artery or princeps pollicis became clotted and the digit was salvaged with repeated stellate blocks. After the second week the flow stabilized, and after 2 years the patient had flow that was over 50% when compared to the opposite thumb. Cold intolerance lasted for $2^1/_4$ years, however.

the adjacent or opposite digit, and the third on a dressing to determine ambient temperature. They can be easily monitored by nursing personnel. Normal digital temperatures range from 30° to 35° C. When the arterial and venous anastomoses are patent, the temperature of the replanted part will approximate within two to three degrees that of the control digit. If the temperature of the replanted part falls several degrees or especially below 30° C, thrombosis either on the arterial or venous side is likely.

Both the digital plethysmograph and the temperature gauge can also be used to monitor the response to vasoactive agents. For instance, if there is decreased flow in the postoperative period, this will appear as a decrease in flow on the pulse volume flowmeter and a decrease in temperature below 30° C. The administration of an axillary or stellate block, an increase in intravenous heparin, and correction of any constricting dressings will, if successful, result in an increase in flow and in temperature.

Clinical evaluation, of course, is most important. However, experienced surgeons cannot always be present on the ward, and we have found that

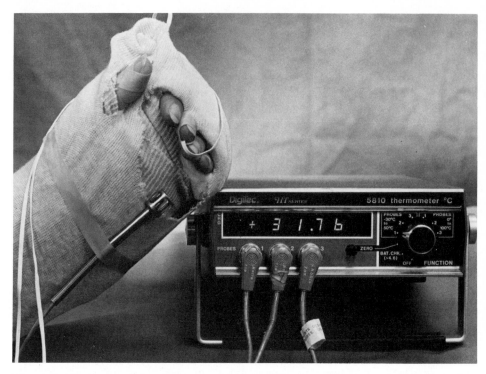

Fig. 6-4. Thermistor is battery operated and is used continually in the postoperative period at the patient's bedside and monitored by the nurses on an hourly basis. One probe is placed on the amputated part, the second probe on the adjacent or opposite normal digit, and the third probe on the dressing to record ambient temperature. In ideal flow situations, the amputated part is within 2 to 3 Celsius degrees of the normal part. If there is a decrease of 2 to 3 degrees or if there is a decrease below 30° C depending on ambient temperature, then there may be a precarious situation. Measures are then instituted to increase flow.

experienced ancillary personnel using well-calibrated instruments can, in many instances, avert difficulty early.

PHYSIOLOGIC CONSIDERATIONS
Generalized flow considerations

There are, in general, three phases after microvascular repair. The underlying causes are not well understood, but we have often observed these phases.

Phase I. Phase I includes the intraoperative period when the surgery is done under axillary block with decreased sympathetic tone. Vessels are probed, local vasodilating agents are used, and anastomoses are carried out. The initial flow is usually good, there being no sympathetic tone, and local spasm can usually be overcome by mechanical means, proximal dissection, or

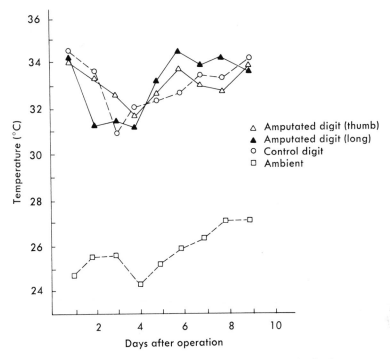

Fig. 6-5. A patient with complete amputation of the thumb who had consistently high temperatures in the postoperative period. His postoperative course was uncomplicated, and he has done well since then.

vasoactive agents. In many patients, because of a relatively clean cut, a good approximation of the vessel, and decreased pain and sympathetic tone, the replanted part will continue to have excellent flow.

Phase II. In other patients, however, there will be a second phase lasting from 1 to 10 days when there will be a general decrease in flow. The decrease in flow is rather phasic; that is, if the flowmeter is allowed to run over a 24-hour period, there will be variations in flow over time in a gentle, undulating pattern. As flow reaches a low point, certain patients will clot their arterial or venous anastomosis with resulting loss of viability of the replanted part. We believe that three areas are responsible for this: (1) compression from the dressing, (2) increased sympathetic tone, and (3) local factors.

Compression from the dressing. Constricting dressings will cause decreased flow. This is obvious when there is circumferential plaster or when a blood-soaked bandage is allowed to dry in conjunction with swelling of the amputated and replanted part. For this reason, daily checks are made of the bandage; if in the early postoperative period excessive bleeding is present, the bandage is changed while wet.

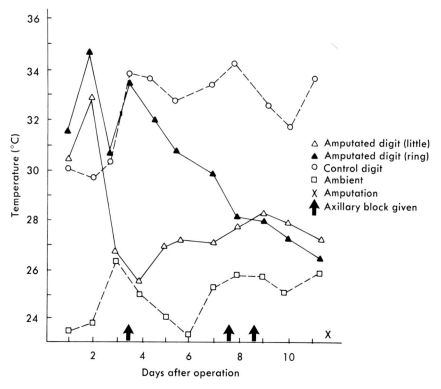

Fig. 6-6. A patient with complete amputation of the long, ring, and little fingers. He had replantation of the ring and little fingers. In the postoperative period the patient had a decreased temperature as evidenced on the graph. This was unresponsive to axillary blocks and increased use of heparin. The patient had failure of the replantation and underwent amputation of both replanted digits.

Increased sympathetic tone. The amputated part, of course has no sympathetic tone. The proximal vessels are strongly affected by sympathetic tone, and we believe that this tone is one of the most important deterrents to successful replantation. We have observed that increased sympathetic tone in the postoperative period is caused by four major factors:

1. DIMINUTION OF EFFECTS OF ANESTHETIC. The axillary or stellate block wears off and there is a concomitant increase in tone to the level that existed before block was administered.

2. PAIN. Pain in the intraoperative or postoperative period contributes significantly to sympathetic tone. We have noted in several instances during an operative procedure that as the axillary block wears off, the flow through the vessels decreases. When general anesthesia is instituted to relieve the pain, flow increases. For this and other reasons, repeated axillary blocks and administration of adequate pain medication are important.

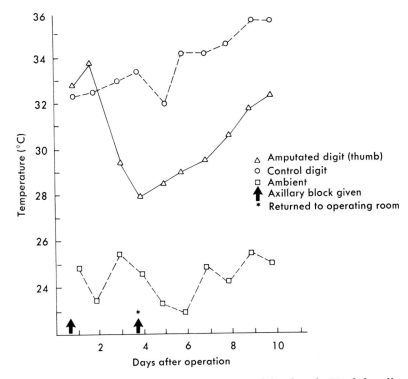

Fig. 6-7. Patient with amputation and replantation of the thumb. He did well until the third postoperative day when he developed gastroenteritis and dehydration. Heparin was stopped because of potential bleeding in the gastrointestinal tract. The patient then had decreased temperature and cessation of flow to the thumb. He was taken back to the operating room after proper hydration where under regional anesthesia arterial anastomosis was redone. The patient subsequently continued to have viability of the thumb, and evaluation 4 months postoperatively showed patency of at least one of the arterial anastomoses.

3. DRESSING CHANGES. Direct measurements in 25 patients have confirmed that within the first 10 days of replantation if an adherent dressing is removed, there is an immediate decrease in blood flow. We, as well as most other groups working in replantation surgery, have had the unfortunate experience of having a replanted part lost in the early postoperative period because of dressing changes. If the dressing change is carried out when the dressing is not adherent, there is no decrease in flow. This phenomenon is probably secondary to both painful stimuli and the well-recognized increased response to circulating catecholamines exhibited by sympathetically denervated vessels.

4. PSYCHOLOGIC STRESS. On multiple patients we have observed that psychologic stress (for example, the person who originally caused the loss of the part coming into the room) will cause an immediate and often sustained de-

crease in flow. This has been observed both with temperature monitoring and with pulse volume flowmeter monitoring. We also have noted that our success in children, especially hyperactive children, has been much less than that in the general population.

Local factors. Flow in phase II is also believed to be affected by local factors. These would include the accumulation of thrombin at the anastomosis site or the sites of unrecognized intimal damage, and edema of the injured tissues, both proximal and distal to the replantation, thus causing an increase in extravascular pressure and decreased flow.

Measurements carried out with the pulse volume flowmeter, the temperature gauge, and the Doppler scanner, as well as clinical evaluations, have confirmed that this decreased flow in phase II has been a significant problem in 30% of our 200 replantations to date.

Phase III. The third phase after replantation surgery lasts from about 3 weeks until 2 to 3 years after replantation. During this period there is a gradual increase in the measured flow in the digit or hand, a gradual decrease in cold intolerance, and stabilization of alterations in flow pattern.

Measurements in individual patients taken over a 3-year period after replantation show that although in the early postoperative period the pulsatile flow may be decreased, this will gradually increase.

Cold intolerance is usually a problem the first year after replantation. Cold pressor tests indicate that in the early postoperative course the replanted digit will have lower temperature. After several months autonomic control becomes hyperactive. When subjected to cold stress, the digit will become cooler and remain cooler over longer periods of time with a much longer warm-up time than adjacent normal digits. This is the period of most uncomfortable cold intolerance, and it will often take several hours for the patient to warm up his digit after a particularly cold encounter.

After 2 to 3 years, however, the measured response to the cold pressor test and the subjective response return to normal.

Alterations of decreased flow

Postoperative management is designed to monitor flow alterations, to prevent situations or events that decrease flow, and, in the event that there is decreased flow, to use physiologic means to increase flow.

One way to increase flow is by depression of the replanted part when there is decreased arterial inflow or elevation of the replanted part if there is venous congestion.

Removal of the constricting part of a dressing will also increase flow. If circular plaster is used, if a blood cast occurs, or if a certain amount of swelling is not allowed for in the dressing, there is relative constriction and decreased flow. If the constriction can be removed, good flow often will resume.

Avoidance of pain is another means of increasing flow. The feedback loop between pain and increased sympathetic tone has been observed by us in many instances. If pain can be relieved during surgery and in the postoperative period, there is a decrease in sympathetic tone and an increase in flow.

Hypotension must also be avoided. Early in the replantation program large volumes of blood were given, and this was important to avoid orthostatic hypotension. This is not as much a problem today, although patients are kept in bed for several days postoperatively.

Sympathetic blocks increase flow. In 25 of our early replantations we monitored the flow to the replanted digit during administration of a sympathetic block. In all but two instances, there was an immediate increase in flow. This finding has been confirmed in subsequent patients. If a sympathetic block is needed today, we will usually do an axillary block using a long-acting anesthetic (bupivacaine), which also relieves pain. Sympathetic block is only used when the viability of the replanted part is precarious. Earlier in our replantation program these blocks were used routinely, but we now reserve them for patients in whom there is observed difficulty.

Heparin is a controversial subject. Of the first 150 replantations performed in our Center, heparin was used routinely on most. Because we believe that we see clinical results from heparin, we have continued its use in certain patients. Other investigators have not found it particularly helpful. At the present time there is general agreement that (1) in vessels larger than 2 mm and in replantations involving vessels at the wrist or proximal area, heparin is not usually necessary; (2) in some replantations of digits in which there is a relatively clean cut, no difficulty with surgery, and excellent flow to the digit, heparin is probably not of benefit. In avulsion injury and injuries where there is marginal flow, we still believe that heparin is indicated and have continued to prescribe it.

POSTOPERATIVE MANAGEMENT
In the operating and recovery room

1. Management in the operating room includes stellate block, a long-acting axillary block at the beginning of the case, or a stellate block at the end if further decreased sympathetic tone is needed.

2. We loosely close the skin and avoid large open areas when possible.

3. A loose dressing is applied and continued to above the elbow. This includes a Dacron fluff (Polyfill) that will not be as constricting when wet.

4. Plaster is put on only one side of the extremity, usually the volar side.

5. Monitoring is begun in the operating room. At the termination of arterial anastomosis, the pulse volume flowmeter assesses the flow into the digit. In complete amputations, we prefer to have greater than 50% to 75% of the flow of the opposite digit. If this is not present, we will often redo the anastomosis, resecting any damaged intima. We believe that a vigorous flow in the operating room is necessary for a good postoperative course.

6. Temperature monitoring is begun as soon as the patient comes to the recovery room. We have found temperature to be a simple, effective measurement of postoperative flow. In complete amputations we have found that if the flow is good, the temperature of the replanted part will be within one to two degrees of the normal part, around 30° to 35° C. If there is a problem with flow, the temperature will fall. If the temperature falls below 30° C, there is a good chance that the flow is inadequate for continued viability. Although we recognize that there is a time lag between a decrease in flow and its reflection in decreased temperature, we have found that the nursing personnel can easily use the thermistor and that the time lag has not in general been a problem. Temperature monitoring is continued until discharge from the hospital.

On the ward

After removal from the recovery room to the ward, the following steps are taken to continue optimal management of the patient:

1. There is general elevation of the part, vital signs are checked every 4 hours with circulation checks every hour, and the hematocrit is obtained every 3 days. Platelet counts, activated partial thromboplastin time, and electrolytes are obtained as needed.

2. Approximately 1 unit of dextran is given daily, and aspirin is given in doses of 600 mg orally twice daily. Smoking is not allowed to avoid any possible vasoconstrictive effects.

3. The patient is kept quiet for 3 to 4 days and then ambulated slowly with continued monitoring.

4. Meperidine HCl (Demerol) and morphine are given as needed for pain.

5. Sedation is used (chlorpromazine HCl 25 mg t.i.d. in adults or appropriately less in children) to decrease anxiety.

6. The dressing is checked for constricting areas.

7. Heparin is given in selected cases. If a patient had uneventful surgery and excellent flow, heparin is generally not given. If, however, there is intimal damage or difficulty with postoperative flow, heparin is given in anticoagulating doses. We use approximately 500 to 1000 units per hour in a continuous drip. If there is bleeding into the dressing, the heparin dosage is decreased and the dressing is changed so that it will not become constricting.

8. In regard to psychologic factors, we have found that patients who have amputations and replantation are under considerable stress. This stress is unpleasant to the patient and detrimental to his postoperative course. We feel that efforts by both the nursing staff and the physician can help alleviate anxiety. This requires setting aside time to explain the injury, the attempts at repair, and the expected postoperative course. Since we have a relatively large population of replantations and a large follow-up clinic, we often bring a patient who is a year or so beyond replantation to the room of the acutely injured patient to help with further explanations. The returning patient brings

another dimension of assistance to the patient in the immediate postoperative period.

The involvement of nursing personnel is most important. Informed nurses can take the extra time necessary to help a patient understand his problem, his forced inactivity for a period of time, and his eventual return to work.

In the clinic

In single-digit and often in multiple-digit replantations the dressing is not changed until the patient returns to the clinic 3 weeks after the surgery. The hospital stay is usually from 3 to 10 days after surgery or until flow has stabilized. The patient is sent home with the original dressing on; in some cases the outer dressing is removed so that it does not go above the elbow.

At the initial clinic visit the dressing is slowly removed after soaking. Good healing is usually present where the skin was opposed and some epithelialization has taken place in areas left open. The patient is instructed in dressing changes three times daily and continues his care at home. Also at this visit, the hand therapist initiates the splinting program either by making a holding splint or by starting active and passive flexion and extension.

Splinting and therapy

The participation of an interested and well-trained hand therapist is essential in returning the severely (Fig. 6-8) injured patient to work and recreational activities. The necessary aspects of the hand therapist's participation are several.

First, the therapist is present to evaluate the patient with the surgeon at the initial dressing change. The therapist is either present at the hand clinic or there is a close line of communication.

Second, the splints are fabricated and instructions given on the day they are needed, not several days or weeks later.

Third, the therapist is another professional to take the necessary time to explain the expected postoperative course, to give encouragement, to monitor the progression in strength, motion, and sensibility, and to suggest intervention if these do not proceed as expected.

Finally, the therapist is needed to ensure that the use of the splints and active therapy do not cause undue pain to the patient, since pain in the postoperative period is not beneficial.

After the initial dressing change, approximately 3 weeks after replantation, the patient requires a supervised passive range-of-motion exercise to maintain and increase joint motion distal and proximal to the replantation, distal to the anastomotic site. This can be accomplished through dynamic splinting, individually constructed of Orthoplast with Velcro straps, which allow for easy application and removal. The patient obtains a set of splints, which usually consists of a volar metacarpal phalangeal joint flexion outrigger, a volar prox-

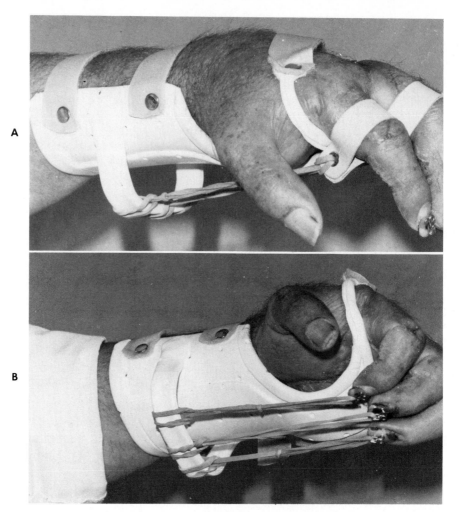

Fig. 6-8. Fifty-year-old man with complete amputation and replantation of index, long, and ring fingers. Here 8 weeks after replantation flexion splints are applied. **A,** Leather loops at proximal phalangeal level assist metacarpophalangeal flexion. **B,** Surgical rubber bands attached to hook on the nails assist proximal and distal interphalangeal flexion.

imal interphalangeal joint flexion outrigger, and a dorsal interphalangeal joint extension outrigger with a metacarpal phalangeal stop or lumbrical bar.

Various lengths and strengths of surgical rubber bands are attached to the outrigger and motor the digit either by leather loops or by hooks glued to the fingernails with rapid-setting glue. Only leather loops are used on the extension outrigger.

In some instances, static Orthoplast splinting is indicated to protect the internally fixed replanted digit and allow the patient to remove the splint and change the dressing at home. This is especially important since many of our patients come from many miles away.

Construction of all necessary splints is completed during one visit after the patient is seen in the hand clinic for dressing changes. The patient is instructed in the application of splints and given a strict wearing schedule. Generally the schedule would be to alternate flexion and extension splints hourly during the day for approximately 4 to 6 hours. In addition to splinting, the patient is given a program of active range-of-motion exercises to enhance the progress made by the splinting. This includes wooden blocks in three sizes to exercise the proximal interphalangeal and distal interphalangeal joint, various sized sponges, and the use of clay to obtain maximum active flexion.

Once an active range-of-motion exercise program is instituted, the patients can decrease the time of splinting. The patients are instructed to wear the splints alternately at night if pain is not a problem.

As the splints are applied, the patients are seen for follow-up on a weekly and biweekly basis and routine checks on (1) progress of active and passive range of motion, (2) proper splint fit and adjustment, (3) need for additional splinting, (4) additions to active range-of-motion exercises. If the patient's progress is not significant over a period of time, increased visits and encouragement are given or surgical intervention may be necessary.

ACKNOWLEDGMENT

Work in this chapter was partially supported by NIH Grant no. 1 RO1 GM25666.

7. Management of bone in microvascular surgery

Michael George Hayes
James R. Urbaniak

Replantation of partially or totally severed digits, transfer of vascularized bone grafts to bridge segmental loss of bone, and the transfer of composite grafts of skin, subcutaneous tissue, and bone are a few of the major advances brought about by the application of microsurgical techniques. In all these procedures, the successful repair of bone is an important factor in the final outcome. The procedures are difficult and time consuming and must only be performed in selected cases where more contemporary methods of treatment are not applicable.

MANAGEMENT OF BONE IN REPLANTATION SURGERY

Successful replantation of amputated digits is dependent on reanastomosis of adequate vessels that are of suitable caliber and have a normal intimal lining at the site of repair. In addition, the repair must be performed without tension across the anastomotic site.[7,14]

Most injuries causing amputation have a crushing element, and this area must be excised if successful revascularization is to be achieved. There are two alternatives to obtain tension-free repairs. The bone may be shortened, or the vascular defect can be grafted.

If the vascular defect is grafted, the number of anastomoses required is increased and this may compromise the result. In addition, the duration of surgery is extended, and in the situation where vessels are grafted because of extensive damage, there is concomitant injury to nerves and other soft tissues, which do not function well if repaired under tension. In most cases, bone shortening is preferable, since in the long term it allows a more functional result.[7,15]

In general, the amount of shortening depends on the type of injury. In a crush or avulsion injury, a greater amount of bone must be removed until normal intimal coaptation is possible without tension. In the digit, usually between 0.5 and 1.5 cm of bone is removed, whereas in amputations at the proximal hand and wrist level, 2 to 3 cm is excised. In the case of thumb amputations, it is important to preserve as much of the proximal stump as possible. Bone shortening, if indicated, should be performed on the distal segment, and if replantation fails, adequate bone stock is available to allow further reconstruction.

Joints

Amputations that occur through the distal interphalangeal joint or through the proximal interphalangeal joint require excision and fusion of the joint. In cases of amputations distal to the proximal interphalangeal joint with a superficialis tendon intact, the preservation of that joint results in a "sublimis" finger, which gives good long-term function.

Amputations in the region of the metacarpophalangeal joint are best managed by metacarpal head resection and leaving the base of the proximal phalanx with the cartilages intact, resulting in a resection arthroplasty. These joints can later be reconstructed using silicone or silicone-Dacron implants. Wrist amputation is best managed by resection of one or both of the carpal rows, or in cases with severe local soft-tissue damage, wrist arthrodesis is a more functional result. However, in avulsion types of amputation where poor nerve recovery is likely to occur, wrist motion may be desirable to allow a tenodesis function.

Bone fixation

Many methods are available to obtain solid, immediate fixation of bone, and these include small compression plates, screw fixation, and staples. We have found that a single, intramedullary Kirschner wire inserted by use of a motorized, cordless drill is the most satisfactory method. This simple technique is less time consuming and requires minimal exposure and less skeletal mass for fixation than more elaborate types of fixation. In addition, it has the distinct advantage of allowing rotation of the replanted digit if realignment of the vessels is required (Figs. 7-1 and 7-2).

The insertion of cross-pins for improved stabilization may result in damage to the repaired neurovascular bundle or tethering of other soft tissues that may compromise the long-term functional result.

In amputations through the forearm, where ischemia time is of critical importance, fixation with intramedullary Rush pins is timesaving and satisfactory. If this technique still allows sliding, then a heavy wire mattress suture in the bone can prevent this situation and therefore prevent stretching of the repaired structures (Fig. 7-3).

Summary

From a replantation point of view, several important points emerge with reference to the management of bone. It is important to ensure that adequate

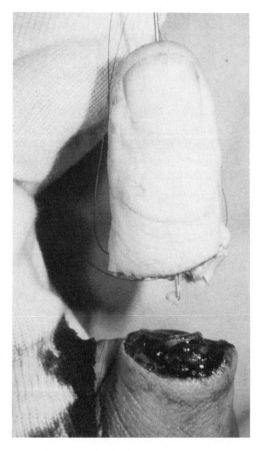

Fig. 7-1. Guillotine amputation of the right thumb has been debrided and the bone from the distal segment shortened. An intramedullary Kirschner wire has been passed in a retrograde fashion, and the digit is about to be stabilized to the proximal stump.

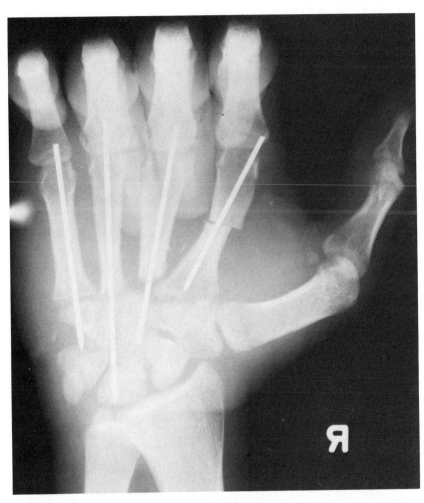

Fig. 7-2. This patient sustained multiple amputations and bone stabilization was achieved with multiple intramedullary Kirschner wires. This technique allows rapid and satisfactory stabilization of the fractures.

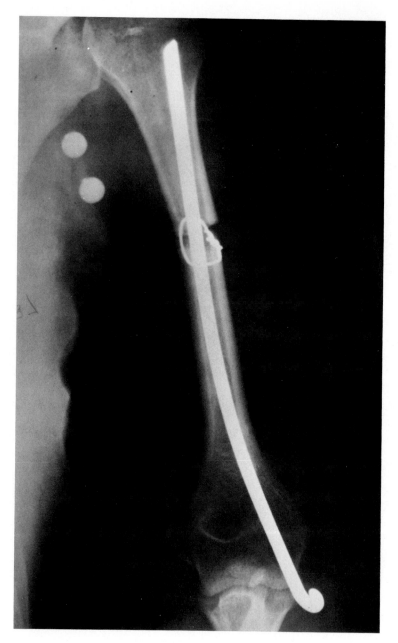

Fig. 7-3. An intramedullary Rush pin has been used to stabilize the major bone segment and an interrupted wire mattress suture is shown. This combination prevents sliding of the bone segments and protects the soft-tissue repairs.

shortening of the bone allows soft-tissue repair without undue tension. Stabilization must be achieved as rapidly as possible and with minimal soft-tissue exposure. The above technique has been used in over 200 replantations without serious problems from delayed union or malunion.

FREE VASCULARIZED BONE GRAFT

Conventional methods of bone grafting in the management of large skeletal defects from trauma or after the excision of benign bone neoplasms are unpredictable with slow healing postoperatively and a high rate of failure. Major injuries to the lower extremities involving bone loss frequently occur in the young and often both lower extremities are involved, which compounds the reconstructive problem. The use of vascularized bone grafts in certain situations has been experimentally evaluated and applied clinically. From the experimental findings, it became apparent that maintenance of the endosteal supply to the bone graft was of critical importance if the technique was to succeed and to prove to be more valuable than conventional techniques of bone grafting.[1,2,6,8]

Human anatomy has been reexamined from a microvascular point of view, with particular emphasis on the blood supply to bone. The removal of a segment of bone with its periosteal and endosteal blood supply intact and transferal of it to a different site in the body, to breach a segmental loss of bone, with reanastomosis of the graft vessels to vessels of similar caliber in the recipient site has been investigated. Several criteria for the technique emerged. The vessels supplying the graft had to be 1 mm more in size and the variations in the anatomy understood by the microvascular surgeon. In addition, it is important that excision of the bone from the donor site did not cause significant morbidity.

Two areas met this criteria. The fibula, whose major endosteal supply comes from the nutrient artery, provides up to 30 cm of bone, and because of its triangular cross section, it is able to resist angular and rotational stresses better than the other donor site, which is the rib.[11,12,15] In addition, the diameter of the fibula is such that it approximates the shafts of the radius and ulna and fits comfortably into the medullary cavity of the femur, tibia, or humerus into which it may be doweled.

The rib provides about an equal length of bone, but the posterior intercostal artery, which supplies the endosteal blood supply, is usually only 1 mm or less in diameter, a size that makes reanastomosis difficult (Fig. 7-4).

The key to successful transfer of a vascularized bone graft is careful preoperative planning, angiographic evaluation of the donor and recipient sites and, if necessary, cadaveric rehearsal by the surgical teams.

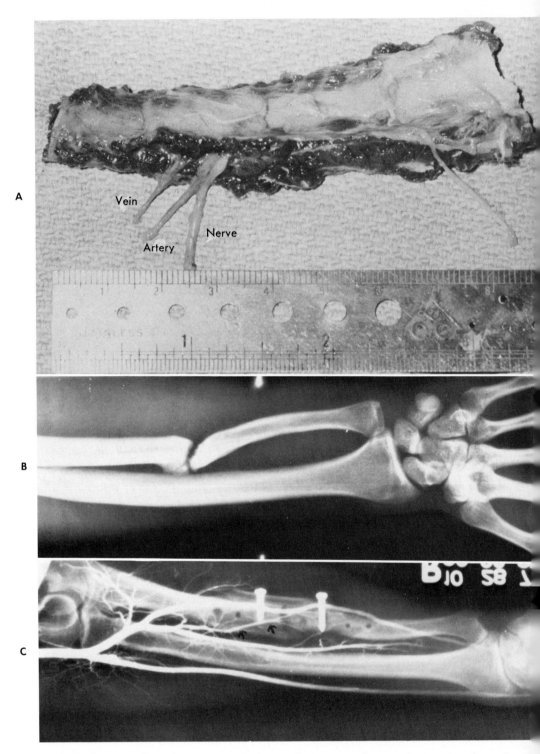

Fig. 7-4. A, Rib with its intercostal vessels is a satisfactory donor area for a free vascularized bone graft, and this specimen illustrates the vascular pedicle. *N,* Nerve; *A,* artery; *V,* vein. **B,** Roentgenogram demonstrates a nonunion in an adult male after two attempts at plating and bone grafting. **C,** Four months after vascularized rib graft to nonunion of ulna demonstrates bone union and patent donor vessel *(arrows).*

Case studies
CASE ONE

S.M. was involved in an automobile accident in April 1974 and sustained a fracture of his left femur and right ulna. He was treated in a cast for eight weeks and underwent compression plating and bone grafting of his ulna fracture. His femoral fracture went on to union. Two years later, the ulna remained ununited and he underwent further bone grafting and compression type of fixation, which then failed. He was readmitted complaining of pain in the region of the nonunion, tenderness over the plate, and obvious motion of the ulna (Fig. 7-4, *B*). After preoperative arteriography, the nonunion site was exposed and the plate removed. The graft bed was prepared for a segment of his eighth rib with the intercostal vessels. The rib was fixed across the nonunion site with an intramedullary pin, and the intercostal vessels were sewn to the ulna artery with use of an end-to-side anastomosis and vein graft. After the arterial anastomosis was complete, there was bleeding from the distal intercostal vein, and this was reanastomosed distally to a branch of the cephalic vein.

The wound was partially closed primarily but required skin grafting to complete closure some 5 days postoperatively. Follow-up four months later indicated evidence of bone union (Fig. 7-4, *C*).

CASE TWO

A.V., a male laborer, sustained a compound fracture with segmental loss to his dominant humerus. The soft tissue healed, but the humerus went on to persistent nonunion despite four attempts at bone grafting and fixation. He had 7.5 cm of shortening in the arm with a functional shoulder, elbow, and hand.

The middle third of the fibula with its vascular supply was isolated and transferred to the humerus, and the vessels were anastomosed to the brachial artery. The graft became united at both ends, but unfortunately several months later, the patient fell and sustained a fracture through the bone-graft site.

COMPOSITE TISSUE TRANSFER

The successful transfer of vascularized skin flaps and vascularized bone grafts led to the concept of composite tissue transfer where skin, subcutaneous tissue, and bone were isolated on a vascular pedicle and transferred to a distant graft site where segmental loss of bone and soft tissue had occurred.[3-5,9,10] Once again, this procedure is exceedingly complex and time consuming and needs careful preoperative planning, team rehearsal, and coordination of the surgical teams at the time of surgery.

Experience is limited in these procedures, but the concept of restoring bone and soft-tissue continuity in a single, one-stage procedure has great theoretical appeal.

Two areas of the body have been used for this type of transfer. The free groin flap based on the superficial circumflex iliac and superficial inferior epigastric vessels and including a large piece of bone from the iliac crest has been transferred to a large bone and soft-tissue defect in the tibia. In addition, a composite flap taken from the interdigital space between the great and second toe and based on the dorsalis pedis artery with a segment of bone removed from the second toe has also been used. The major problem encountered is discrepancy in the size of vessels for anastomosis at the graft site. A preoperative angiogram is imperative both to help selection of the most convenient vessel for anastomosis and to ensure that the distal circulation will not be compromised when the anastomosis has been completed.

Case studies

CASE ONE

I.J., a 17-year-old white male, sustained a severe avulsion type of injury to the ulnar aspect of his dominant index finger (Fig. 7-5). In the injury he sustained loss of the following structures: ulnar skin from the web space to the distal interphalangeal joint,

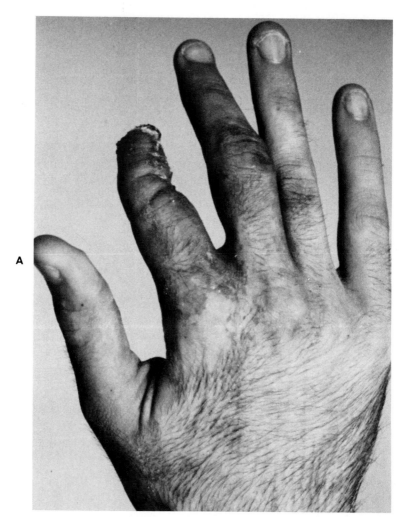

A

Fig. 7-5. A, Preoperative damage to index finger. **B,** Preoperative radiologic appearance.

entire middle phalanx and distal half of the proximal phalanx, and the neurovascular bundle of the ulnar side. The radial neurovascular bundle was intact. The flexor and extensor mechanisms were also intact.

He was initially treated with débridement and distraction with a pin and outrigger through the distal phalanx. The skin wound healed by primary intention, and the patient was readmitted 3 months after the initial injury for reconstruction of the finger. Two surgical teams were used and a composite graft consisting of the entire proximal phalanx of the second toe with the skin, subcutaneous tissue, and neurovascular structures was taken. The donor vessels used were the dorsalis pedis artery and saphenous vein. This area of skin is supplied by the superficial branch of the deep peroneal nerve, which accompanies the dorsalis pedis artery. This cutaneous nerve was also carefully identified and prepared for anastomosis.

Composite bone and skin grafts taken from this area are dependent on the dorsalis

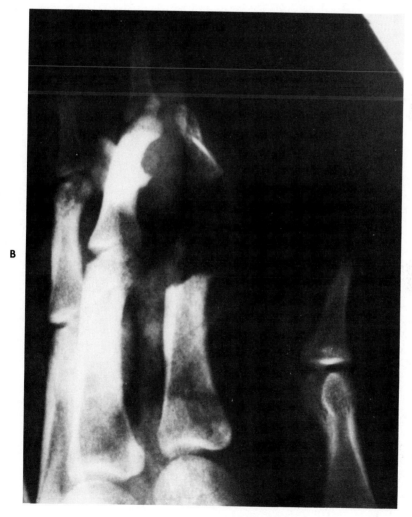

Fig. 7-5, cont'd. For legend see opposite page.

pedis artery and, in particular, by the first metatarsal branch, which is the feeding vessel to the interdigital space. This vessel is approximately 1 mm in diameter and has a variable relation to the first interosseous muscle.[5] Commonly, it passes through a muscular tunnel in the substance of the interosseous muscle for a distance of 15 mm and then becomes subcutaneous again. It may cross through the entire muscle or, rarely, run on the plantar aspect of the muscle, becoming superficial at the level of the web space. It usually courses superficially to the deep transverse ligament.

The least common variation is where the artery is a branch of the plantar arterial arch. This uncommon variation, which occurred in this patient, prolongs the dissection as it is more difficult.

The proximal phalanx was dissected free from the metatarsophalangeal and inter-phalangeal joints and the composite graft of skin, artery, vein, nerve, and proximal phalanx was transferred to the ulnar side of the finger and fixed in place with a central Kirschner wire (Fig. 7-6). The artery and vein were anastomosed and the digital nerve was connected to the deep peroneal nerve, which was present in the graft. The skin of the composite graft was sewn into place, and the donor site was closed primarily with intramedullary stabilization on the second toe. A functional digit with 10 mm two-point sensation has been obtained (Fig. 7-7).

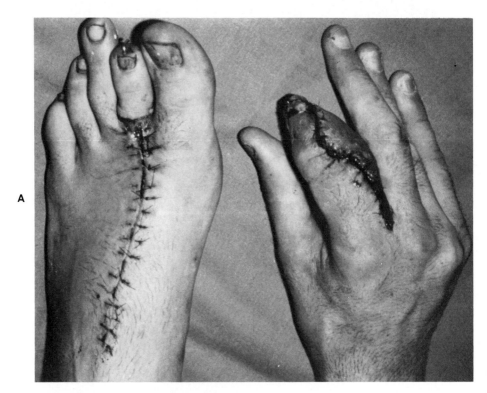

A

Fig. 7-6. A, Postoperative appearance of the donor and composite graft sites. **B,** Post-operative radiologic appearance.

B

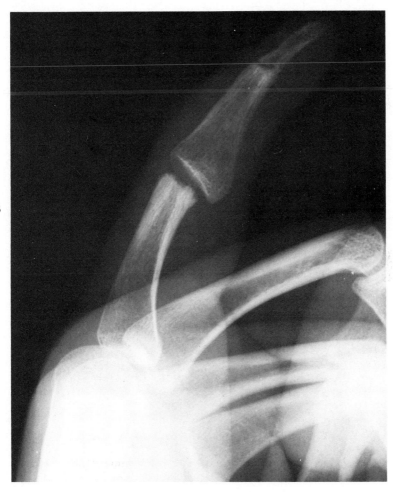

Fig. 7-6, cont'd. For legend see opposite page.

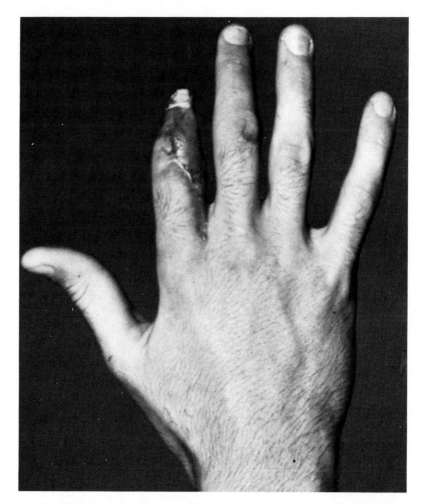

Fig. 7-7. Result with a functional digit with 10 mm two-point sensation.

CASE TWO

J.B., a 23-year-old white male, fell off a lawn mower and sustained a compound fracture to his right tibia with segmental loss of 12 cm of bone and soft tissue from the anteromedial aspect of his leg. The fibula was intact. The skin defect measured 12 cm in its long axis and approximately 8 cm in width. Initial treatment was débridement and cast fixation. In view of the extensive bone and soft-tissue loss, a composite bone graft from the iliac region was planned and discussed with the patient. At operation, one surgical team stabilized the tibia with a Rush rod and the ends of the disrupted anterior tibial vessels were identified and isolated. Concurrently, another operative team took a large skin and bone flap, based on the superficial circumflex iliac and superficial inferior epigastric artery and vein; included in the flap was a large, lozenge-shaped graft from the iliac crest.

The composite flap was transferred to the recipient site and the bone was stabilized with a thin Rush pin through the medial malleolus, across the bone graft, and into the proximal end of the fractured tibia. The artery and vein were anastomosed with microvascular techniques, and the skin portion of the graft was sewn into place. Unfortunately, 10 days postoperatively, the skin portion of the graft necrosed because of arterial thrombosis. However, the bone graft has remained in place and was covered with a cross-leg flap.

DISCUSSION

Free vascularized bone grafting and composite tissue transfer including skin, subcutaneous tissue, and bone is one of the major advances in orthopedic surgery, which has resulted from the application of microsurgical techniques. Experience in this field is limited and vessel discrepancy is the major problem encountered. Interposition vein grafts and side-to-side anastomoses were used in some cases in order to overcome this problem. Taylor[11] emphasized the importance of preoperative arteriography in the planning of these procedures and, in particular, to avoid the use of a vessel that is the solitary supply to the distal part of the limb.

CONCLUSION

Management of bone is an important facet in replantation surgery where the major factor is obtaining rapid bone stabilization and, at the same time, allowing tension-free anastomosis of vessels with normal intimal lining. Perhaps the more exciting aspects of microvascular surgery include transfer of vascularized bone grafts to areas where conventional methods have failed or are inappropriate and in cases of severe trauma where there is segmental bone and soft-tissue loss. The concept of a one-stage restoration of bone and soft tissue is an exciting advance, but the procedure is complex, difficult, and time consuming and requires careful preoperative planning including arteriography, preoperative team rehearsal and coordination, and meticulous microsurgery technique.

REFERENCES

1. Adelaar, R. S., Soucacos, P. N., and Urbaniak, J. R.: Autologous cortical bone grafts with microsurgical anastomoses of the periosteal vessels, Surg. Forum **25:**487, 1974.
2. Brookes, N.: The blood supply of bone, London, 1971, Butterworth & Co. (Publishers).
3. Conley, J.: Use of composite flaps containing bone for major repairs in the head and neck, Plast. Reconstr. Surg. **49:**552, 1972.
4. Conley, J., Cinelli, P. B., Johnson, P. N., and Cross, M.: Investigation of bone changes in composite flaps after transfer to the head and neck region, Plast. Reconstr. Surg. **51:**658, 1973.
5. Gilbert, A.: Composite tissue transfers from the foot: anatomic basis and surgical technique, Danillier, A. I., and Strauch, B., editors: Symposium of Microsurgery, St. Louis, 1976, The C. V. Mosby Co.

6. McCullough, D. W., and Fredrickson, J. M.: Neurovascularised rib grafts to reconstruct mandibular defects, Can. J. Otolaryngol. **2**:96, 1973.

7. O'Brien, B. M.: Microsurgery in the treatment of injuries, Recent Adv. Orthopaed. London, 1975, Churchill Livingstone, pp. 235-274.

8. Ostrup, L. T., and Fredrickson, J. M.: Distant transfer of a free living bone graft by microvascular anastomoses, Plast. Reconstr. Surg. **54**:274, 1974.

9. Strauch, B., Bloomburg, A. E., and Lewin, M. L.: An experimental approach to mandibular replacement: island vascular composite rib grafts, Br. J. Plast. Surg. **24**:334, 1971.

10. Snyder, C. C., Bateman, J. M., Davis, C. W., and Warden, G. D.: Mandibulo-facial restoration with live osteocutaneous flaps, Plast. Reconstr. Surg. **45**:14, 1970.

11. Taylor, G.: Tissue defects in the limbs: replacement with free vascularised tissue transfers, Aust. N.Z. J. Surg. **47**:276, 1977.

12. Taylor, G. I., Miller, G. D. H., and Ham, F. J.: The free vascularised bone graft, Plast. Reconstr. Surg. **55**:533, 1975.

13. Taylor, G. I.: Microvascular free bone transfer, Orthop. Clin. North Am. **8**:425-447, 1977.

14. Urbaniak, J. R., Soucacos, P. N., Adelaar, R. S., Bright, D. W., and Whitehurst, L. A.: Experimental evaluation of microsurgical techniques in small artery anastomoses, Orthop. Clin. North Am. **8**:248, 1977.

15. Urbaniak, J. R., Hayes, M. G., and Bright, D. W.: Management of bone in digital replantation of free vascularised and composite bone grafts, Clin. Orthop. **133**:184, 1978.

8. Vascular defects and salvage of failed vascular repairs

Jack W. Tupper

Vascular defects occur in a variety of situations in which the orthopedic surgeon may find himself: (1) replantation of amputated parts, (2) repair of partially or completely devascularized parts without amputation, (3) free flaps with short recipient vessels, (4) ulnar artery thrombosis at the wrist (hypothenar hammer syndrome), and (5) thrombosis of larger vessels subjected to direct trauma.

REPLANTATION OF AMPUTATED PARTS

After general soft-tissue débridement, bone is shortened only if necessary to obtain easy skin closure. Internal fixation is then carried out. During débridement (with a loupe), arteries, veins, and nerves are tagged with small suture material but are not specifically trimmed. After the bone, tendon, and nerve repairs have been accomplished under the microscope, the vessels are specifically debrided to an uninjured level. Because avulsion is a part of many injuries and is especially inimical to tubular structures, vessel damage often extends beyond that to other soft tissue. Signs of damage to a vessel are (1) hemorrhagic adventitia, (2) an adventitia that is loose from the media (from concussion), (3) a vessel with recurrent severe or persistent spasm of more than the very end, and (4) torn or hemorrhagic intima.

After definitive vessel débridement, there is often a gap so that a direct anastomosis cannot be accomplished. No attempt should be made to secure apposition by an awkward amount of flexion or by excess tension. A technically difficult anastomosis will usually be a poor one.

Fortunately, a readily available vein graft will function very well for either arterial or venous defects. Two technically easy anastomoses are better than one that is difficult. Donor sites are the dorsum of the hand or foot and the volar or dorsal forearm. Preoperative skin marking of visible veins followed by a zig-zag incision will allow choice of a vein of appropriate diameter and length (Fig. 8-1). Small branches should be identified and ligated prior to excision of

111

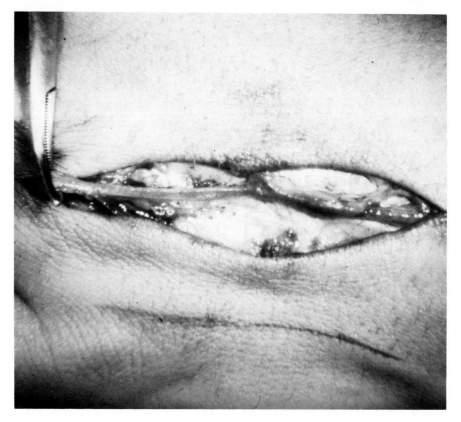

Fig. 8-1. Dorsal hand vein donor site.

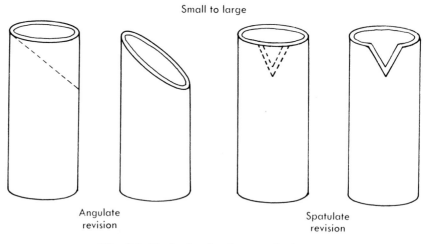

Small to large

Angulate
revision

Spatulate
revision

Fig. 8-2. Methods of enlarging the lumen.

graft. Most veins will have valves and, therefore, should be reversed for arterial defects. Valves are usually visible externally as a slight enlargement. Anastomosis should obviously not be at the site of the valve.

There are several ways of equalizing luminal size if vessels do not match. The circumference of a smaller vessel may be increased by about 30% by having its end sectioned at a 45-degree angle. The end of a smaller vessel may also be spatulated to increase the luminal size (Fig. 8-2). A larger vessel may be coned by excision of a V and primary closing of it to make a smaller lumen (Fig. 8-3). One may also carry out an end-to-side anastomosis if a smaller recipient artery is jointed to a larger donor vessel (Fig. 8-4). Repair or vein grafting of smaller vessels is greatly aided by a double clamp on a frame, especially if there are cleats to put tension on the initial two sutures. The Acland frame with two fixed clamps is ideal for this (Fig. 8-5). There is no need for clamps to slide, since one should not make an anastomosis under tension and the slide mechanism adds weight to the device. My preferred suture material for small vessel anastomosis is 18-micron nylon with a short (3 mm), straight needle 50 to 70 microns in thickness.* The initial sutures are placed at about 180 degrees from each other, tied, and then anchored to the appropriate cleat under slight tension. Sutures pass through the entire wall and are usually placed a distance from the edge of the vessel opening approximately equal to slightly more than the thickness of the vessel wall. This is true whether or not the vessels being joined have the same wall diameters. After the initial two stay sutures, three or four additional interrupted sutures are then placed evenly between the two stay sutures, the frame is turned over and the backside of the closure finished in like manner. When the repair is finished, the clamp is removed and the tourniquet released. If the vein graft

---

*S & T Chirurgische Nadeln, 7893 Jestetten, Baden (BRD), Allmend Strasse 2, Postfach 93 Germany. Also Ethicon, Inc., 3640 Allendale Drive, Somerville, N.J. 08876.

Large to small

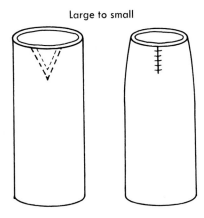

Fig. 8-3. Method of decreasing the lumen.

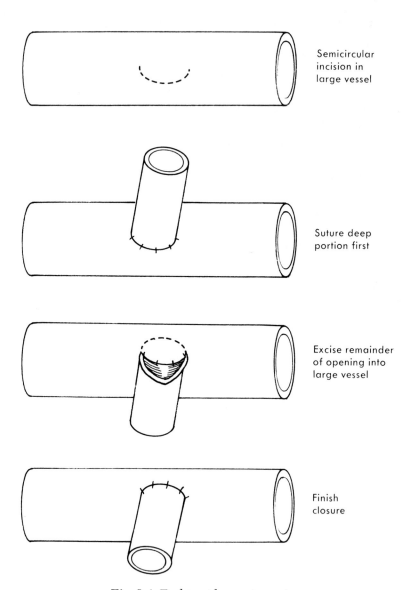

Semicircular
incision in
large vessel

Suture deep
portion first

Excise remainder
of opening into
large vessel

Finish
closure

Fig. 8-4. End-to-side anastomosis.

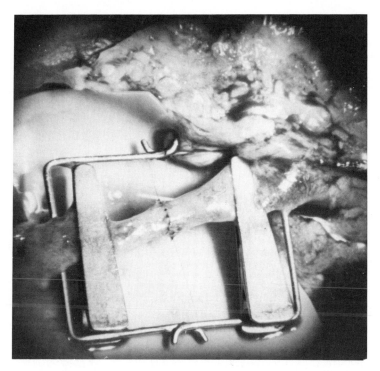

Fig. 8-5. Acland frame with two fixed clamps and cleats.

is a very long one, it is advisable to finish the proximal anastomosis first and then release the tourniquet, for this will allow the vein graft to elongate some back to its previous normal length. This will prevent the use of too long a graft with possible subsequent buckling. After release of the tourniquet, if immediate flow does not occur, one should check the blood pressure. If a long area of spasm is present on the proximal end, there has been insufficient débridement of the vessel. Ooze through the suture line will spontaneously stop, but if any of the gaps permit spurting, this will frequently require one more suture. After visual flow begins through the anastomosis, there will be a short delay followed first by an increase in pulp volume and then a bit later by return of pink color. Capillary refill is more easily evaluated in the eponychial tissue than in the nail bed.

Other techniques that may occasionally be of value in making up a vascular defect involve (1) arterial transfers (such as the radial indicis on a proximal pedicle to a recipient thumb vessel), which require only one distal anastomosis (Fig. 8-6, *A*), and (2) arterial grafts, which may occasionally be taken from the other artery on the finger if both have been injured and it is feasible to repair only one or short sections may be taken from a nonreplantable digit (Fig. 8-7).

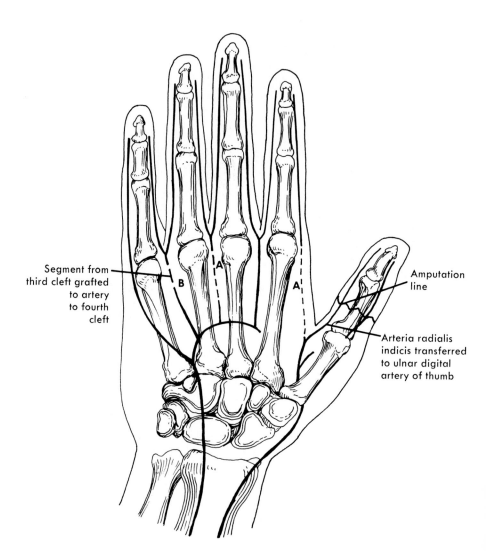

Segment from
third cleft grafted
to artery
to fourth
cleft

Amputation
line

Arteria radialis
indicis transferred
to ulnar digital
artery of thumb

Fig. 8-6. *Dotted lines,* **A,** Sections of artery used as arterial graft. *Dotted line,* **B,** Arteries may be spared to contribute to an essential vessel. One would usually use vein grafts for this.

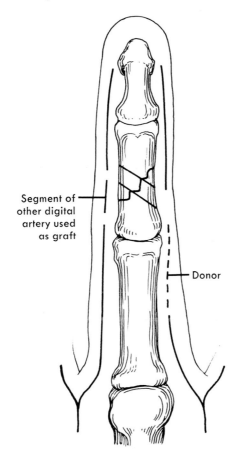

Segment of
other digital
artery used
as graft

Donor

Fig. 8-7. Arterial graft from one side of amputated digit to the other.

FREE FLAPS

Occasionally, a short trunk on the recipient artery requires a graft to accomplish an easy anastomosis to the donor vessel.

ULNAR HAMMER SYNDROME

Thrombosis of the ulnar artery at the wrist usually destroys an inch or so of the ulnar artery. Collaterals allow the arteries distal to this to remain patent, but many patients have claudication or cryalgia if this vessel is not patent. This may be easily replaced by a similar-sized vein from the back of the hand reversing it so as to have no trouble with the valves.

LARGE VESSEL DEFECTS FROM DIRECT TRAUMA

Larger veins of appropriate size may be used for any vessel. The saphenous vein from the fossa ovalis to the knee will adequately replace a long segment of brachial artery.

SALVAGE OF FAILED VASCULAR ANASTOMOSES

A surgeon embarking upon this type of surgery must be willing to bail himself or herself out if thrombosis occurs. Early arterial failures then may be saved and as long as 12 hours later by aggressive excision of the thrombotic zone and vein grafting. If a technically perfect anastomosis is done on a well debrided vessel, with free use of vein grafts to reduce tension and to reduce the temptation of insufficient débridement, anastomoses rarely fail. Failure of venous anastomoses is a more difficult problem, for it tends to occur more slowly and there is usually secondary arterial thombosis at the same time. If there is obviously insufficient venous drainage at the end of the initial operative procedure, the procedure is not yet ended, and additional revisional anastomoses should be done at that time.

No systemic heparin is used at any time. Preoperative and postoperative aspirin is used, and postoperatively low molecular dextran is given.

9. Thrombosis of ulnar artery at the wrist

L. Andrew Koman
James R. Urbaniak

Von Rosen, in 1934, first described thrombosis of the ulnar artery at the wrist as a distinct pathologic entity, recognizing its relationship to blunt trauma of the hand.[14] Clinical diagnosis was made possible by Edgar Allen, who described a simple bedside method for the determination of patency of the arterial channels at the wrist in 1929.[1] Since Leriche's classic paper in 1937, the mainstay of orthopaedic treatment has been excision of the involved segment and ligation of the artery.[6,8,10,15] In 1965 Kleinert advocated the use of direct surgical repair.[9] Using microvascular technique, he described excision and direct repair, as well as multiple arteriotomies and thrombectomies to reestablish ulnar artery flow, with evidence of continued patency at follow-up. The term "hypothenar hammer syndrome" was coined by Conn in 1970 who proposed cervical sympathectomy as the treatment of choice.[4]

Thrombosis of the ulnar artery at the wrist is a relatively common and often misdiagnosed problem whose treatment at this point in time is controversial. The availability of dependable microsurgical techniques enabling the surgeon to vein-graft large defects prompted our review of the management of this problem.

CLINICAL MATERIAL

Between 1966 and 1977, 20 arteriograph-proved and symptomatic thrombosed ulnar arteries were seen at Duke University Medical Center and the Durham Veterans Administration Hospital. Patients and charts were reviewed. Evaluation included thermography, temperature probes, digital plethysmography, Doppler-flow studies, Allen testing, and arteriography.

Sixteen patients had unilateral involvement. Both females included in the study had bilateral disease. Sixteen patients were male and two were female. The average age was 45 years, with a range from 14 to 70 years. Of the three patients below the age of 35 years, two had significant episodes of trauma.

The dominant hand was involved 81% of the time and tended to occur in males with work-related trauma. The only cases of bilateral involvement were in women. The history of a specific episode of trauma could be elicited in five patients, whereas 12 had histories compatible with repeated minor trauma.

The most common symptoms were pain, cold intolerance, numbness, and gangrene. All patients had pretreatment pain. Most patients (16) had cold intolerance. Four patients had evidence of skin necrosis, with two patients losing portions of their fingers. Only three patients had palpable masses over Guyon's canal.

There were no specific laboratory findings. The sedimentation rate in all but two patients was less than 10. The average hemoglobin, however, was elevated to 16.5, with the range from 13.9 to 21.

Associated medical problems included smoking, alcoholism, hypertension, polycythemia, hemophilia, anticoagulant therapy, and heart disease. Of these, only smoking had a significant association, with 15 of the 18 patients being classified as heavy smokers.

Initial diagnosis was ulnar artery thrombosis in less than half of the patients. Other diagnoses included unilateral Raynaud's disease, four; arterial insufficiency, two; carpal tunnel syndrome, two; and arterial sclerotic cardiovascular disease, one. Treatment was quite diverse, with 13 patients receiving interarterial reserpine and four patients receiving interarterial tolazoline HCl (Priscoline). In most instances, the intra-arterial reserpine and tolazoline were given in conjunction with the arteriogram. In seven patients, intra-arterial reserpine and tolazoline in conjunction with other conservative treatment was the only treatment received. Of these patients, almost all had significant cold intolerance and pain at follow-up. Four patients had sympathectomies after symptomatic relief from stellate ganglion blocks. Two of the four had gangrene, which resolved after sympathectomies. Six patients had resection of the involved segment and ligation. Two patients had resection of the involved area and vein grafting. One patient was treated with biofeedback techniques, in conjunction with intra-arterial reserpine and discontinuation of smoking, and he had some relief of pain, enabling him to return to work, despite persistent mild cold intolerance and numbness.

After treatment, most patients had persistence of cold intolerance and pain. Less than half had persistent numbness, and there was no progression of gangrene after stabilization of symptoms with any treatment. All four patients with sympathectomies had bothersome symptoms (Horner's syndrome) secondary to treatment.

ANATOMY

Proximal to the wrist, the ulnar artery in company with the ulnar nerve lies radial to the flexor carpi ulnaris muscle and then its tendon (Fig. 9-1). The artery enters Guyon's canal, which is bounded dorsoulnarly by the pisohamate ligament and its respective carpal bones, volarly by the dorsal fascia of the palmaris brevis muscle as it blends into the volar carpal ligament, and dorso-

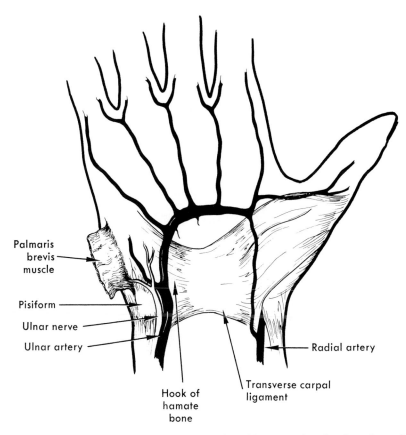

Palmaris
brevis
muscle

Pisiform

Ulnar nerve

Ulnar artery

Radial artery

Transverse carpal
ligament

Hook of
hamate
bone

Fig. 9-1. Classic superficial palmar arch completed by superficial palmar branch of the radial artery.

radially by the fibers of the flexor retinaculum and transverse carpal liga-ment.[12] After its emergence from Guyon's canal, the ulnar artery gives off the deep palmar branch to the hypothenar musculature and changes its name to the superficial palmar arch. The superficial palmar arch continues across the flexor retinaculum deep to the palmaris brevis muscle accompanied by its two paired veins, which constitute the superficial venous arch. The arch pene-trates the central palmar compartment and crosses the palm superficial to the branches of the median nerve and deep to the palmar aponeurosis. Its course and branching are variable, with its main contributions being the four common digital arteries. Several small and variable cutaneous and muscular branches are present. The first major branch is the proper palmar artery to the ulnar side of the little finger, which exits under the palmaris brevis muscle and before the artery's entry into the deep compartment of the hand. In most cases, three remaining common palmar digital arteries then branch from the deep arch.[3] Classically, the arch is completed by the superficial palmar branch of the

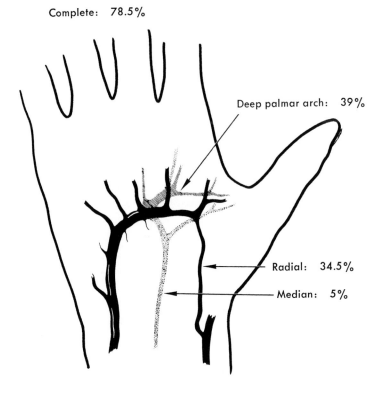

Fig. 9-2. Variations of superficial palmar arch. Arch defined as complete if direct anastomosis with palmar arch, or radial or median artery. In 650 patients, Coleman found 78.5% were complete; 39% from the deep arch or princeps pollicis; 34.5% from the radial artery; 5% from the median artery; and 21.5% were incomplete.[3] (Adapted from Coleman, S. S., and Anson, B. J.: Surg. Gynecol. Obstet. **113**(4):409, 1961.)

radial artery. The arch is complete 78.5% of the time, if direct connections exist with either the radial artery, a large branch from the deep palmar arch, or the median artery[3]; 21.5% of the time the arch is incomplete without direct connection to another major vessel (Fig. 9-2).[3] This absence of a direction connection may be of clinical significance if the ulnar artery becomes occluded.

PATHOGENESIS

The anatomic predisposition for trauma to the ulnar artery in the confines of Guyon's canal is evident. Some protection is afforded by the action of the palmaris brevis muscle,[12] but repeated trauma at its exposed position with subsequent intimal damage, subintimal hematoma, and disruption of the internal elastic membrane leads to organized thrombus formation by the classic

Table 3. Differential diagnosis of ulnar artery thrombosis

Systemic disease	Mechanical causes
Arteriosclerosis	Thoracic outlet
Thromboangiitis obliterans	Direct trauma
Giant cell arteritis	Embolic occlusion
Scleroderma	Radial artery occlusion
Polycythemia	Ergot poisoning
Raynaud's disease	

pattern.[4,11] Patients with a poor collateral circulation and an underlying small-vessel pathologic condition have increased symptomatology. Ischemia may also lead to a reflex increase in sympathetic tone and generalized spasm.

CLINICAL SYNDROME

Thrombosis of the ulnar artery at the wrist occurs in males much more frequently than in females. A history of acute or chronic trauma is usually elicitable. The typical patient presents with the acute onset of pain, numbness, and cold sensitivity. The hand may be pale or cyanotic, and blisters, ulcerations, or gangrene may exist. The ulnar portion of the hand is usually cool, and decreased sweating and sensation may be present. The Allen test is usually positive.

DIFFERENTIAL DIAGNOSIS

The differential diagnosis includes systemic diseases—scleroderma, thromboangiitis obliterans (Buerger's disease), giant cell arteritis, arteriosclerosis, polycythemia, Raynaud's disease, and mechanical causes—and other problems such as thoracic outlet, direct trauma, embolic occlusion, radial artery occlusion, and ergot poisoning (Table 3). Scleroderma is usually bilateral and associated with classic skin changes, esophageal motility abnormalities or the CRST syndrome (calcinosis, Raynaud's phenomenon, sclerodactyly, and telangiectasia).

Buerger's disease presents most frequently to young cigarette-smoking males. Upper-extremity symptomatology is rare, without bilateral lower extremity involvement. Digital artery occlusion and severe ischemic pain often with ulceration are not unusual. This is in contradistinction to ulnar artery thrombosis where symptoms are usually isolated to the upper extremity, rarely bilateral, and infrequently result in gangrene not localized to the tip of a digit. Polycythemia is easily confirmed by routine blood testing, and generalized arteriosclerosis has other associated classical findings.

Ergot, or methysergide poisoning, may induce vasoconstriction, with resultant intimal hyperplasia and thrombosis of both large and small vessels. Thoracic outlet obstruction may cause arterial or venous occlusion with thrombosis or an embolus to distal vessels. Embolic occlusion is rarely isolated to the upper extremity, and changes in fundi, and so forth, are prevalent.

EVALUATION

The evaluation of suspected ulnar artery thrombosis must include a detailed history and physical examination as well as routine and special laboratory tests. Specialized evaluation includes the following.

Thermography. We have found this to be a useful noninvasive technique, which if obtained prior to management, provides a quantitative method of follow-up. Information is similar to that obtained by temperature probes. The right side of Fig. 9-3 represents a normal thermogram with evenly distributed heat patterns. The picture obtained is that of the mirror image of the subject. The left side of Fig. 9-3 represents a patient with ulnar artery thrombosis. Note the absence of detectable heat over the ulnar digits. Fig. 9-4 is the arteriogram of the same patient showing the decreased blood flow to the ulnar side of the hand.

Temperature probes. YSI 427 small surface temperature probes are used to

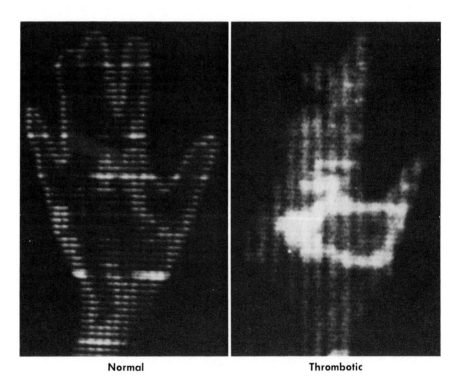

Normal   **Thrombotic**

Fig. 9-3. Normal thermogram contrasted with abnormal thermogram obtained with ulnar artery thrombosis *(right)*. The absence of any detectable pattern in the ulnar distribution reflects poor arterial perfusion.

measure the surface temperature of involved digits and have been found to provide a reliable and quantitative reflection of digital perfusion.[13] Portable battery-powered telethermometers allow easy preoperative, intraoperative and postoperative monitoring. Consistent temperature depression of greater than 2.5° C. compared to that in a noninvolved digit is indicative of insufficient perfusion and may be indicative of cold intolerance.[7]

Digital plethysmography. Pulse volume recordings have been of great value in our evaluation of ulnar artery thrombosis. Use of this technique provides quantitative and reproducible documentation of pulsatile blood flow. Figs. 9-5 and 9-6 represent the patient in case 1. At the time of this recording, the ulnar two digits were potentially nonviable. Note that occlusion of the radial artery obliterates pulsatile blood flow to the index and long fingers. Fig. 9-6 shows the arteriogram confirming the diagnosis. A pulse volume recording of less than 75% correlates well with cold intolerance in our series of replanted digits.[7] In our experience with ulnar artery thrombosis, the absence of pulsatile flow represents symptomatology warranting further intervention. Digital plethysmography is especially useful in the operating room with the patient

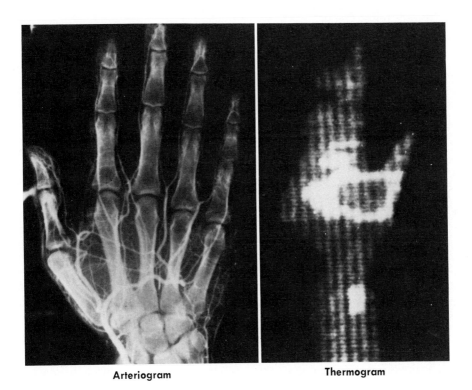

Arteriogram   **Thermogram**

Fig. 9-4. Arteriogram of the patient in Fig. 9-3 with ulnar artery thrombosis. Although there is some collateral flow to the little and ring fingers, it is insufficient to fully perfuse the digits as evidenced in the thermogram and confirmed in the arteriogram.

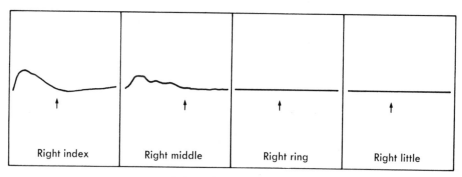

**Pulse volume recording
Radial artery occluded**

Fig. 9-5. Pulse volume recording of patient in case 1. No pulsatile flow is recordable in the little or ring fingers. Note complete absence of pulsatile flow in hand after occlusion of the radial artery.

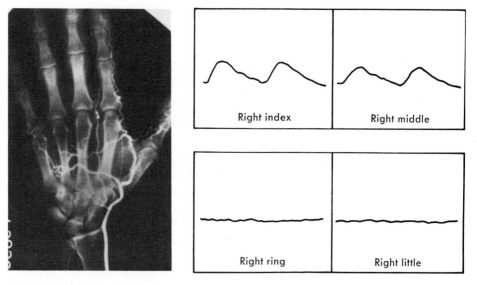

Fig. 9-6. Arteriogram of case 1 compared with pulse volume recording of the patient's digits. At the time of this recording, little and ring fingers were potentially nonviable.

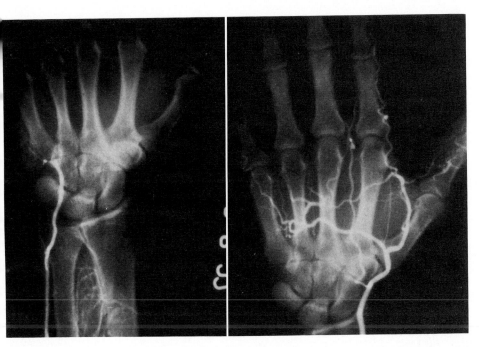

Fig. 9-7. Arteriogram of case 1. The superficial palmar arch is partially filled by the radial artery with a complete block of the ulnar artery at Guyon's canal. The ulnar artery originated from the brachial artery 12.5 cm above the elbow.

asleep. Excision of the thrombosed segment is done; and if insufficient pulsatile flow in the involved digits is present, vein grafting is performed. If the flow is satisfactory after resection of the involved portion of the ulnar artery, then excision and ligation is favored over vein grafting.

Doppler mapping. Doppler mapping of the arterial flow in the hand is routinely performed and correlates with arteriography. Digital vessels as well as larger arteries are audible, and the exact level of thrombosis can be identified.

Arteriography. Arteriography remains the definitive study and, we believe, should be performed prior to surgery. Although Doppler mapping correlates well, it does not allow as accurate an estimate of intimal damage and associated arteriosclerotic changes. Only with an arteriogram can the potential for surgical reconstruction be accurately predicted prior to operative exposure.

During arteriography, intra-arterial medications may be administered and may eliminate the need for further intervention. Femoral arteriograms are recommended to eliminate possible confusion arising from a superficial radial or ulnar artery having separate origin high on the brachial artery. Patient H. T. is an example (Fig. 9-7). His ulnar artery originated 12.5 cm proximal to the elbow and a standard brachial injection would have failed to show the existence of an ulnar artery demonstrating only the arteries visualized on the right of Fig. 9-7. The left is the arteriogram of the selective injection of the ulnar artery.

In the following case reports, a different method of management was used for each patient.

Case reports

CASE ONE

H. T. is a 38-year-old white male right-handed automobile mechanic. Fifteen years prior to admission, he sustained a Monteggia fracture of his right arm with nonunion of the ulna and dislocation of the radial head. He presented with a 1-day history of numbness, pain, and cyanosis of the ulnar side of the right hand. No specific trauma was noted, but he used a pneumatic hammer in his daily work.

In the emergency room the hand was cold and cyanotic with decreased capillary refill in the ulnar distribution. Allen test showed no filling on the ulnar side. Grip strength was diminished.

Pulse volume recorder showed that he had diminished flow to the little and ring fingers (Figs. 9-5 and 9-6). Doppler mapping showed no flow from the level of Guyon's canal to the proximal palmar crease or in the digital arteries to the ring or little fingers.

In the emergency room, a stellate ganglion block was done with decreased symptoms and increased capillary refill. His arm was observed in the emergency room overnight and had deteriorated to the point that he had a potentially nonviable little finger. He was taken to the vascular radiology section where an arteriogram was done confirming the ulnar artery thrombosis (Fig. 9-7). Intra-arterial reserpine was given with no result. He was taken to the operating room where the affected segment was excised and a vein graft placed (Fig. 9-8). At the conclusion of the procedure his pulse volume recording showed that there was pulsatile flow in all digits with the radial artery occluded. Postoperatively, he was treated with heparin followed by sodium warfarin (Coumadin). Prior to discharge he had repeat Doppler studies, which showed patency of his ulnar artery, and the Allen test showed the ulnar artery filled. He had good relief of pain in his hand and excellent capillary refill. After his discharge from the hospital, he resumed smoking and returned to work against advice. Working without his splint, his wound dehisced and his ulnar artery thrombosed. A superficial infection occurred, but responded well to local care. After dehiscence of the wound, the patient's cold intolerance returned.

CASE TWO

J. P. is a 37-year-old electrician who was admitted for cyanosis, pain, paresthesias, and cold intolerance of the right hand of 8 months' duration. The original diagnosis was Raynaud's disease. Prior to symptoms, he sustained a crushing injury to his right hand. The patient's main complaint was cold intolerance. He smoked one to two packs per day. He had decreased sensation in the ulnar distribution and a positive Allen test. Flow studies showed decreased flow in the little and ring fingers. Arteriogram confirmed occlusion of the ulnar artery with no communication between the superficial and deep arches. With help from the Biofeedback Division of the Psychology Department, he was able to stop smoking and voluntarily increase blood flow to his hand (as determined by pulse volume recordings and temperature studies) and did return to work.

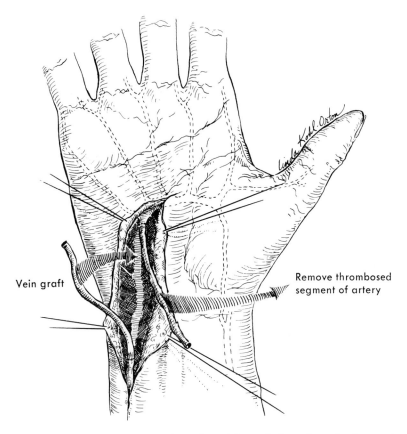

Fig. 9-8. Diagrammatic representation of excision of thrombosed ulnar artery and replacement with vein graft.

CASE THREE

L. L. is a 45-year-old telephone company lineman with a 2-month history of numbness and cold intolerance in the ring and little fingers of his left hand. He smoked two packs per day. He had decreased sensation on the ulnar side of the hand and a positive Allen test. Temperature was 2 Celsius degrees cooler in the left ring and long fingers. The flow to the left ring finger was 30% of normal. Arteriogram confirmed the diagnosis. Stellate ganglion block gave no relief. Intra-arterial reserpine, however, provided much improvement. Hematocrit was 55 with a hemoglobin of 15.4. He was able to decrease his cigarette smoking and the symptoms, except for the cold intolerance, were relieved.

CASE FOUR

B. J. had ulnar nerve symptoms and documented thrombosis of the ulnar artery at the wrist. He underwent decompression of the ulnar nerve at the wrist and excision of the thrombosed ulnar artery. Good pulsatile backflow was evident from the superficial palmar arch; therefore the open ends were ligated. Follow-up showed symptomatic improvement, and he returned to work without significant cold intolerance.

DISCUSSION

A review of the literature and examination of the patients presented provides support for almost any treatment modality. Upper-extremity sympathectomy,[4] stellate and brachial blocks, excision of the thrombosed segment and ligation,[6,8,10,15] arteriotomy and thrombectomy,[9] intra-arterial reserpine and tolazoline (Priscoline), discontinuance of smoking and biofeedback techniques, and excision and vein grafting have all been employed with varying results. Of importance are two observations. First, regardless of treatment, if the acute episode can be overcome and the patient's symptoms can be made tolerable by minor environmental modifications, there is no progression of gangrene and the patient can usually return to work. Second, regardless of treatment, including vein grafting and reconstitution and maintenance of flow, residual symptomatology can be expected. We have adopted an approach that is individualized to the patient employing potentially any of these treatments.

The initial diagnosis is made by history, physical exam, Allen test, thermography, Doppler mapping, and digital plethysmography with elimination of other processes in the differential diagnosis. In acute thrombosis with jeopardized digital survival, a stellate ganglion block is given by a member of the anesthesia department or under controlled conditions in the emergency room. This will often provide relief of pain by blocking reflex vasospasm. Success is judged clinically and confirmed with Doppler mapping, plethysmography, or thermography. Since sympathetic blocade sometimes accompanies complete motor and sensory blocade, if the vascular status of the hand is still compromised, brachial block is performed.

If symptoms persist, arteriography is done. The definitive diagnosis, exact level of block, and potential operability are obtained and intra-arterial medications may be given. Tolazoline (Priscoline) and reserpine have been used occasionally with dramatic results. Relief with diminution of symptoms requires observation in the hospital, discontinuation of smoking, and possible benefit from biofeedback techniques.

Rarely does occlusion of the ulnar artery at the wrist compromise digital survival, but when it does, surgical intervention may become an emergency. If symptoms persist, with objective evidence of inadequate blood flow by Doppler mapping, thermography, or digital plethysmography, then operative intervention is indicated.

The vessel is exposed under tourniquet, the thrombosed segment resected and the proximal portion clamped. If there is good backflow from collateral circulation and pulse volume recordings of the digits are normal in the operating room, the artery is ligated and the wound closed. Continued symptoms should be controlled conservatively (cessation of smoking, biofeedback, warm temperature, and so forth) or by sympathectomy as a last resort.

If after clamping, there is poor backflow and no pulsatile flow by digital plethysmography, then vein grafting should be considered if the hemoglobin is normal. Erythrocytosis is a contraindication to vein grafting. If the symptoms persist, the above conservative regimen is followed.

Vein grafting is performed if the hemoglobin is normal, and there is inadequate perfusion with clamping of the ends of the ulnar artery and superficial palmar arch. The entire thrombosed segment is resected until normal intima as judged under the operating microscope is seen, and the defect is grafted by use of a vein graft from the forearm. Vein grafting is contraindicated if there is no peripheral "run off" on the arteriogram. Postoperative persistence of symptoms is treated as before.

Sympathectomy should be employed only when all else has failed. It is a significant surgical undertaking with expected morbidity (Horner's syndrome) and with variable results. Conn, the principal proponent of sympathectomy, believed it preferable because of the "risk of poor or delayed healing of an incision in an ischemic extremity".[4] This risk has been proved negligible.[6,8,10,15] Kleinert reported one case with progression of gangrene after thrombectomy, which responded to sympathectomy.[9]

CONCLUSION

Ulnar artery thrombosis generally occurs in males in the fifth decade of life with an occupational predisposition to trauma. Symptoms are those of nerve compression and arterial insufficiency and are related, in part, to the individual's vascular anatomy of the hand. Diagnosis is on the basis of suspicion, positive Allen test, and confirmatory studies. Treatment must be individualized and depends on the analysis of history, physical examination, and laboratory and diagnostic data. All patients do not need surgery. In some instances, simple resection and ligation is favored over the more difficult vein-grafting procedure.

The treatment of ulnar artery thrombosis is a complex problem requiring individualized management. The minor cold intolerance occurring after ligation of a carpenter's ulnar artery is a fair exchange for return to full employment but may be unacceptable for a housewife with grown children. The business executive with emphysema and polycythemia may respond well to intra-arterial reserpine followed by biofeedback techniques but would be hampered by the Horner's syndrome associated with upper-extremity sympathectomy. More than technical skills are required for management of this entity, and any operative procedure must be coupled with identification and removal (if possible) of the underlying cause of the problem.

REFERENCES

1. Allen, E. V.: Thromboangiitis obliterans: methods of diagnosis of chronic occlusive arterial lesions distal to the wrist with illustrative cases, Am. J. Med. Sci. **178:**237-244, 1929.
2. Benedict, K. T., Chang, W., and McCready, F. J.: The hypothenar hammer syndrome, Radiology **3:**57-60, April 1974.

3. Coleman, S. S., and Anson, B. J.: Arterial patterns in the hand based upon a study of 650 specimens, Surg. Gynecol. Obstet. **113**(4):409, Oct. 1961.
4. Conn, J., Jr., Bergan, J. J., and Bell, J. L.: Hypothenar hammer syndrome, Surgery **68**(6):1122, 1970.
5. Dale, W. A.: Management of ischemia of the hand and fingers, Surgery **67**:62-79, Jan. 1970.
6. Eguro, H., and Goldner, J. L.: Bilateral thrombosis of the ulnar arteries in the hands, Plast. Reconstr. Surg. **52**(5):573-578, 1973.
7. Gelberman, R., Urbaniak, J. R., Bright, D. S., and Levin, L. S.: Digital sensitivity following replantation, J. Hand Surg. 3(4):313-320, 1978.
8. Herndon, W. A., Hershey, S. L., and Lambdin, C. S.: Thrombosis of the ulnar artery in the hand, J. Bone Joint Surg. **57-A**:994-995, 1975.
9. Kleinert, H. E., and Volianitis, G. J.: Thrombosis of the palmar arterial arch and its tributaries: etiology and neuroconcepts and treatment, J. Trauma 5(4):447, 1965.
10. Leriche, R., Fontaine, R., and Dupertuis, S. M.: Arterectomy with follow-up studies on 78 operations, Surg. Gynecol. Obstet. **64**:149-155, 1937.
11. Little, J. M., and Ferguson, D. A.: The incidence of the hypothenar hammer syndrome, Arch. Surg. **105**:684, Nov. 1972.
12. Shrewsbury, M. M.: The palmaris brevis: a reconsideration of its anatomy and possible function, J. Bone Joint Surg. **54-A**(2):334, 1976.
13. Stirrat, C. R., Seaber, A. V., Urbaniak, J. R., and Bright, D. S.: Temperature monitoring in digital replantation, J. Hand Surg. 3:342-347, 1978.
14. von Rosen, S.: Ein Fall von Thrombose in der Arteria ulnaris nach Einwirkung von stumpfer Gewalt, Acta Chir. Scand. **73**:500-506, 1934.
15. Zweig, J., Lie, K. K., Posch, J. L., and Larsen, R. D.: Thrombosis of the ulnar artery following blunt trauma to the hand, J. Bone Joint Surg. **51-A**:1191, 1969.

GENERAL DISCUSSION

Dr. Urbaniak: There are some important points about microsurgical instruments and their use. We have the problem that everyone desiring to perform microsurgery uses the same instruments. Do you separate your instruments in the operating room? I know Jack Tupper does, but does anyone else? Dr. Kutz, how do you keep them separate? Does everyone try to use the same set of instruments?

Dr. Kutz: We have two sets for the hand fellows and each staff man has his own set of instruments that he uses on his own patients.

Dr. Wilgis: That's essentially the way we do it, each staff man has his own set and we have one or two sets for the residents.

Dr. Urbaniak: Dr. Bright, I know that half the people in the audience use your sets.

Dr. Bright: We have probably the worst of the world. Everybody uses our sets including our loupes, but it has its advantages, we get more people trained. It's bad for the instruments; so I concur with the others.

Dr. Urbaniak: In this particular discipline, I really believe, for optimal performance, the individual surgeon should have his own instruments, which he alone uses. Until a year or so ago, our instruments never worked, if you want to know the truth. Not only did they not function, we never could find them. We would have six or more of the little microclips in the hospital and have a replant at night and could not find one. This used to happen frequently. With the reorganization of our operating-room personnel with selected nurses to scrub on the microsurgical team, this situation has been corrected. Our morale was improved tremendously. This brings up the next question—the OR nurse for microsurgery. Jack, do you have a specialist?

Dr. Tupper: Yes, we have two nurses who alternately call for replants, and they are the only ones that handle the instruments. They know they are the ones that will get into trouble, and there is a certain tolerance for breakage, and I think this is one of the reasons why a friend doesn't exist who is good enough to borrow my instruments. You just have to make this decision and stick by it, because the friend himself might take care of them but he is then working with a different nurse who couldn't care less. She may want to go home, and they all get dropped in a pan and that's the end of them. So the fewer people who have responsibility for the instruments the better.

Dr. Kutz: I have to agree with Jack. Fortunately, in the Institute we have several people working. We do have nurses in charge of the hand unit and under her about one half of the girls can rotate and scrub in. We have fortunately one or two on each shift who seem to be more concerned about the instruments and take care of them. They see the instruments and take care of them personally. As far as other people using the instruments are concerned, we believe there are so few that you really need that the expense of buying them for each individual person is not so great. If they do have their own instruments, they take care of them much better. As Jack said, lending them to a friend can be difficult at times. I have Designs for Vision and the pupillary distance is exact, but once in a while you'll find someone the same size. We have a urologist on the staff who was putting the vas deferens together, and I walked in on a case one day and couldn't find any glasses. He borrowed them without telling me.

Dr. Urbaniak: Dr. Wilgis, what about your nurses; are they specialists in microsurgery?

Dr. Wilgis: We have three OR nurses who are responsible for all microsurgery cases. One important thing that we do is that we rotate these individuals through the lab. This allows them to get into the lab and see the actual work and participate in microsurgery. I think this increases the interest level, and it's been a helpful maneuver for us.

Dr. Urbaniak: Don, what about your feelings on OR nurses?

Dr. Bright: In general, we get whoever is on at that particular time. Since replants are almost routine, we now have people on each shift who have scrubbed with us and who do know the instruments very well. Generally, our help in the OR is good with these experienced individuals. If, however, you get somebody who is not experienced, it lengthens your case and increases your fatigue and irritability. This is exactly what you don't need in the middle of the night when you are on a case. After the instruments leave the OR, however, they are put into a general pile, and I have seen them dumped on a stainless steel tray for washing and then on another tray for drying. I can attest that not only is that terribly expensive as far as replacing instruments, but makes many instruments useless after one use. I would take the advice of the other panelists and learn by our own bad experience. Thankfully our situation has improved during the past year, but it has been difficult to convince the operating supervisors of the importance of experienced microsurgical scrub nurses.

Dr. Urbaniak: A few quick questions. Jack, what kind of background material do you use?

Dr. Tupper: Ordinary latex blue. I like blue for nerves and yellow for vessels. The best thing about the latex in preference to plastic is that it has no shiny surface and you don't get light reflected back.

Dr. Kutz: I like Carolina blue.

Dr. Urbaniak: Microsurgery is the only place I can tolerate Carolina blue, for Duke blue is too dark! What about yellow?

Dr. Wilgis: We generally use yellow.

Dr. Urbaniak: Joe made a very important point about irrigation solution. Keep it at 37° C. We don't always get it that way, and you certainly notice the difference when you use cold solution. Don, what solution do you use for irrigating the vessel while you are repairing it?

Dr. Bright: I believe it is important to have heparinized saline or Ringer's lactate solution for irrigation. That should be almost after every suture you use. The instruments should be washed with a solution because any dried blood will prevent them from properly working. I believe the suggestion to have plain water for the instruments is probably better than saline.

Dr. Wilgis: I try to use every little advantage that I can, and although saline is universally available, I believe a buffered solution is better. Physiologically, the pH is more correct. We happen to use a preparation called "V-Sol," which is a buffered electrolyte balance. There is some evidence that saline does destroy surface cells so we like a buffered solution.

Dr. Urbaniak: Joe, you use a bland solution for irrigation, don't you?

Dr. Kutz: No, we use the buffered solution for irrigating, but we do not allow this to stay on the instruments. Instead of wiping them off, we use a water solution for the instruments. If the nurse sees the instruments soaking in the buffer, she will wipe them off and place them in the proper solution before they corrode. This is why we use a water solution for the instruments and a buffered solution for irrigation.

Dr. Urbaniak: Jack told us he uses the heparin solution.

Dr. Tupper: We use the buffered salt solution that comes already packaged in a little plastic bottle and is very controlled. I believe the débridement should be carried out under water, and you can more easily debride the fascicles of the nerve with them floating under water. There usually is a large enough cavity in the palm where you can do this. It lets all these little things (fascicles) float up to the surface. I've become so accustomed to doing things under water that I have an entire débridement tank now, so that the entire repair can be performed under water while I view through the operating scope.

Dr. Urbaniak: The size of the needle and suture is important. The panel generally uses something in the 10-0 line for suture and a needle of 50 to 75 microns for digital vessels. If we move proximally to the wrist, Jack, what size needle and suture do you use for an ulnar artery?

Dr. Tupper: I use the same sizes.

Dr. Kutz: We often use 8-0 suture and a corresponding needle size (150 microns).

Dr. Wilgis: I agree with Joe. With the very small needle sometimes I have trouble getting it through the bigger vessel wall.

Dr. Bright: We've done it both ways, either way depending on the thickness of the vessel. The 10-0 will hold the anastomosis fine; there is no problem with strength. Passing the needle is the important thing.

Dr. Tupper: I'd like to mention a recent case we had. Our hospital doctors were injecting gel foam pellets into a vascular anomaly in the leg; apparently this is something the radiologists do now. Somehow these pellets backed up and the patient would wind up with a cold foot. Arteriograms showed the pellets caused a complete block of posterior tibial and anterior tibial arteries. Vascular surgeons get a little panicky when they are confronted with this caliber of vessel and I was consulted. We removed these pellets actually without any trouble at all. We were used to a fine suture on those particular vessels. 7V (10-0) was a little bit too fine. Larger suture such as 8-0 or 9-0 suture would have been more appropriate.

Dr. Kutz: There is just one point I'd like to make and that is on vascular clamps. Now most of these were made so that they have spring action, and I noticed yesterday in the lab and I believe you'll share my concern when you start using them. If you get to the point where the vessels start sliding out of the clamp, this is the point where you have too much tension and this is an indication that you have too much of a gap and you should do a vein graft.

Dr. Urbaniak: This is a good point. Don't depend on any clamps to do the approximations. It is like repairing a nerve or tendon. You have to get the vessels mobilized and approximate the ends without tension. If tension exists, don't hesitate to insert a vascular graft.

• • •

Dr. Urbaniak: I'm sure we have all experienced the situation when we have performed the best anastomosis technically possible, and no blood will flow through it. What happens here? You do a "perfect anastomosis," but no blood flows into the finger at all. Joe Kutz, what is the problem when you do a technically great anastomosis and it doesn't work? When you are looking at it and there is no backflow or no blood returning through the veins?

Dr. Kutz: I imagine that in this situation what we are dealing with is capillary damage. Dr. Tupper brought a clue about this when he came back from China; that is, when you examine an amputated finger and you see the so-called red line, the Chinese thought that this was not a finger to put back on. This is not completely true, because we have salvaged a lot of these fingers since then. I believe the biggest problem is the spasm, that is, spasm of the arterioles and capillaries that can occur in some of these severely injured fingers. When we reattach a crushed digit, or sometimes even after prolonged cooling, we notice that the finger will not bleed as well or will not return to normal color. As near as we can tell, it is caused by poor capillary perfusion. If the tissue is not perfused, it is not going to survive.

Dr. Tupper. I think if you've made your anastomosis at surgery and it is your usual beautiful anastomosis and no blood comes, the first thing you ought to do is wake up the anesthesiologist and see what the blood pressure is because all it takes is a little hypotension down to about 80 and the blood just does not flow. If the pressure is up, then I think you just haven't debrided the artery enough. You've got to cut out more artery proximally until it bleeds. I think if I've had good blood flow before I started the anastomosis, I've never seen one that then refused to flow once I had completed the anastomosis.

Dr. Urbaniak: I've seen it a number of times; there is something abnormal distally. Don, you've been there many times. We never attempt to anastomose a vessel if the blood doesn't squirt across and hit somebody. But there must be something wrong distally, perhaps in the capillary-tissue exchange or perfusion level.

Dr. Bright: We went almost a year one time without a failure. They all worked and we thought there was nothing we couldn't do, but that's not true. I mean you're always going to have periods of time, well, at least for a little while, that 100% of the digits are replantable, but remember there's always going to be the digit that was overcooled or that was too traumatized. After all, the whole digit is dependent upon more than just the integrity of the artery. The vessel may flow distally to the nail, but if capillary extravasation occurs, it may work fine for an hour or two, or even 24 hours, and then fail to survive despite a technically good anastomosis. If you are engaged in replanting a large number of amputated parts, there will always be a small number that, despite all variations or repeated attempts at anastomoses, you will not be able to keep alive. You must remember these are patients. The digit is important, but it's not the whole patient. When we take them back to the OR, we end up spending about as long as we did on the original replant. When you have somebody in surgery for 9 hours and then add another 9 hours, plus blood, cost, and a certain amount of danger to the patient, you must critically evaluate the decision to return the patient to the OR. Even though you can use a brachial block in adults, in a child it usually requires general anesthesia. General anesthesia is not unsafe, but it's not always without complications. You have to decide how much you are going to put into this individual digit. If there is something you can go back and remedy, fine, but if you've done the best job initially you can and it doesn't make it, then it's no use fooling yourself and the patient.

Dr. Urbaniak: What Dr. Bright and I are saying is that the replants that have failed despite our returning them to the OR are the ones we were suspicious or less confident about at the conclusion of the initial procedure. We spent a lot of time and did everything we could, but they apparently had some distal problem, some problem that as of today we don't know how to solve. The ones that we've done are working very well at the end of the primary procedure, and they just keep on doing well. I think that may explain some of the discrepancy.

Joe, do you prefer vein grafts or bone shortening if you've got the choice? Jack says never shorten the bone—he doesn't want any "stubby fingers."

Dr. Kutz: I prefer to vein graft at this point. I shorten if it's necessary to debride the soft tissue. If the bone is too long to get back to good soft tissue, then I would debride the bone. If the soft tissue is adequate with very minimal débridement, then I would use a vein graft, because I believe that your problem is going to be tension. You really must judge it properly and give yourself a bit of security. When you're going to shorten the bone and think you're going to take tension off the vessel, you often shorten the bone a centimeter and you still end up having to put in a vein graft. If you shorten another centimeter, you've really done the patient a disfavor. Many times you will have a big bulge of excess tissue, which will produce edema, swelling, and compression at the anastomosis site and prevent adequate backflow, which may result in the loss of a digit.

Dr. Urbaniak: I might comment that we usually take the opposite view. Many times when you need a vein graft because the vessels are too short, the nerves are damaged and are too short and the tendons may be damaged. Therefore, I would prefer bone shortening. We don't hesitate to do it. We have 25 thumbs that have been replanted now, and I don't have one patient complaining of a short thumb. We've shortened many of them over a centimeter and I don't notice any gross deformity; it's hard to see in a thumb. In an index finger you're doing the patient a favor by shortening it because you're getting it "out of the way" more. What I'm saying is that other tissues may need to be grafted too, and you can't graft them all. That's another view. Jack, I'm sure you have a comeback on that, don't you?

Dr. Tupper: I think the one point of validity to what you're saying is in terms of nerves because I think we're all surprised early in the game when we were all shortening bone and we were all surprised how much return of sensation we got. Again, now I would nerve-graft too. I think the thumb is probably the best one to shorten. I agree a little shortening of the thumb does not make any difference. There is one other point. If you don't have this sophisticated equipment to tell whether it's alive or not, I think the nail bed is a poor place to press on. You can push the blood back and forth in the nail bed and think something good is happening. The eponychial fold just above the nail is far better, and you can determine in any race what's happening with the distal perfusion.

Dr. Urbaniak: The good results of nerve repair in children were emphasized in the presentation on vessels. We know we get good results in everything in children we do in surgery. But this has not been our experience with replants in children. I notice that when Dr. Kutz and Dr. Kleinert show their slides on their many replants, the little bar graph that represents children under 10 years has the worst results. How do you explain that, Joe?

Dr. Kutz: I think the problem was that initially when we first started doing these, we began doing them in children. My first attempt was in a child in 1961 with the naked eye and it lived for a while. But as we've been improving our techniques and using more sophisticated instruments over a period of time, I believe that the best functional results are in children. Now if we break down our results in the last 3 years, I'd say our children's results are probably equal or better than the adults. The results that we've been showing are everything that we've done since we first started in 1961.

Dr. Tupper: I think your percentage of viability and my percentage of viability will always be lower in children than it will be in adults because I'll try anything in a child simply because I know that if I succeed in making it viable the child will succeed in making it useful. So my percentage of viability will be less on small children; however, the percentage of usefulness in the ones that survive is better than that in adults.

Dr. Urbaniak: I agree with that. Our percentage in children has been worse for that reason. We have some feeling about vasospasm in children. We may be off course, I'm not sure. This is why we do like the temperature recording. This is an inexpensive and simple method of monitoring the replanted part postoperatively. The nurse can check it through the night. Just turn the dial, and it reads 32° C or so, and as Don mentioned, if it stays above 30° C we feel pretty good. If it goes below 30° C (the normal digit is somewhere between 34 and 35 depending on the ambient temperature), we become concerned. It is simple and doesn't disturb the child. It avoids contacting and squeezing the digit in the sensitive and anxious child. We've actually almost lost fingertips from the staff pinching on them too frequently.

Joe, how do you want the part managed when the patient is sent to you?

Dr. Kutz: I missed the point that you made between the different methods, but basically what we recommend is to have the parts put in a plastic bag and sometimes with or without dressing around and then immerse that in ice, which I think is essentially the same way. I don't like direct contact with ice.

Dr. Urbaniak: We instruct the referring physician to place the amputated part in saline solution which is in a plastic bag. The bag is then placed in ice. Maceration of the tissue by immersion of the part in the solution has not been detrimental to our knowledge.

Dr. Kutz: Do you use the same suture material in all replants?

Dr. Urbaniak: Well, I believe everyone is using monofilament nylon. Now Prolene (polypropylene) is on the market. There have been studies to show that it is less reactive on nerves, but we don't know whether it is or not. It is more difficult to keep knotted. Do you use anything different?

Dr. Kutz: We don't use nylon on tendons or on the other structures. We use Dacron and we've used Dexon on a lot of periosteal sutures and things like that—if that's what you are referring to as far as all structures are concerned.

Dr. Urbaniak: No, I'm sorry I missed the question then. We do the same thing, really. On tendons we use a polyester suture.

10. Microsurgery in the anterior approach to the cervical spine

Richard S. Kramer

The following indications favoring the anterior surgical approach to the cervical spine, and the frequency with which this exposure is employed, have increased substantially in the past decade:

1. Symptomatic cervical osteoarthritis (spondylosis) involving one or two levels, with or without foraminal osteophyte formation, is perhaps the best example of a disorder for which the anterior approach is most widely used and for which the operation was indeed designed.
2. Simple posterolateral extrusions of "soft" disk fragments, secondary to degenerative disk disease, are now commonly relieved by anterior diskectomy and root decompression.
3. Traumatic injuries of the cervical spine, including central disk herniations as well as selected cases of compression fracture, often require this approach.
4. Vertebral body tumors, either primary or metastatic, may be resected anteriorly, with necessary stabilization provided by a rib or iliac crest graft.

Indeed, among experienced surgeons the anterior approach to the cervical spine has become routine and ordinarily quite safe. Certainly intraoperative magnification is not *required* for most of these procedures, and indeed one may question the wisdom of lengthening and otherwise "complicating" a straightforward operation by introducing a surgical microscope into the field. However, our experience and that of others[2,4] suggest that routine use of the operating microscope during the critical stages of nearly all anterior cervical operations not only enhances the surgeon's technique, but also provides significant benefits to operating room personnel, residents, and students. For these and other reasons to be enumerated, magnification has become a valuable adjunct to anterior cervical surgery at Duke University Hospital.

GENERAL OPERATIVE APPROACH

Regardless of the disease process or the indications for operation, anterior cervical spine surgery at Duke University is performed jointly by the orthopaedists and neurosurgeons: the orthopaedist assumes responsibility for the exposure and the earliest stages of resection of either disk or vertebral body, as well as for any fusion procedure required; the neurosurgeon takes over as the posterior longitudinal ligament is approached, removing the last few millimeters of disk or bone, osteophytes, or the ligament itself when appropriate, and performing any required operative manipulation within the vertebral canal or the foramina.

With few exceptions, the Smith-Robinson approach[5] is employed in all cases requiring diskectomy, whether the goal is removal of a "soft" disk fragment, a foraminal spur for primary radiculopathy, or a transverse osteophyte for prevention or treatment of myelopathy; these three problems comprise the primary indications for over 90% of the anterior cervical spine procedures performed at Duke University.

After induction of general anesthesia, the patient is positioned supine in head-halter traction with 3 to 5 lb. of weight. A transverse incision (concealed in a natural skin crease) is preferred for cosmetic reasons, but an oblique incision along the anterior border of the sternomastoid may be required when the surgical objective is below C6 or if fusion of more than two levels is contemplated. We generally prefer to approach the anterior cervical spine through a right-sided exposure, so as to minimize any risk associated with retraction of the carotid artery supplying the dominant hemisphere. On the other hand, the necessarily oblique character of the approach is such that lesions encroaching on the right intervertebral foramen will be better visualized if the approach is from the left.

After the platysma is incised, the natural plane between the sternomastoid and the strap muscles is developed; the carotid sheath is gently retracted laterally and the viscera medially, so that the anterior aspect of the spine and the longus colli muscles are exposed. During the course of the dissection, the carotid (Chassaignac's) tubercle of C6 provides a reliable and easily palpable landmark; nevertheless, I routinely confirm the location radiographically. After coagulation of the numerous small vessels that are found on the surface of the anterior longitudinal ligament, a window is created in the ligament by sharp dissection; disk material is then removed with the pituitary rongeur and orthopaedic curettes.

At this point the sterile-draped operating microscope is introduced, equipped with a 250 or 300 mm objective. Additional weight is added to the traction device as the neurosurgeon removes the remaining disk material, exposing the full breadth of the posterior longitudinal ligament. The ease and safety with which this phase of the operation can be accomplished under conditions of stereoscopic magnification and high-intensity illumination, as provided by the operating microscope, can hardly be overemphasized. The posterior longitudinal ligament may be examined in detail for any defect suggesting possible extrusion of disk material. Where indicated, the ligament

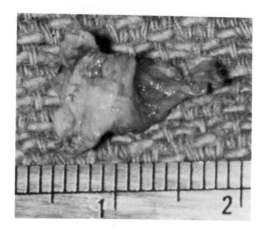

Fig. 10-1. Free fragment of disk material discovered laterally in the foramen after removal of the posterior longitudinal ligament.

itself is readily removed under magnification, with the surgeon generally moving from one side or the other (rather than from the midline), since the ligament is attenuated laterally and can be lifted away from underlying veins and dura with a blunt hook during sharp dissection.

Removal of large, herniated "soft" disk fragments is readily accomplished by use of the anterior approach (Fig. 10-1). Furthermore, magnification aids in the recognition of herniated disk material in those occasional instances where the extrusion occurs as a free fragment impacted laterally in the foramen.

After introduction of an interspace spreader, foraminal and transverse osteophytes are removed with the high-speed drill, equipped with a diamond bur (for protection of the dura); the angled handpiece provides optimal visualization. A variety of small curettes, particularly those developed by Dr. Frank Mayfield, prove extremely useful in removing small osteophytes. One should keep in mind the location of the vertebral artery when introducing such instruments laterally into the foramina.

Although anterior cervical diskectomy *without* fusion has numerous adherents,[1,2,4] the long-term consequences of this procedure are uncertain. We currently employ an autogenous bone graft, taken from the iliac crest, in virtually all cases. A single small drain is left in the depths of the operative field (to be removed within 8 to 12 hours); the anatomic closure is a simple matter indeed.

CASE STUDY

The singular benefits to be derived from routine use of the operating microscope are perhaps best appreciated in those cases where degenerative or traumatic osteoarthritis at a single level in the cervical spine has resulted in foraminal spurs with secondary radiculopathy. Although it is generally be-

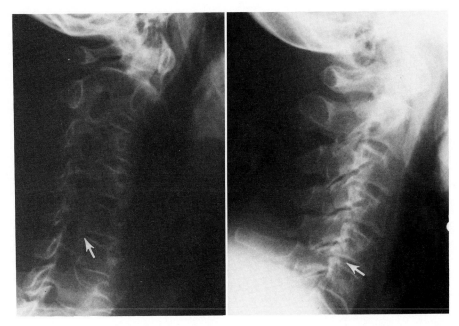

Fig. 10-2. Plain radiographs of the cervical spine reveal degenerative changes localized to the C5-C6 interspace, with a prominent foraminal osteophyte on the right *(arrow).*

lieved that osteophytes will regress after simple fusion alone,[3] we have observed this phenomenon in only 60% to 70% of our patients and therefore prefer to surgically remove symptomatic spurs prior to fusion.

W. J., a 57-year-old hospital administrator, presented with a 2-year history of recurrent low-grade posterior cervical aching pain with occasional radiation into the right shoulder. In the 3 months prior to first evaluation his neck pain had increased in intensity, coincident with development of right arm pain in a C6 root distribution. Examination revealed cervical mechanical signs with development of radicular pain and paresthesias upon Spurling's maneuver on the right-hand side. Paravertebral spasm and limitation of motion were noted. There was slight weakness of the right biceps, diminution of the right biceps reflex, and mild hypalgesia in a C6 root distribution. Routine radiographs revealed degenerative changes at the C5-C6 interspace (Fig. 10-2), with a prominent osteophyte projecting into the intervertebral foramen on the right. A cervical myelogram confirmed that nerve root involvement was isolated to a single level (Fig. 10-3).

Anterior cervical diskectomy and fusion were undertaken through a left anterior approach in order to improve visualization of the right intervertebral foramen. The operation was performed as described above; complete removal of the offending spur and direct confirmation of nerve root decompression were readily accomplished under magnification. An autogenous bone graft from the iliac crest was gently impacted into the interspace to provide interbody fusion. The patient was virtually asymptomatic with respect to radicular

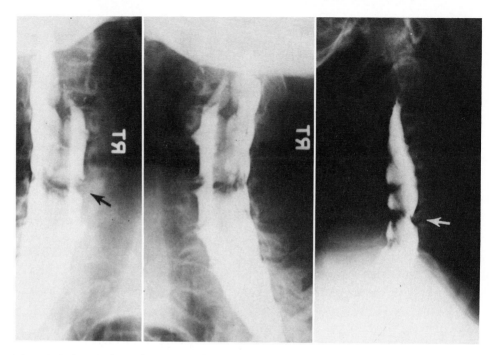

Fig. 10-3. Cervical myelogram confirms that the pathosis is limited to the C5-C6 level (*arrow*).

pain upon awakening in the recovery room; his subsequent recovery was uneventful, and satisfactory fusion was confirmed radiographically at 3 months.

DISCUSSION

The advantages provided by routine use of the operating microscope in anterior cervical spine surgery are substantial. Most significant, in my judgment, is the provision of stereoscopic visualization of structures situated deep within the interspace (such as spurs, "soft" disk fragments, and posterior longitudinal ligament). The interpupillary distance in the average adult surgeon absolutely precludes simultaneous binocular observation of this area unless the operator suffers from spasmodic torticollis. Obviously, when one is working with sharp instruments scant millimeters from the spinal cord, nerve root, or vertebral artery, a three-dimensional view of the operative field is highly desirable.

Additionally, of course, the operating microscope provides superb illumination in the depths of the operative field, as well as low-level magnification (3× to 6×).

When equipped with one of the new lightweight television cameras and video tape capability, the operating microscope tends to capture the attention and enhance the morale of the operating room team. In teaching hospitals, the ability to simultaneously transmit and record the intimate details of the operation expands training opportunities immeasurably.

The simple movement of the instrument in and out of the operative field (and its intraoperative adjustments) should add no more than 10 minutes to the average operating time. Properly draped, the risk of wound contamination from the overhanging microscope is trivial.

Most of us associate the operating microscope with a limited number of unique and very specialized operations, for which it was designed. The purpose of this presentation is simply to suggest that a considerable variety of "routine" procedures, particularly the anterior operative approach to the cervical spine, are substantially enhanced by application of this exciting development in modern surgery.

REFERENCES

1. Boldrey, E. B.: Anterior cervical decompression (without fusion). Presented at the 25th annual meeting of the American Association of Neurological Surgeons, Key Biscayne, Fla., Nov. 12, 1964.
2. Hankinson, H. L., and Wilson, C. B.: Use of the operating microscope in anterior discectomy without fusion, J. Neurosurg. 43:452, 1975.
3. Johnson, R. M., and Southwick, W. O.: Surgical approaches to the cervical spine. In Rothman, R. H., and Simeone, F. A., editors: The spine, Philadelphia, 1975, W. B. Saunders Co., vol. 1, p. 116.
4. Robertson, J. T.: Anterior removal of cervical disc without fusion, Clin. Neurosurg. 20:259, 1973.
5. Smith, G. W., and Robinson, R. A.: The treatment of certain cervical spine disorders by anterior removal of the intervertebral disc and interbody fusion, J. Bone Joint Surg. 40-A:607, 1958.

11. Microneurosurgery

Robert H. Wilkins

HISTORICAL BACKGROUND

The surgical microscope has been used by neurosurgeons for only about 20 years.[4] Clinical microsurgery was developed initially by otolaryngologists; the problem of sterility had to be solved before this approach could be used successfully in neurosurgery.

In 1957, Kurze began to use the operating microscope in neurosurgical operations, especially those performed for the removal of acoustic neurinomas.[4] Two years later, Guiot and Thibaut reported their initial experience with the transsphenoidal removal of pituitary adenomas.[6] During the early 1960s, Hardy further developed transsphenoidal hypophysectomy and tumor removal.[8,9] Jacobson, Donaghy, Chou, and others used microsurgical techniques in performing cerebral arteriotomies and embolectomies.[4,20] In the middle of that decade, Rand[4] and Pool and Colton[15] first employed the operating microscope in the direct treatment of intracranial aneurysms. In 1966, Jannetta began to perform microvascular decompression of the trigeminal nerve for tic douloureux[10] and of the facial nerve for hemifacial spasm.[11] Then in 1967, Yaşargil and Donaghy initiated the procedure of extracranial-intracranial arterial bypass grafting for the treatment of cerebral ischemia.[4,21]

Thus, modern microneurosurgery was introduced largely during the decade between 1957 and 1967.[5,14,16,17,21] Many basic advancements in instrumentation and techniques within the same time period permitted the rapid growth of this and the other types of microsurgery. Since 1967, microneurosurgery has matured by technical refinements and widespread usage.[7,13] The one individual who probably has been more influential than any other in developing and popularizing microneurosurgery over the past 20 years has been Dr. M. Gazi Yaşargil, Professor at the Neurochirurgische Universitätsklinik in Zürich, Switzerland.

CURRENT PRACTICE

At the present time, microneurosurgical equipment and techniques are used to extend the abilities of the surgeon in standard neurosurgical opera-

146

tions. It has also permitted the reintroduction of outmoded procedures and the development of new ones.

Standard neurosurgical operations

The operating microscope has allowed the neurosurgeon to perform standard operations with greater finesse and better results. For example, the operative mortality associated with the direct treatment of intracranial aneurysms has fallen during the past decade from 20% to 35%[19] to 5% to 10%,[22] largely because of the introduction of microsurgical techniques. Arteriovenous malformations of the brain and spinal cord can be resected with greater precision, and divided cranial and peripheral nerves can be brought together with increased accuracy. Benign intracranial tumors, such as craniopharyngiomas, can be resected more completely, with better preservation of adjacent structures. Microsurgical techniques now allow the neurosurgeon to save the facial nerve frequently during the complete resection of an acoustic neurinoma and have even permitted him on occasion to keep the cochlear portion of the eighth cranial nerve intact.[18] Finally, the neurosurgeon finds the operating microscope a great help in removing intramedullary neoplasms of the spinal cord; the planes of dissection are more easily identified, and there is less risk of damage to the adjacent spinal cord.

Reintroduction of transsphenoidal operations

During the first decade of the twentieth century, a number of surgeons contributed to the development of transsphenoidal operations for pituitary tumors.[12] However, these lesions were not usually diagnosed until they were quite large. The transsphenoidal approach afforded only limited visibility, and it was soon discovered that a more complete tumor resection could be carried out with increased safety by a transfrontal approach. This then became the standard neurosurgical approach to the pituitary gland.

Because of recent advancements in neuroendocrinology and neuroradiology, pituitary adenomas are now frequently diagnosed when they are still confined to the sella turcica. This fact and the discovery that hypophysectomy is of value in the treatment of some patients with carcinoma of the breast have stimulated renewed interest in the transsphenoidal approach to the pituitary gland. As mentioned previously, in the late 1950s and early 1960s Guiot of France and Hardy of Canada responded to this need by developing microsurgical transsphenoidal procedures that are now used throughout the world.

New procedures

Patients with cerebral ischemia from extracranial atherosclerosis can frequently be helped by carotid endarterectomy or a related procedure involving the major arterial trunks in the neck. However, such procedures are of no value to patients with complete occlusion of the internal carotid artery or stenosis of

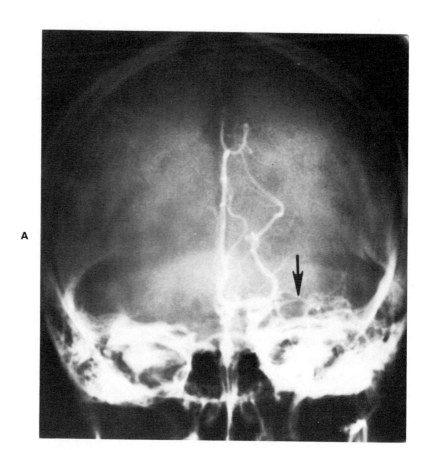

Fig. 11-1. Preoperative, **A**, and postoperative, **B**, anteroposterior left carotid arteriograms in a patient with occlusion of the proximal portion of the left middle cerebral
artery *(larger arrow)*. Before operation the patient had left cerebral transient ischemic
attacks despite anticoagulant therapy. A branch of the left superficial temporal artery
was sutured end to side to a branch of the left middle cerebral artery *(smaller arrow)*,
and the patient has had no further attacks.

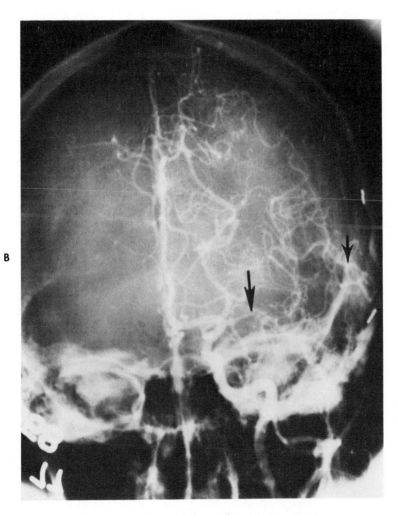

B

Fig. 11-1, cont'd. For legend see opposite page.

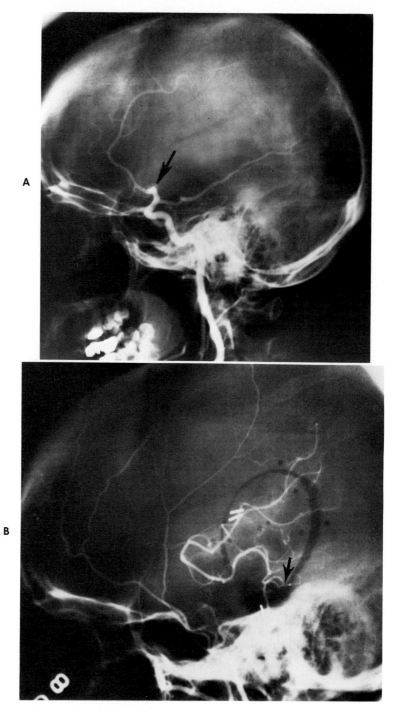

Fig. 11-2. Same patient as shown in Fig. 11-1. Preoperative, **A**, and postoperative, **B** left lateral arteriograms. Arteriogram **A** demonstrates the obstruction of the left middle cerebral artery *(arrow)*. **B,** Selective external carotid arteriogram showing filling of the middle cerebral artery from the superficial temporal artery through the anastomosis *(arrow)*.

this vessel above the neck, or with stenosis or complete occlusion of a cerebral artery.[20] In 1967, after appropriate animal experimentation, Yaşargil and Donaghy introduced the technique of anastomosing an extracranial artery directly to an intracranial artery to provide an extra source of blood to an ischemic area of the brain.[4,21,23] More than 2000 of these operations have since been performed.[1,2,23] Usually a branch of the superficial temporal artery (STA) is sutured to a branch of the middle cerebral artery (MCA), although other vascular combinations have also been used (Figs. 11-1 and 11-2).

It appears that STA-MCA bypass grafting is quite effective in reducing the transient cerebral ischemic attacks resulting from the types of arterial stenosis or occlusion mentioned previously. Such bypass grafting has also been shown to be of value as a preliminary step before the permanent surgical occlusion of an intracranial artery, as might be required during the resection of a giant aneurysm of the middle cerebral artery or internal carotid artery.

Another new procedure that has been developed during the past decade has been that of microvascular decompression of certain cranial nerves for treatment of several clinical syndromes. During the period from 1920 to 1940, Dr. Walter Dandy of Johns Hopkins Hospital frequently divided the fifth cranial nerve at the pons for the treatment of tic douloureux. He therefore had a unique opportunity to inspect this area carefully in such patients. Dandy noted, "Since the writer has been dividing the sensory root by the cerebellar route, tumors and aneurysms have been found in 10 per cent of the cases, over 500. And in almost every additional case a large arterial branch . . . lies upon or under the sensory root. . . . This I believe is the cause of tic douloureux."[3]

Jannetta, using microsurgical techniques, has confirmed Dandy's observations and has devised a method of separating the vessel(s) from the trigeminal nerve, without dividing the nerve.[10] This approach has proved reasonably successful in relieving the pain of tic douloureux without producing significant facial hypesthesia.

Jannetta has also found vascular compression of the seventh cranial nerve at the pons in patients with hemifacial spasm.[11] He has devised an analogous technique involving the separation of the offending vessel from the facial nerve by microsurgical methods; the results have been excellent. Jannetta is currently investigating patients with other cranial nerve syndromes that may have a similar etiology and pathogenesis. This entire line of investigation has been made feasible by the development of microneurosurgery.

SUMMARY

Microsurgical technology has revolutionized neurosurgery. It allows greater precision in the performance of standard neurosurgical procedures, leading to better results. It has stimulated the reintroduction of transsphenoidal operations on the pituitary gland. And it has permitted the development of the new techniques of extracranial-intracranial arterial bypass grafting and microvascular decompression of the trigeminal and facial nerves.

REFERENCES

1. Austin, G. M.: Microneurosurgical anastomoses for cerebral ischemia, Springfield, Ill., 1976, Charles C Thomas, Publisher.
2. Chater, N., and Popp, J.: Microsurgical vascular bypass for occlusive cerebrovascular disease: review of 100 cases, Surg. Neurol. **6:**115-118, 1976.
3. Dandy, W. E.: The brain, New York, 1969, Paul B. Hoeber, Inc., Harper & Row, Publishers, p. 170 (a classic reprint).
4. Donaghy, R. M. P.: A history of microsurgery. In Yaşargil, M. G., editor: Microsurgery, applied to neurosurgery, Stuttgart, 1969, Georg Thieme Verlag, pp. 4-11.
5. Donaghy, R. M. P., and Yaşargil, M. G.: Micro-vascular surgery, St. Louis, 1967, The C. V. Mosby Co.
6. Guiot, G., and Thibaut, V.: L'extirpation des adénomes hypophysaires par voie trans-sphénoïdale, Neurochirurgie **1:**133-150, 1959.
7. Handa, H.: Microneurosurgery, Baltimore, 1975, University Park Press.
8. Hardy, J.: L'exérèse des adénomes hypophysaires par voie trans-sphénoïdale, Union Med. Can. **91:**933-945, 1962.
9. Hardy, J.: Transsphenoidal microsurgery of the normal and pathological pituitary, Clin. Neurosurg. **16:**185-217, 1969.
10. Jannetta, P. J.: Microsurgical approach to the trigeminal nerve for tic douloureux, Prog. Neurol. Surg. **7:**180-200, 1976.
11. Jannetta, P. J., Abbasy, M., Maroon, J. C., Ramos, F. M., and Albin, M. S.: Etiology and definitive microsurgical treatment of hemifacial spasm. Operative techniques and results in 47 patients, J. Neurosurg. **47:**321-328, 1977.
12. Johnson, H. C.: Surgery of the hypophysis. In Walker, A. E., editor: A history of neurological surgery, Baltimore, 1951, The Williams & Wilkins Co., pp. 152-177.
13. Koos, W. T., Böck, F. W., and Spetzler, R. F.: Clinical microneurosurgery, Stuttgart, 1976, Georg Thieme Verlag.
14. Kurze, T.: Microtechniques in neurological surgery, Clin. Neurosurg. **11:**128-137, 1964.
15. Pool, J. L., and Colton, R. P.: The dissecting microscope for intracranial vascular surgery, J. Neurosurg. **25:**315-318, 1966.
16. Rand, R. W.: Microneurosurgery, St. Louis, 1969, The C. V. Mosby Co.
17. Rand, R. W., and Jannetta, P. J.: Microneurosurgery: application of the binocular surgical microscope in brain tumors, intracranial aneurysms, spinal cord disease, and nerve reconstruction, Clin. Neurosurg. **15:**319-342, 1968.
18. Rand, R. W., and Kurze, T.: Preservation of vestibular, cochlear, and facial nerves during microsurgical removal of acoustic tumors. Report of two cases. J. Neurosurg. **28:**158-161, 1968.
19. Sahs, A. L., Perret, G. E., Locksley, H. B., and Nishioka, H.: Intracranial aneurysms and subarachnoid hemorrhage. A cooperative study, Philadelphia, 1969, J. B. Lippincott Co.
20. Tew, J. M., Jr.: Reconstructive intracranial vascular surgery for prevention of stroke, Clin. Neurosurg. **22:**264-280, 1975.
21. Yaşargil, M. G.: Microsurgery, applied to neurosurgery, Stuttgart, 1969, Georg Thieme Verlag.
22. Yaşargil, M. G., and Fox, J. L.: The microsurgical approach to intracranial aneurysms, Surg. Neurol. **3:**7-14, 1975.
23. Yaşargil, M. G., and Yonekawa, Y.: Results of microsurgical extra-intracranial arterial bypass in the treatment of cerebral ischemia, Neurosurgery **1:**22-24, 1977.

12. Microsurgery and the technique of lumbar laminectomy

Richard H. Rothman

Forty years have now passed since Mixter and Barr delivered their classic address at the Massachusetts General Hospital delineating for the first time the surgical cure of sciatica, by excision of a herniated lumbar disk. During these four decades we have come to understand, not only the precision and beauty of this operation, and its ability to promptly and dependably eradicate the pain of a compressed nerve root, but we have also come to understand the misery and suffering that can be wrought by the misapplication of this surgical technique. One need only suffer through a typical afternoon in a spine clinic where six to eight new patients are seen with failures of spinal surgery, to understand and respect the exacting limitations and techniques that must be used with this treatment modality. It is as though the gods of ancient Greece who punished Prometheus for stealing the secret of fire and had him bound to a rock to have his liver torn from him by eagles, are now watching us ready to inflict their terrible punishment if we abuse this power of laminectomy.

To the patient observer it has become a truism that conservative therapy will cure the majority of patients with lumbar disk protrusion. Fortunately the modalities that have shown themselves to be effective are both safe and inexpensive. Bed rest and aspirin during the acute phases of sciatica, followed by the use of a lightweight flexible corset during the subacute phases and finally the use of isometric flexion exercises during the chronic phase will usually suffice. Because of the self-limiting nature of sciatica, caused by disk compression, many bizarre types of treatment have found their advocates. It is the self-limiting nature of disk herniation that leads to the almost fanatical support of treatment plans ranging from honey and vinegar to the copper bracelet. Of new patients seen in our office with low-back disorders, secondary to disk degeneration, the surgical therapy is rarely necessary and in recent years has been indicated in only one out of 20 new patients evaluated by us.

In terms of surgical success, patient selection remains the most critical factor. This principle cannot be underlined with sufficient vigor. Selection is

153

aimed specifically toward the diagnosis of frank mechanical nerve root compression. There are many causes and forms of sciatica, but only that sciatic pain attributable to mechanical compression lends itself to surgical treatment and cure. It is ironic that relief of leg pain not back pain is the achievable goal of spinal surgery.

Of those patients, who are properly selected and properly treated, perineural fibrosis and scar remain the leading causes of surgical failure. It has been our experience with salvage surgery that neurolysis is a futile exercise. Those patients whom we have tried to salvage and in whom perineural fibrosis was the primary pathosis, surgery was uniformly a failure. Neurolysis, no matter how carefully and expertly performed, in the long run, has shown itself to be a fool's errand. It is the prevention of this perineural and intraneural scarring that must be the key to success.

It has been shown by both clinical and laboratory studies that perineural scar is related to three factors:

1. Mechanical trauma
2. Epidural hematoma
3. Contact between the dura and skeletal muscle.

TECHNIQUE

Efforts must thus be directed in our surgical technique toward the prevention of contact between muscles and neural tissue after decompression has been accomplished. We have used two techniques to minimize the contact between muscle and nerve, through the use of an interposition membrane. The first of these has been an absorbable membrane of gelatin (Gelfoam). These gelatin membranes have been shown not only to inhibit scar tissue formation but also are completely resorbed by the end of 6 weeks. During the past year, we have substituted autogenous fat grafts for the Gelfoam membrane and have been quite pleased with the result. These fat grafts have been shown experimentally to remain viable in their new intraspinal location and to be a permanent barrier to scar. The graft is carefully fashioned, so as to completely cover all exposed dura and nerve root, where it might come into contact with the muscle, through the laminectomy opening.

The dexterity and technique of the surgeon is, in and of itself, quite critical to the success rate of the procedure. All other factors being equal, it has been shown that the experienced and adept spinal surgeon will be rewarded with a higher rate of success.

Absolute hemostasis and atraumatic technique are also of fundamental importance in the prevention of perineural fibrosis and scarring. Our house staff and fellows are now taught that preservation of the longitudinal intraspinal veins is a reasonable and achievable goal (Fig. 12-1). Not only the internal vertebral veins are preserved but also the small arteries and veins coursing along the nerve root itself are preserved, and a conscious effort is

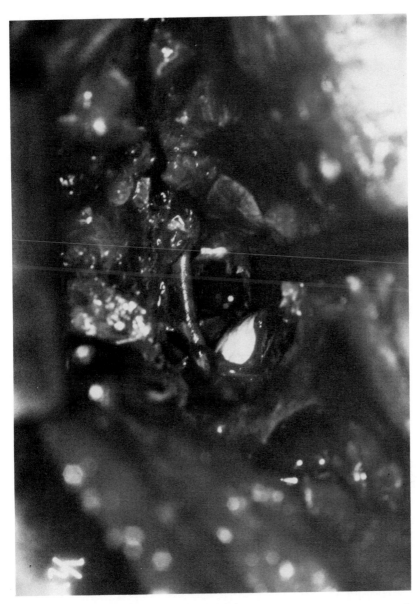

Fig. 12-1. Absolute hemostasis and preservation of the integrity of the internal spinal veins after completion of a radical disk excision. The nerve root is retracted to the right, and the anterior internal vertebral vein is seen coursing to the left.

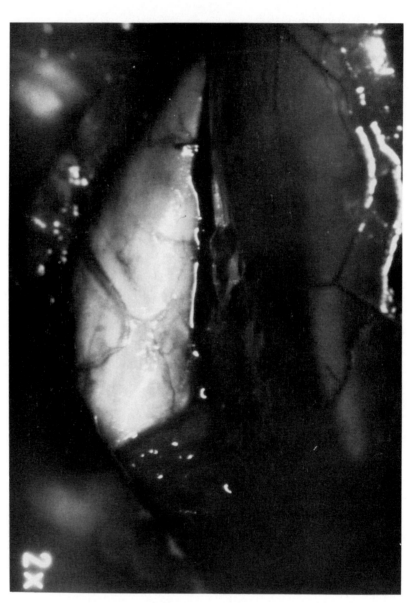

Fig. 12-2. Preservation of the arterial and venous blood supply to the intraspinal portion of the lumbar nerve root and the degree of hemostasis expected. The light structure to the left-hand portion of the slide is the nerve root, and the dural sac is the larger structure to the right.

made not to "strip" the nerve root (Fig. 12-2). At one time it was simply believed that one could handle these intraspinal vessels with impunity and simply pack the torn vessel off during surgery without causing harm. We now know that this type of approach leads to significant postoperative intraspinal hematoma and the proliferation of scar tissue during the healing phase. As seen in Fig. 13-1 it is possible to perform a radical disk excision, removing a large window of annulus, and completely decompressing the root with adequate preservation of the intraspinal veins.

The position used during surgery is quite critical (Fig. 12-3). We believe that a modified kneeling position, as shown here, allows even the most pendulous and obese abdomen to hang free, creating a negative intra-abdominal pressure. It has been demonstrated, through the use of catheters in the vena cava, that the traditional laminectomy frames are grossly inadequate in terms of lowering the venous pressure. Any lateral compression of the abdomen will be transmitted to the vena cava, heighten the pressure in the intraspinal veins, and cause excessive bleeding. The position shown here is quite comfortable and physiologic. We have had no episodes of thromboembolism and have used this routinely for both spinal fusions and laminectomies. Although the patient shown here had inhalation anesthesia, we routinely use spinal anesthesia for

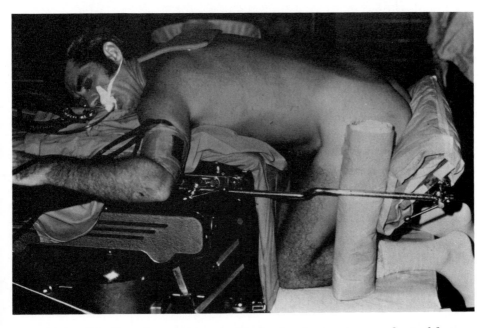

Fig. 12-3. Modified kneeling position used for lumbar laminectomy and spinal fusions. Note that the hip and knee are not fully flexed. The arms are not elevated beyond 90 degrees and an ECG monitor is used. The abdomen is completely free of external compression.

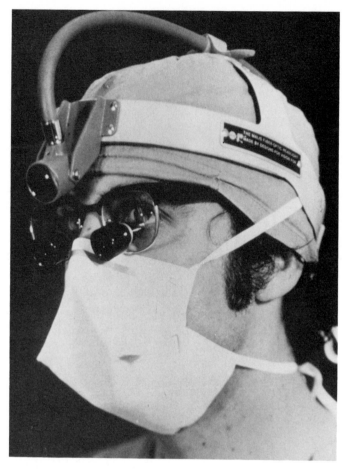

Fig. 12-4. Fiberoptic headlamp and binocular magnification of the type used in intraspinal surgery.

both laminectomies and spinal fusions. In this position it is important not to elevate the arm above 90 degrees in order to prevent brachial plexus traction symptoms. We also consider it advisable to use ECG monitoring in this position.

Fiberoptic lighting is a must for adequate visualization during intraspinal surgery (Fig. 12-4). Overhead operating room lights simply do not illuminate the lateral recesses where the majority of disk pathosis is found. Lightweight headlamps such as this give excellent illumination.

The use of magnification has been a great adjunct in the performance of lumbar disk surgery not only in terms of minimizing trauma, but also in terms of preventing damage to intraspinal vessels. After using both the operating microscope and binocular loops, we have found that binocular loop

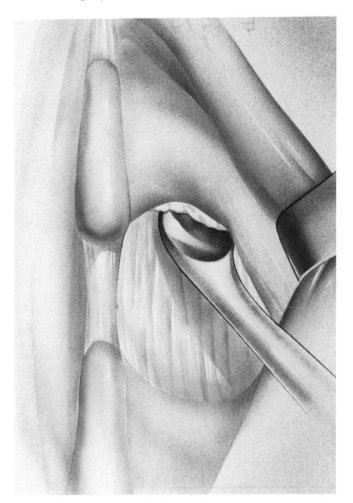

Fig. 12-5. Lamina and interlaminar space are cleaned of all soft tissues with sharp curettes.

magnification has proved most satisfactory. A 3.5 magnification provides adequate detail and yet maintains a good depth of field.

The technique of laminectomy that I will outline has allowed for the performance of several hundred nerve root decompressions by our attending and house staff without damage to a single nerve root during the past 5 years.

The first stage in this laminectomy is stripping of the paraspinal musculature and then careful delineation of the bony landmarks. With the use of extremely sharp curettes, all soft tissues are removed from the lamina above and below the interspace to be entered (Fig. 12-5). Careful delineation of these structures will allow for increased safety and increased certainty in terms of identification of the proper level of laminectomy.

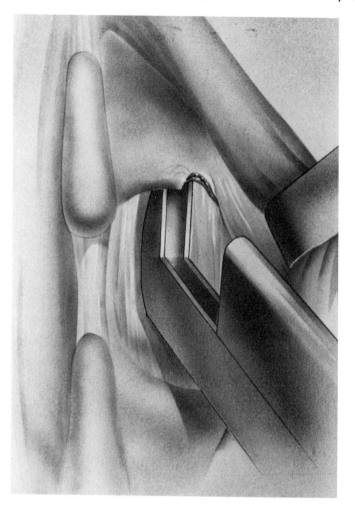

Fig. 12-6. Half of the upper lamina is removed with a Kerasin punch to expose the free upper border of the ligamentum flavum.

After cleaning of the soft tissues from the spine and identification of the proper level, approximately one half of the superior lamina is removed with either a Lexel rongeur or Kerasin punch (Fig. 12-6). Bony structure is removed in a cranial direction until the upper border of the ligamentum flavum is identified.

Once the free upper margin of the ligamentum flavum is found, this structure can be sharply excised (Fig. 12-7). In the midline there is usually a defect that is easily identified, and then the ligamentum flavum is opened like a book with a scalpel to sharply free the lower margin from the lamina. The ligamentum can then be lifted free.

Then, and this is a most critical step, additional bone is removed laterally

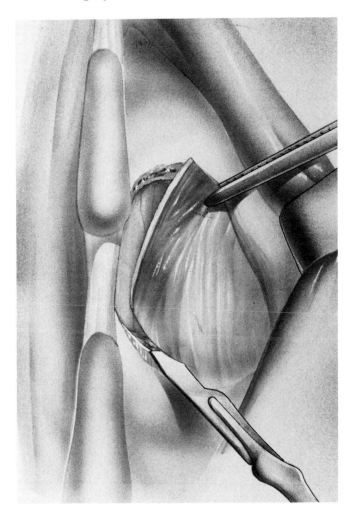

Fig. 12-7. Ligamentum flavum is turned laterally, as one dissects free its lower margin and lateral margin with a scalpel. This is done with the point of the knife under direct vision.

until we are able to clearly visualize the lateral border of the nerve root. This often necessitates removal of the medial half of the facet joint. This can be done with impunity. I believe the single most important measure of safety involved during this phase of the laminectomy is clear identification of this lateral border of the nerve root (Fig. 12-8). This root is often stretched and tightly compressed over an extruded disk fragment, an appearance that makes this identification difficult. Additionally the root may be enmeshed in scar tissue provoked by a free fragment of disk material and its surrounding granulation tissue (Fig. 12-9). If any doubt exists as to the true margin of the root, the dissection should be carried in a cranial and caudal direction to more

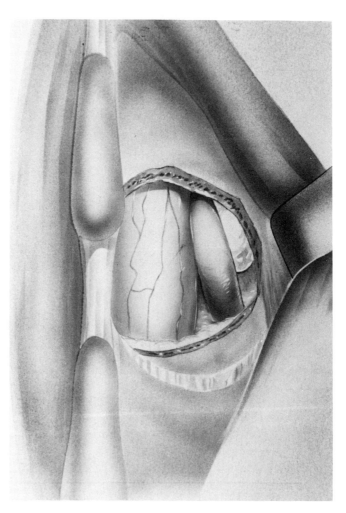

Fig. 12-8. Lateral border of the nerve root is visualized clearly before the nerve root is retracted.

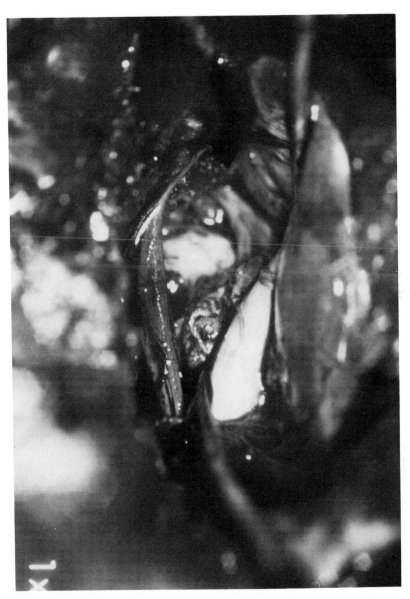

Fig. 12-9. Clear delineation of the lateral border of the nerve root, which is retracted medially so that a free fragment of disk material beneath the root is exposed. The fragment is surrounded by granulation tissue. Note preservation of the internal vertebral vein in the left-hand portion of the photograph.

normal anatomy. Fig. 12-9 illustrates how clearly one can demonstrate the edge of the dura and edge of the nerve root with a large free fragment of disk material sitting beneath the root and medial to the internal longitudinal vein.

The nerve root is clearly identified and absolute hemostasis achieved. Excision of the extruded fragment can be easily performed with a pituitary rongeur. Retraction of the root may be necessary and performed either with a root retractor or preferably with cotton paddies only (Fig. 12-10).

Once the free fragment is excised, we remove a large rectangular window of annulus centered beneath the nerve root. The purpose of the resection of this large window of annulus is to prevent late nerve root compression caused by collapse of the disk space and further buckling of the annulus.

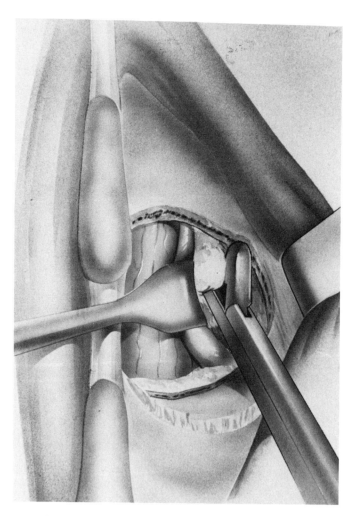

Fig. 12-10. Once the nerve root is retracted medially, the extruded fragment is easily excised with a pituitary rongeur.

Through this large window in the annulus a radical disk excision can be performed, with excision of the majority of the nuclear material. Large heavy-tipped pituitary rongeurs are used to prevent inadvertent instrument breakage. With good lighting and magnification, the interior of the disk space can be visualized and excision of the nucleus performed under direct vision. The surgeon should always be able to feel his instrument against the bony end plate if he is to avoid inadvertent puncture of the anterior annulus and great vessels.

Once excision of the nucleus has been completed, attention is turned to the course of the nerve root through the foramen and a complete exploration of the

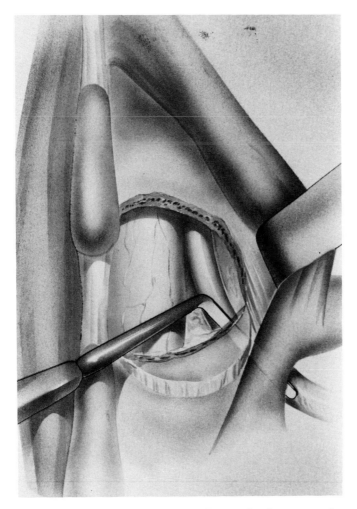

Fig. 12-11. One explores the spinal nerve well into the foramen to be certain that compression is not present in this lateral portion of the spinal canal. A Fraser or uterine sound is used for this purpose.

foramen performed (Fig. 12-11). This is done by palpation rather than direct visualization. A short and long Fraser elevator can be used or preferably a malleable uterine probe. With this technique one should be able to recognize compression in the foramen either by osteophytic overgrowth, pedicle migration, bulging of the annulus, or lateral disk extrusions.

Once this has been performed, the disk space and entire operative wound are irrigated with antibiotic solution and the autogenous fat graft transferred from the subcutaneous tissues to cover all exposed dura and nerve root.

In conclusion, it is my belief that no operation in orthopaedic surgery is more dependable and rewarding than a well-executed lumbar laminectomy in a properly selected patient. The relief of pain is prompt, dramatic, and gratifying to both the surgeon and his patient. If these methods and techniques are adhered to, I believe that the gray veil of apprehension that has clouded spinal surgery in the past will be lifted and a new more optimistic era of spinal surgery begun.

GENERAL DISCUSSION

Dr. Bright: Dr. Rothman, do you use any special instruments in doing spine surgery?

Dr. Rothman: Special instruments? Well, I believe the thing that's most special about them is that we have them sharpened every 2 or 3 days, either by our technicians or our residents. The curette is probably the most helpful instrument for working around the spine, for removing osteophytes, or for cleaning the soft tissues. I think the most common difficulty is trying to use old curettes. We insist that the instruments be sharpened and our residents learn how to perform this task in the same way that we did. We do use uterine probes for exploring foramina. They are mallable and give you a good feeling for whether there is adequate room in the foramen. You don't want to have to open every foramen that you are interested in. If you use a 2 mm or a 1.5 mm uterine probe, you can follow the nerve root with it and rest assured that there is no foraminal encroachment.

Dr. Bright: Bob, I notice that in the neurosurgical lab the microinstruments have much longer handles than the ones that we use in extremity surgery. Could you comment on this? Is there much difference? Do you have difficulty working at longer distances with the longer instruments?

Dr. Wilkins: Yes, it does introduce another factor in microsurgical technique. This, I believe, is especially true in work where the instruments are going down this long cylinder that you are trying to see through. You can get around this to a certain extent by using instruments so that your hand is out of the way. The barrel of the instrument will frequently be in the field of vision and you have to work around it. As far as suturing is concerned, its much easier to suture on a flat surface like the cerebral surface, rather than in depth such as when you are suturing a facial nerve after the removal of an acoustic neuroma.

Dr. Bright: Dr. Rothman, could you describe a little bit more about the fat graft that you talked about? Does it make reexploration easier and have there been any problems with infection?

Dr. Rothman: We have not had a problem with infection using the subcutaneous fat grafts. One technical problem is that a very slender patient may be hard pressed to find adequate fat to transfer. In our Philadelphia society, obesity is endemic; so we don't run into that problem frequently. We have not found it necessary to reexplore any of the patients in whom we have used a fat graft. As a matter of face, we haven't had to explore very many we used Gelfoam in either. Based on the findings of the two centers doing laboratory work on interposition grafts, I believe that fat is the more effective barrier.

Dr. Kramer: A neurosurgeon in Cincinnati, Dr. Mayfield, has been using autogenous fat grafts for years, perhaps intuitively. He has had the experience of reexploring some of these patients. He's also done research work in laboratory animals, and he says the reexploration is inordinately easier. He has been doing it for years; other neurosurgeons have also but have not reported it.

Dr. Bright: Now, when I scrub with the neurosurgery staff at Duke, you all seem to be using fat grafts. Is this correct? Will you comment on this?

Dr. Kramer: I think most of us are. I've been using fat grafts for about a year, in response to hearing Dr. Mayfield discuss this subject at a meeting about a year ago.

Dr. Bright: Dr. Kramer, several authors have noted that after anterior cervical fusion, there is a diminution in the step-off and osteophyte formation. Do you agree, and if so, why do the posterior dissection?

Dr. Kramer: We have a mixed bag of findings here. In the Duke series there are patients who have been followed more closely postoperatively by Dr. Urbaniak. Some of these patients, in the Duke series, show resolution of osteophytes as a consequence of simple fusion and limited diskectomy. We also have patients in the series who quite clearly are not resolving osteophytes in follow-up radiographs. Of course, the neurosurgeon, if the patient is brought to the neurosurgeon's attention, in many cases can't exclude soft disk rupture as a cause of radicular pain. It seems to me a very straightforward matter to remove the osteophytes, be they transverse or posterolateral, prior to fusion. Then you know where you stand, and you don't have to work from statistics.

Dr. Bright: Dr. Rothman, would you like to comment on that?

Dr. Rothman: I could not agree more wholeheartedly. There have been many speakers who have advocated not decompressing the nerve root. I think you have to differentiate those series that were done for neck and referred arm pain secondary to osteoarthritic changes without objective evidence of root conduction defect from patients operated on for radiculopathy with neurologic deficits. It is the latter group that deserves spinal decompression and fusion. In these patients, only 70% resorb their osteophytes. That's shown both in our series and by Dr. Robinson. It seems to me not to be intelligent to count on a 70% spontaneous resorption rate, when we can remove 100%. Our primary goal should be decompression of the cervical root.

Dr. Bright: I think I can speak for the orthopaedists here in that we agree. The first 100 or 200 that were done here were done by fusion alone. Since then most of the procedures have been done in conjunction with the neurosurgery department; and, I believe, the results are definitely better. We would agree.

Dr. Kramer and Dr. Wilkins, do you agree that only patients with frank disk extrusion, as opposed to protrusion of the annulus, are relieved by lumbar laminectomy?

Dr. Kramer: I think that was a terribly pertinent point. By virtue of the years I am not as experienced a lumbar disk surgeon as some, but I see a lot of these patients. If I get in there and don't find a free fragment, I ask myself why I am there. I know that I have set in motion, in many cases, a chain of events that is going to lead to pain clinics and this and that and the other thing. I really couldn't agree more that, if we could, we should select the free fragment disk and leave the rest to conservative therapy.

Dr. Wilkins: I agree with that overall statement. In the older patient, there is always the possibility that the nerve root is being compressed laterally by osteophytes or with spinal stenosis that may not be apparent on myelography. Perhaps body scanning, in the future, will help us in making differentiations of this sort. I think that the patients in this category can frequently be helped by decompression of a nerve root without necessarily dissecting it. As far as simple disk disease is concerned, I agree with Dr. Rothman that those with free fragments do much better than those without.

Dr. Bright: I would like to ask the panel about cervical disease. If the patient has a soft disk or fresh protrusion with nerve root signs, in general it has been approached from posteriorly, but surgeons in some places, at times, approach them anteriorly. I visited Ed Simmons in Toronto, and he stated that he had done a lot of these soft disk extrusions from the front and could get to them better. At Duke, they are done from both directions. Do you have any feeling about this, that you could convey to the audience? Do you use the operating microscope in the posterior approach to the cervical spine?

Dr. Kramer: I believe we held on longer to the posterior approach to soft disk extrusion than many centers for traditional reasons. It has always been a very dependable operation, and I've done one as recently as 3 weeks ago. I must say, everyone on our staff is increasingly impressed with the decreased morbidity. You are all familiar with an approach from the front. If you retrieve a soft disk from the front, that patient, as far as the neck is concerned, is going to feel well within 2 or 3 days. If you have gone through the extensive manipulation of muscle and soft tissues required for a posterior approach, the postoperative period of discomfort can extend 3 to 5 weeks. I must say that I am about ready not to approach any more posteriorly. I believe the anterior approach seems to be adequate. Now you are always concerned that there is a laterally placed fragment that you simply aren't going to recognize from the front and in those instances I would be very selective.

Dr. Rothman: We've looked at our data for cervical radiculopathy managed by anterior and posterior approaches. Both come out to about 92% good results, if you have had correlative neurologic deficit and myelogram. We can't espouse one over the other in terms of the quality of the result. I believe it depends on what your own morbidity is with the approach used and what you feel most comfortable with. I do them from the front; other surgeons do them posteriorly. I think the key is to make the correct diagnosis, have the right indications, and then be able to execute the decompression well whether you do it from the front or the back.

Dr. Wilkins: It does help if you are doing this from the back though to have illumination and magnification. We use loupes and a head lamp rather than the microscope.

Dr. Bright: Just one more question. Dr. Rothman, with facet osteoarthritis and some instability after laminectomy, what are your indications for fusion?

Dr. Rothman: In the neck or the back?

Dr. Bright: In the low back.

Dr. Rothman: When you see those elements, low back pain is not very responsive to surgery. I believe the older patient with spinal stenosis, degenerative disk changes, facet joint encroachment on the lateral recess, and neurogenic claudication (sciatic pain worse with walking and relieved by rest) is an excellent operative candidate. Our older patients who have demonstrable compression of the neural elements from osteoarthritis do extremely well. We operate under spinal anesthesia. There is very little trauma involved, and even if they are 60 or 70 years old, I would not hesitate to do a decompression. In this kind of patient, obviously, you do not expect a soft disk herniation. I didn't mean to imply that the neural compression had to be from a soft disk. In the older patient it's going to be from hypertrophy of the ligamentum, bulging of the ligamentum, enlarged facet joints, and narrowing lateral recess, and you rarely take out the disk, but do a thorough dorsal and lateral decompression. I think they do extremely well in terms of ridding them of their leg pain and neurogenic claudication. They do not do well in terms of relieving their back pain. We point out to the patient that your operation will help your leg but not your back, and if you're not content with that concept, then you really should not go through the surgery.

13. Internal neurolysis

E. F. Shaw Wilgis

In dealing with the peripheral nerve lesion associated with intraneural fibrosis, the operative technique of internal neurolysis has proved valuable. This technique was introduced by Babcock and perfected by Curtis[1] in 1972 and consists of the release of the individual fascicles from interfascicular scar tissue in these peripheral nerve lesions. Such lesions may be induced by trauma or chronic nerve entrapment in the upper extremity at the elbow or wrist. The procedure must be performed with the aid of a suitable magnification system, such as a 3-power eyeglass or the operating microscope, in order to preserve the fascicles and interfascicular plexus.

Lundborg,[2] in 1976, studied intraneural tissue reactions caused by internal neurolysis and found in this experimental model that after internal neurolysis, endoneurial vessels were unaffected by internal neurolysis, and their endothelium constituted an effective blood nerve barrier. This, in effect, causes an improved intraneural microcirculation and provides the opportunity for return of function of the nerve. He also found that the perineurial barrier remained unaffected, which means that the internal milieu around the nerve fibers is not altered by the procedure. He did find, however, that the internal neurolysis produced strong tissue reaction and extensive fibrosis in the epineurium and endoneurial areas, but this did not interfere with either the perineurial barrier or the blood nerve barrier. This important study, therefore, supports the concept that although internal neurolysis does cause scarring, the important physiologic state of the nerve is unaffected. It can be further postulated that the physiologic state of the scarred nerve will be improved.

ACUTE COMPRESSION SYNDROMES

We have seen and treated several patients who have benefited from an early operation on the nerve and opening of the epineurium and separating the fascicles before the chronic scarring phase. One such patient recently treated sustained a knife wound to the lower brachial plexus. Despite having function in his median nerve, over a period of 8 hours he developed a total median nerve deficit. Operated upon 1 day later, the epineurium of the

170

median nerve was found to be extremely thickened and edematous. The epineurium was split, the fascicles were teased apart and the patient showed early recovery of median nerve function.

One other patient developed an intraneural hematoma after blunt mechanical trauma to the median nerve at the wrist. With internal dissection of the nerve under suitable magnification, the hematoma was removed and nerve function restored.

These examples illustrate that internal neurolysis can be employed in the acute situation much like a fasciotomy of a muscle group to prevent the chronic scarring that inevitably will result from internal hematoma or swelling within the closed nerve sheath.

CHRONIC COMPRESSION SYNDROMES

Curtis[1] reported a series of 96 operations for carpal tunnel syndrome in which there was either motor or sensory deficit, using internal neurolysis as an adjunct to carpal tunnel treatment. He noted that sensation and motor power improved in over 90% of these patients. These statistics have held up in our personal series, the results of which are in Table 4. We have followed 47 patients who have undergone internal neurolysis of the median nerve, and in 43 of these patients we have noticed excellent recovery of motor and sensory function after the operation.

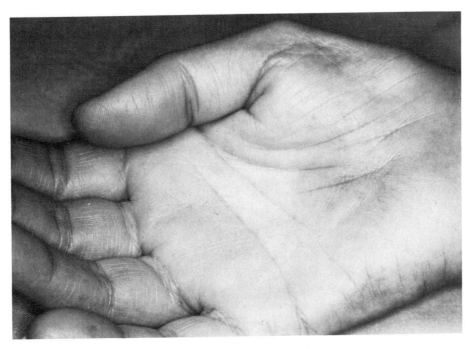

Fig. 13-1. Showing thenar atrophy in a patient with carpal tunnel syndrome.

Table 4. Internal neurolysis of peripheral nerves

Median nerve at wrist	47	Improved 43
Ulnar nerve at elbow	15	Improved 14
Digital nerve	12	Improved 12

Other sites of chronic nerve entrapment lend themselves to the application of the technique of internal neurolysis as well. Ulnar nerve entrapment at the elbow with motor and sensory changes is a condition in which internal neurolysis is applicable. We have found the nerve most commonly entrapped beneath the origin of the flexor carpi ulnaris muscle and the transverse band of fascia described by Osborne.[3] In Table 4, 15 patients with ulnar nerve entrapment at the elbow with definite motor involvement and intrinsic weakness were operated upon. Internal neurolysis of the ulnar nerve was carried out under suitable magnification. In all cases, after internal neurolysis, the nerve was transposed beneath the flexor muscle mass anteriorly. We found 14 of these 15 patients showed significant motor recovery and improvement in the intrinsic power.

Another group of patients who have benefited from microscopic internal neurolysis had trauma to common digital or digital nerves. These nerves are very superficial. They are normally surrounded by the fascia of Cleland and Grayson. Scarring in these fascial layers from superficial blunt or open trauma, causes a severe compression of the digital nerve for a distance of several millimeters. This can totally disrupt the digital nerve function. Another group of patients may have had a sharp injury to one fascicle of the normal five fascicles in the digital nerve and thereby develop severe scarring in a short segment of the nerve. Table 4 shows 12 patients who have had microscopic internal neurolysis with interfascicular dissection of the digital nerves with considerable improvement in all 12. Internal neurolysis in this group can sometimes improve digital causalgia and severe hypersensitive states in the finger.

INDICATIONS AND TECHNIQUE

The indications for internal neurolysis are as follows:
1. In the acute situation, a progressive loss of nerve function after traumatic incident.
2. In the chronic situation, the indications for the median nerve are constant sensory loss and thenar atrophy or palsy or failure to improve after simple division of the transverse carpal ligament (Fig. 13-1). With reference to the ulnar nerve, one must have motor weakness or beginning atrophy of the intrinsic musculature. I must emphasize that in all entrapment syndromes the transient symptoms of numbness without intrinsic atrophy, is not an indication for an internal neurolysis.

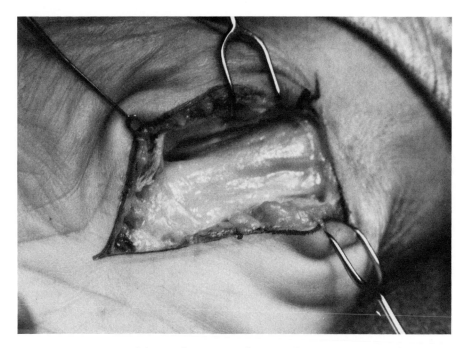

Fig. 13-2. Exposure of the median nerve showing the constriction and scarring.

   3. Scarring about a peripheral nerve such as the digital nerve, secondary to
      blunt or open trauma and resultant nerve dysfunction, is an indication
      for internal neurolysis.
   The operative technique consists of the exposure of the affected nerve (Fig.
13-2). Once the nerve is exposed, a longitudinal incision is made through the
epineurium. The epineurium is dissected gradually and carefully away from
the fascicular structure (Fig. 13-3). The fascicles are then gently teased apart
by the microsurgical technique and sharp instruments. I must emphasize that
the interfascicular plexus of nerves and blood vessels should not be disturbed.
The posterior aspect of the nerve is left undisturbed because this is the origin
of the microcirculation (Fig. 13-4). Careful hemostasis must be ensured after
tourniquet release so that the exposed interfascicular pattern of the nerve will
not be bathed in hematoma. The postoperative management is no different
from the routine of nerve release.
   In summary, internal neurolysis, under suitable magnification, has proved
a useful adjunct in the treatment of acute nerve compression syndromes as
well as chronic entrapment syndromes with severe scarring. It has been of
benefit in the treatment of the traumatic scarring in small nerves, such as the
digital nerves, as well. The indications mentioned above must be rigidly
adhered to and the technique must be meticulous, or the possibility of further
nerve damage must be entertained. However, the results continue to be

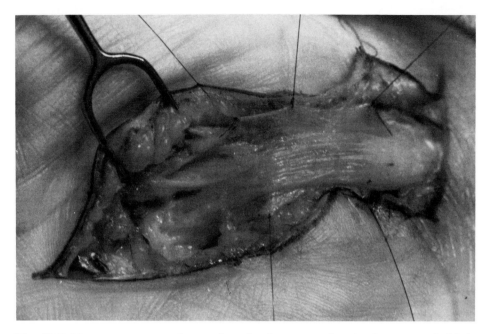

Fig. 13-3. Microscopic internal neurolysis has been completed. The sutures hold the epineurium.

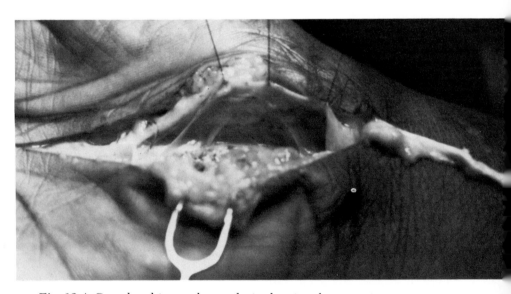

Fig. 13-4. Completed internal neurolysis showing the posterior mesentery intact.

encouraging. With the availability of a suitable magnification system, I recommend that this procedure be included in the surgical armamentarium of surgery of the extremities.

REFERENCES

Curtis, R. M., and Eversmann, W. W., Jr.: Internal neurolysis as an adjunct to the treatment of the carpal tunnel syndrome, J. Bone Joint Surg. **55-A**(4):733-740, June 1973.

Lundborg, B. G., and Nordborg, D.: Intraneural tissue reactions induced by internal neurolysis, Scand. J. Plast. Reconstr. Surg. **10**(1):3-8, 1976.

Osborne, F. V.: Compression lesions of nerve (ulnar neuritis). Presented at the 20th Meeting of the British Society for Surgery of the Hand, London, November 12, 1965.

14. Application of microsurgical techniques in the care of the injured peripheral nerve

James R. Urbaniak
Fredric H. Warren

Refinements in microsurgery have been extremely beneficial in the management of peripheral nerve injuries. If the microsurgeon has the capacity to thread a 50-micron needle with a 20-micron suture through a human hair, then it is reasonable to assume that delicate nerve tissue can be handled and approximated with less trauma than occurs without microsurgical methods. It is not the purpose of this chapter to debate the selection of the type or timing of repair (epineurial versus perineurial repair or nerve grafting; primary repair versus delayed or secondary repair), but rather to emphasize the application of the microsurgical technique in all types of nerve repair. In fact, we believe that the outcome of neurorrhaphy is more dependent on the careful tissue handling, proper alignment, and accurate approximation of the nerve ends than the particular selection of the type of repair.

ANATOMY

The surgeon who engages in the repair of peripheral nerves must be knowledgeable of the anatomy of the peripheral nerve. An awareness of the complex gross and histologic anatomy of the peripheral nerve reinforces the efficacy of magnification in the management of injured nerves.

The nerve cell, like other cells, contains a nucleus, cytoplasm, Golgi apparatus, and mitochondria. Nissl bodies are found in the motor cells, which also contain endoplasmic reticulum and ribosomes. Nerve axons are extensions of the cytoplasm of the neuron and generally contain the majority of the cell's cytoplasm because of their great relative length. The axonal mitochondria are probably responsible for the neural transmission since they are the energy source for this phenomenon. Groups of axons are encased by the Schwann sheath, which consists of a series of attenuated nucleated cells.

In nerve fibers there are two main divisions: (1) myelinated and (2) non-

176

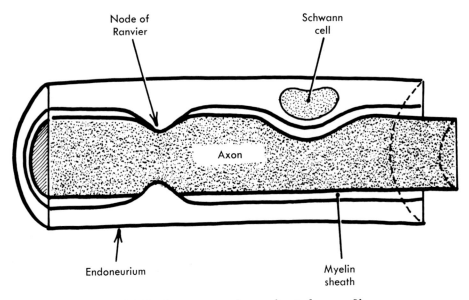

Fig. 14-1. Basic anatomy of a myelinated nerve fiber.

myelinated. Myelinization is dependent on the amount of lipid material in the protein matrix of the nerve sheath. In myelinated fibers the sheath consists of Schwann cells and myelin with an outer connective tissue layer (Fig. 14-1). The myelin layer is divided longitudinally into segments by the nodes of Ranvier, which are narrowed constrictions on the nerve sheath. Unmyelinated fibers consist of ill defined Schwann cells invested by the fibrous endoneurium.

Axons are grouped into bundles called fasciculi (Fig. 14-2). The terms "fasciculus," "funiculus," and "fascicle" are synonymous. Each fascicle is comprised of motor, sensory, and sympathetic nerve fibers of varying proportions. As already noted, each nerve fiber is invested by a fibrous tissue sheath, the endoneurium. Fasciculi are grouped together in varying numbers and separated by another connective tissue layer called the perineurium. Fasciculi are cross-linked with other groups of fascicles, thus forming the fascicular plexus as described by Sunderland (Fig. 14-3). Groups of fasciculi are encased in loose areolar tissue called the epineurium, which is covered by yet another connective tissue layer, the mesoneurium. The mesoneurium is similar to the bowel mesentery because it supports the nerve and contains the blood supply of the nerve itself. If a nerve is stripped of its mesoneurium, it may lose its blood supply and thus function as an in situ nerve graft. As little as 14 cm of nerve divested of its mesoneurium may lead to necrosis of that segment.[3,7]

Lack of appreciation of this ultrastructure of the peripheral nerve and the inability to accurately restore the anatomy of the injured nerve accounts for some of the poor results in neurorrhaphy.

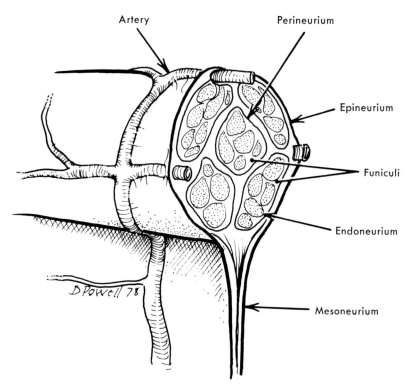

Artery   Perineurium

Epineurium

Funiculi

Endoneurium

Mesoneurium

Fig. 14-2. The surgeon who repairs peripheral nerves should be cognizant of these basic structures of the peripheral nerve.

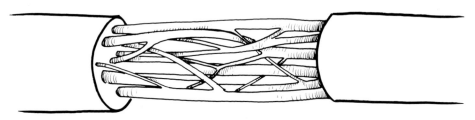

Fig. 14-3. Fasciculi are cross-linked with other groups of fascicles forming the fascicular plexus described by Sunderland.

NERVE PATHOPHYSIOLOGY

Knowledge of the process of nerve degeneration and regeneration is necessary when nerve injuries are treated. Trauma to a nerve in the form of transection causes specific events to occur both in the cell body and in the proximal and distal axons.[7-9]

For 10 to 20 days after transection, the cell body progressively enlarges. It will remain enlarged during the processes of degeneration and regeneration before eventually returning to its normal size. The cell nucleus also enlarges and assumes an eccentric position. Chromatolysis (disappearance of the Nissl bodies) occurs and is now known to be evidence of active regeneration. With this occurrence the cellular RNA is transformed to a more soluble active form. Within 4 days after injury the neural RNA increases as part of the effort of regeneration.[3]

After injury, subtle changes occur in the proximal axon. The elasticity of the nerve fibers and mesoneurium causes retraction from the site of trauma. Edema will occur within the proximal axon within a few hours. The amount of edema will vary according to the extent of the injury. After severe injuries, such as high-velocity missile wounds, the amount of proximal axonal destruction may not be known for several weeks until demarcation occurs.

After injuries, connective tissue proliferation and wallerian degeneration occur in the proximal and distal axons. Neurofibrils disappear and the axonal cytoplasm clumps within 24 to 48 hours after injury.[3,7-9] Axons thicken and Schwann cells begin to digest the fragmented myelin, forming empty spaces within the myelin sheath. Schwann cells also form cords of cells along the degenerated axon cylinders. Although the gross fascicular architecture remains present, the degenerative process continues, emptying the neurilemmal sheaths. This can lead to shrinkage of cross-sectional area to as little as 1% of its normal size within 2 years.[7-9]

Nerve regeneration is related to the capacity of the cell body to synthesize protein.[8] The nerve can replace 50 to 100 times the organic material contained in the cell body during successful regeneration.[3] In the proximal axon during the first 2 or 3 days after injury, proliferation of Schwann cells occurs with varying amounts of retrograde destruction of fascicles and myelin, depending on the severity of the trauma. Destroyed tissue demarcates and is phagocytized within 4 to 6 weeks of injury.[3,8] At this time newly synthesized axoplasm moves down the axonal cylinder to and across the point of injury provided that the nerve gap has been approximated. This axoplasmic flow continues down the distal axonal cylinder, and the axons become remyelinized. With complete axonal regeneration, proper motor nerve end-plate formation and sensory end organ reestablishment must occur for motor and sensory function to return.

TYPES OF NERVE REPAIRS

The goal of any type of nerve repair is restoration of anatomy and reestablishment of function. The most commonly used nerve repair is the *epineurial repair* (Fig. 14-4); however, many surgeons are beginning to use *fascicular repairs* (Fig. 14-5) or a combination of epineurial and fascicular repair (Fig. 14-6). The question of epineurial versus the fascicular repair remains unanswered. We emphasize the use of proper magnification to restore the anatomy as determined by the position of the mesoneurium, small blood vessels, and fascicular identification, grouping, and alignment.

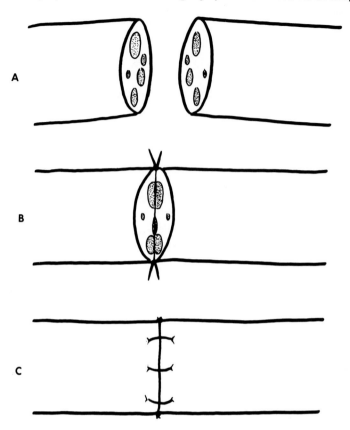

Fig. 14-4. Epineurial repair. The microscope enables the surgeon to critically place the sutures in the epineurium for accurate alignment of the fasciculi. **A,** Nerve ends are trimmed until pouting fascicles are identified. **B,** Corresponding bundles of fascicles are approximated with epineurial stay sutures. **C,** Interrupted epineurial sutures complete the repair.

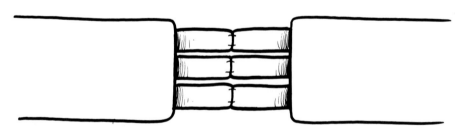

Fig. 14-5. Fascicular or epineurial repair. Microscopic techniques and equipment are mandatory for the repair of nerves by this method.

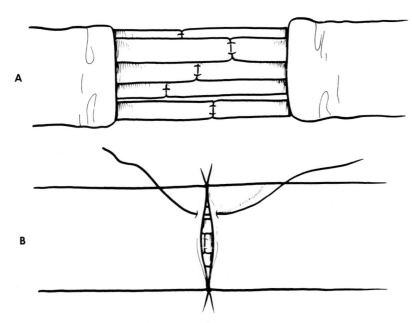

Fig. 14-6. Combination of epineurial and perineurial repair. This method is advocated by some microneurosurgeons to achieve accurate fascicular alignment while obtaining good immediate strength at the suture line. **A,** By use of the microscope, matching fascicles or bundles of fascicles are approximated with 10-0 nylon. **B,** For better strength epineurial sutures of 8-0 nylon are used.

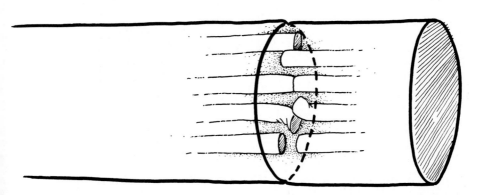

Fig. 14-7. Despite attempts at accurate alignment in epineurial repair, undesirable overriding or buckling of the fasciculi may occur.

Gould demonstrated that digital nerves repaired by delayed epineurial repair using 8-0 or 10-0 suture gave an average recovery of 7 mm of two-point discrimination in adults.[1] He found no significant difference in results in relation to the size of the suture (8-0 versus 10-0 nylon) or the type of magnification (loupes versus the operating microscope). He found the epineurial repair to be functionally as good as the fascicular repair and technically much easier, requiring less operating time.

Performing the fascicular repair requires the use of the operating microscope under high magnification and necessitates accurate placement of the sutures. Of the three repairs mentioned, the fascicular repair comes closest to restoring the normal anatomy. A problem in epineurial repair is that not all the fasciculi are lacerated at the same level. Despite attempts at terminal resection, the fasciculi usually remain uneven, leading to gapping, overriding, straddling, and buckling of the fascicles at the suture line (Fig. 14-7). Fascicular repairs are technically more difficult than present literature indicates. The presence of interfascicular plexus formation may mean that anatomic fascicular alignment is not possible nor even necessary (Fig. 14-3). Additionally, the technical expertise required in this repair is more demanding and requires an experienced microsurgeon.

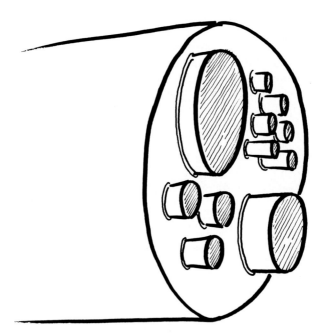

Fig. 14-8. Freshly cut peripheral nerve. Under magnification, the groups of fascicles are mapped on the proximal and distal nerve stumps. Four definite groups of fascicles are identified and will be mated with four similar groups on the other nerve end, either by perineurial repair or four interfascicular nerve grafts.

In the combined type of repair, the larger fasciculi can be anatomically repaired by use of two 10-0 sutures with supplemental epineurial sutures (Fig. 14-6). Perhaps this type of repair is most useful in the larger peripheral nerves such as in a median nerve laceration at the wrist. Most fascicular repairs are done by dissection and identification of *groups of fascicles* rather than individual fascicles on the severed nerve ends and then connection of the anatomically similar groups (Fig. 14-8).

MICROSURGICAL INSTRUMENTS

The topic of microsurgical instruments is discussed in another chapter of this text. Briefly, any standard operating microscope, such as the Zeiss 7-P/H, can be used for microsurgery. Also surgical telescopic loupes of at least 3.5-power magnification are useful. The basic instruments for microsurgical nerve repairs include Beaver surgical blades, tying forceps, jewelers' forceps, spring-loaded microscissors, Barraquer type of needle holders, atraumatic monofilament nylon suture from 8-0 to 11-0 sizes, and a basic hand-tendon surgical set.

INDICATIONS FOR MICROSURGICAL REPAIRS

Microsurgical techniques are useful in the management of peripheral nerve injuries or anomalies of several categories:

Neuroma in continuity

As in all nerve injuries the surgeon must perform a careful preoperative evaluation with special emphasis on two-point discrimination and tenderness. If a patient has good two-point discrimination (10 mm or less), the treatment of choice is internal neurolysis. However, if there is complete loss of sensation or two-point discrimination of greater than 20 mm, the best treatment is resection with direct repair or interposition graft.

The degree of tenderness indicates the need for resection. A minimally tender neuroma would not need the resection required by a painful neuroma. In the past, some cases of neuroma in continuity have been managed by saline neurolysis, particularly in digital nerves, but this method resulted in equivocal results. In our experience, internal neurolysis in *digital nerves* has given gratifying results with elimination of tenderness and improvement of two-point discrimination.

Partial nerve lacerations

Prudent preoperative evaluation is essential in the management of a partial nerve laceration. If the surgeon finds the nerve partially lacerated, the preoperative assessment influences the decision making in the repair. For example, if only a few fascicles of the median nerve at the wrist are found to be severed, are they important ones for supplying critical areas of sensation or motor

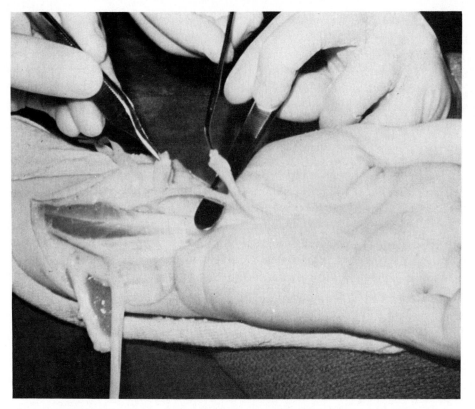

Fig. 14-9. Partial laceration of the median nerve at the wrist. Accurate clinical assessment was important in this patient because he had normal motor function and normal sensation to the thumb index and radial half of the long finger. Careful dissection with magnification permitted repair of the two severed fascicles.

branches to the thumb intrinsics? (See Fig. 14-9.) Using magnification, the injured fascicles can be isolated from the intact fibers and then resected, repaired directly, or grafted, depending on the importance of their destination and the amount of gap.

Very small or distal nerves

In the past small nerves, especially arborized distal digital nerves, were not considered reparable, but with magnification these nerves can be accurately repaired without difficulty (Fig. 14-10). Small nerves, such as the palmar or dorsal cutaneous nerves are now readily repaired, whereas in the past, the recommended treatment was resection. Motor branches to the thumb intrinsics and lumbricals and spinal accessory nerve are also now accurately repaired or grafted with the aid of microsurgery. Small neurilemomas distal to the forearm can even be shelled out by microsurgical techniques without damaging nerve function.

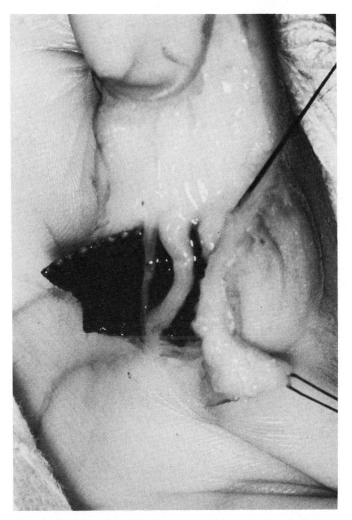

Fig. 14-10. Injured ulnar digital nerve in the thumb was dissected under the microscope, and one fascicle was found to be severed. The single fascicle was repaired with 11-0 Prolene by use of microsurgical technique.

Children

In children's nerve injuries the surgical technique required is more difficult than in adults because of the smaller caliber of the structures. Magnification is therefore essential for these procedures.

Congenital hand problems often require the separation of nerves, as in the correction of syndactyly or pollicization. Magnification makes these procedures considerably easier.

Previously unchallenged complex congenital problems like the lobster-claw hand are now surgically correctable by microsurgical techniques such as transferal of toes to fingers. In addition, various nerve tumors of the digits and hands may be resected by microsurgery without excision of the entire nerve.

Primary repair of severed nerves

Strong arguments against primary repair have been the difficulty of handling the soft delicate nerve tissue of the freshly injured nerve and the inability to assess the amount of injured nerve to resect. Microsurgical techniques permit greater ease in handling the fragile nerve structures in a fresh injury and thereby allow easier immediate repairs. With magnification and microsurgical techniques, the speed of surgery is improved. For example, in the repair of peripheral nerves in replanted hands and digits we are able to accomplish a nerve repair within 5 minutes.

Magnification is an invaluable aid in the initial assessment of any nerve injury. It enables the surgeon to have a more accurate picture of the extent of the injury. If needed, electrical stimulation of the fascicles for motor and sensory function of both the proximal and distal segments can be done within the first 72 hours after injury (described in a previous chapter).

Secondary repair of severed nerves

Regardless of the type of secondary nerve repair—epineurial, perineurial or grafting—microsurgical techniques are valuable for dissection and fascicle identification and alignment. The surgeon using magnification develops a greater appreciation of the large amount of nonaxonal material in the peripheral nerve. The cross section of a peripheral nerve may contain 25% to 75% collagen tissue, with the remaining area composed of axons. In delayed repair, the healing and inflammatory response increases the amount of collagen tissue; therefore magnification is a valuable aid in identification and alignment of the fascicles that have the potential for recovery.

We have demonstrated that by use of microsurgical techniques with replantation of amputated hands and digits, sensibility recovery of 10 mm or less of two-point discrimination can be achieved in over half the patients (Fig. 14-11). Of course, if fascicular repair is elected, magnification is mandatory.

Nerve grafting

The main purpose of nerve grafting is to overcome tension on the nerve at the site of repair. A nerve can be mobilized 15 cm without jeopardizing the mesoneurial blood supply or its ability to regenerate.[7] However, mobilization in the severed nerve reduces the blood supply more than in the intact nerve. The distal nerve stump may be especially subject to loss of its blood supply with mobilization.[3,7]

An alternative to extensive mobilization to provide a tension-free repair is the use of interposition nerve grafts. Interfascicular cable grafts as described by Millesi have provided very encouraging preliminary results in this area[4,5]

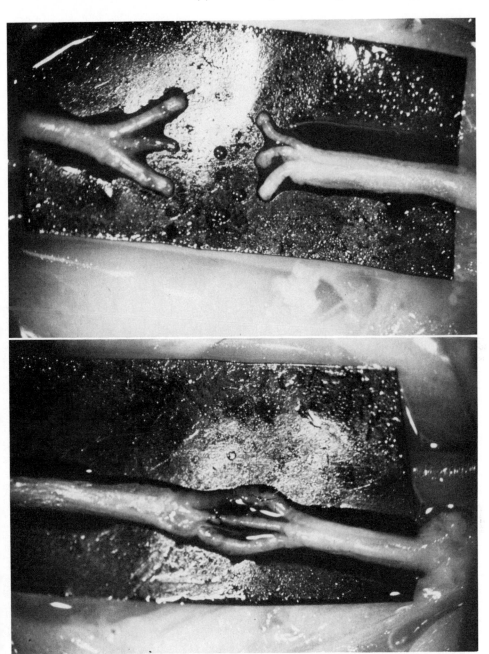

Fig. 14-11. Severed digital nerve with the three fascicles identified on the distal and proximal stumps, **A.** Fascicular (perineurial) repair was performed with 10-0 nylon, **B.** Severed digital nerve, **C,** which has had an epineurial repair with 10-0 nylon after alignment under the microscope, **D.** Epineurial repair is recommended in digital nerves, for the results are good with this method and the technique is easier and quicker.   *Continued.*

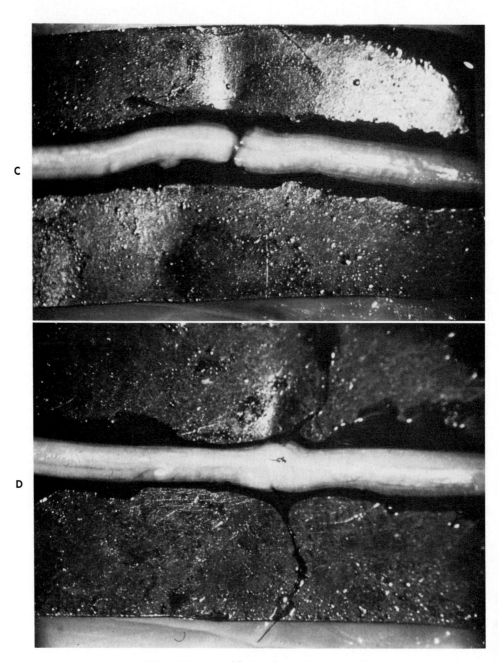

Fig. 14-11, cont'd. For legend see p. 187.

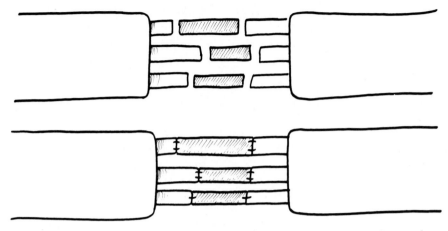

Fig. 14-12. Interfascicular nerve grafting as popularized by Millesi. The sural nerve (*hatched segments*) are used as a graft. This method is used on the patient in Fig. 14-13.

(Fig. 14-12). In general, nerve grafting should be reserved for cases in which the direct repair cannot be done without tension. Although excessive mobilization of a nerve does diminish its blood supply, we must remember that a nerve graft is completely avascular (Fig. 14-13). In addition, when a large segment of a nerve is lost, accurate fascicular identification and alignment for interfascicular grafting does not guarantee that the axons will enter the proper distal tubular sheaths because of the frequent crossovers demonstrated by the fascicular meshwork described by Sunderland (Fig. 14-4).

Our preliminary results have shown that nerve grafting is not as good as direct repair, and we currently use nerve grafting when there is a large defect that cannot be overcome by moderate nerve mobilization and joint flexion. In most severe avulsion injuries, nerve grafting is necessary. Protective sensation can be expected in nerve grafts of 10 to 15 cm. Good motor function does occur but is unlikely when these large defects are bridged. Of course, we must emphasize that our nerve grafts have been performed in the most severely damaged extremities.

Electrical stimulation

The use of electrical stimulation in primary repair is discussed in Chapter 16. This is useful in alignment of fascicles and in isolating motor and sensory components of the nerve prior to repair. Magnification is required in the use of the microelectrode stimulators for this purpose. Magnification is also used in the microimplantation in peripheral nerve stimulators for chronic pain syndromes.

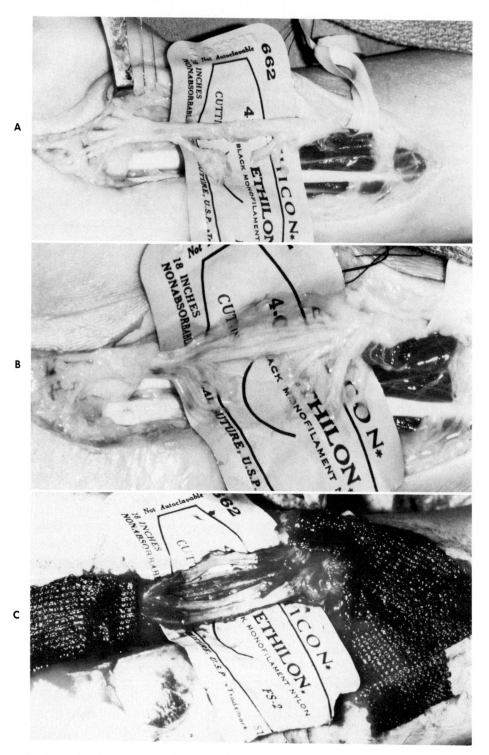

Fig. 14-13. Median nerve at the wrist of a 23-year-old woman that was partially severed by a gunshot wound, **A.** The fascicles were separated into transected fascicles and intact fascicles under the microscope, **B.** The injured ones were repaired by sural nerve interfascicular grafts, which were used to bridge the gaps, **C.**

CONCLUSION

Many technical problems of peripheral nerve repair can be overcome with the application of microsurgery. Accurate preoperative assessment and a knowledge of nerve anatomy and physiology are prerequisites for obtaining good results in nerve repair. However, it is evident that some important factors influencing nerve regeneration cannot be controlled by the surgeon, such as changes in the cell body at the time of injury and reorganization at the junction of the axon and terminal organ or end plate. Nevertheless, the application of microtechniques provides ultimate management at the site of severence. It is our opinion that diligent handling with micromethods influences the outcome more than the particular type of repair (epineurial, perineurial, or grafting).

REFERENCES

1. Gould, J. S.: Digital nerve repair with magnification techniques. Presented at the annual meeting of the Southern Medical Association, New Orleans, Louisiana, Nov. 9, 1976.
2. Grabb, W. C., Bement, S. L., Koepke, G. H., and Green, R. A.: Comparison of methods of peripheral nerve suturing in monkeys, Plast. Reconstr. Surg. **46:**31-38, 1970.
3. Hakstian, R. W.: Funicular orientation by direct stimulation, J. Bone Joint Surg. **50-A:**1178, 1968.
4. Hakstian, R. W.: Perineural neurorrhaphy. Orthop. Clin. North Am. 4(4):945-956, 1973.
5. Kleinert, H. E., and Griffin, J. M.: Technique of nerve anastomosis, Orthop. Clin. North Am. 4:907-915, 1973.
6. Madden, J. W., and Peacock, E. E.: Some thoughts on repair of peripheral nerves, South. Med. J. **64:**17-21, 1971.
7. Millesi, H.: Interfascicular grafts for repair of peripheral nerves of the upper extremity, Orthop. Clin. North Am. 8(2):387-404, 1977.
8. Millesi, H., Meissel, G., and Berger, A.: The interfascicular nerve grafting of the median and ulnar nerves, J. Bone Joint Surg. **54-A:**727-750, 1972.
9. O'Brien, B.: Microvascular reconstructive surgery, New York, 1977, Churchill Livingstone.
10. Peacock, E. E., and Van Winkle, W.: Surgery and biology of wound repair, Philadelphia, 1970, W. B. Saunders Co.
11. Seddon, H. J.: Surgical disorders of peripheral nerves, Baltimore, 1975, The Williams & Wilkins Co.
12. Sunderland, S.: Nerves and nerve injuries, Baltimore, 1968, The Williams & Wilkins Co.
13. Van Beek, A., and Kleinert, H. E.: Practical microneurorrhaphy, Orthop. Clin. North Am. 8(2):377-386, 1977.

15. Nerve grafts to the brachial plexus

E. F. Shaw Wilgis

The history of surgical treatment of brachial plexus injuries is dotted with enthusiastic preliminary reports, but all too often these are followed by rather dismal, long-term results. This is so true that in many centers the direct operative approach to the brachial plexus has been abandoned completely.

With the advent of microsurgery and suitable magnification systems, a new attempt is being made to approach the brachial plexus from the direct surgical point of view and indirect repair by nerve transfers and microscopic nerve grafts to provide axonal regrowth into the distal segments of the plexus. We have seen some encouraging reports and early results. The purpose of this section is to give the current ideas of how to use microsurgery in the direct approach to brachial plexus injuries.

The patient with the total brachial plexus injury and a flail anesthetic arm presents a tremendously difficult problem for management. We must educate the patient to adjust to this useless extremity. The second possibility is to attempt reconstruction by various arthrodeses, tenodeses, and position operations. The results of such surgery can only be classified as cosmetic improvement because without sensibility, the patients usually do not use these extremities. A third approach would be to arthrodese the shoulder, amputate the arm above the elbow, and use a prosthesis. This sometimes gives a satisfactory result, but the acceptance rate in these individuals is very low. If pain is a factor, amputation will not benefit the patient and certainly will not alleviate the pain. It is in these difficult injuries that some attempt at a goal-oriented approach of practical reconstruction by microscopic nerve grafts may be of benefit.

ANATOMY

In any consideration of surgery of the brachial plexus, the anatomy must be considered. The normal anatomy is depicted in Fig. 15-1 and involves the roots of C5 through T1, which form the upper, middle, and lower trunks. These then divide to form the lateral, posterior, and medial cords, which then give off the specific nerves to the upper extremity. The whole brachial plexus

192

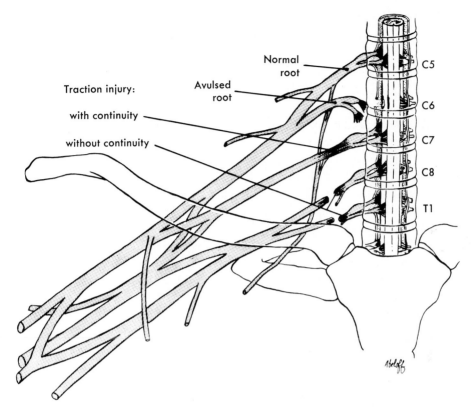

Fig. 15-1. Normal anatomy of brachial plexus and varying types of injury are depicted.

is invested in a strong fascia and the axillary artery is found interposed between the lateral, medial, and posterior cords in the lower portion of the brachial plexus. One must undertake a thorough study of the anatomy before approaching any portion of the structures in this region. One must realize that there are some anatomic variations. I have seen fused posterior and medial cords on one occasion. I recommend that anybody operating in this region have experience with anatomic dissection in the anatomy lab.

OPEN WOUNDS

An open wound to the brachial plexus frequently involves injury to one of the major vessels or pleura. The vascular and thoracic conditions take precedent over the nerve injury, and no attempt should be made to repair a direct injury at the time of vascular repair. There have been reports of unsatisfactory results after primary repair of the nerve structures associated with vascular damage, probably because of abnormal tension on the nerve and hematoma from the vascular injury.

CLOSED INJURIES

The closed traction injuries, most commonly caused by road accidents, are far in away the most common type of injury seen. The varying types of injury are shown in Fig. 15-1. Complete root avulsion from the spinal cord is an irreparable condition and will not improve unless living axons are brought from another nerve to reinnervate the avulsed root. The second injury is a postganglionic injury involving disorganization or rupture of some axons, but the nerve is in continuity. Recovery will often occur in this type of injury but frequently takes a long time, sometimes several years. In this instance, occasionally a well-timed neurolysis would be of benefit. The third type of injury seen is complete rupture of the nerve distal to the root. This is then treated like a nerve division. The patient will present with Tinel's sign in the proximal neuroma and distally have nerve dysfunction. Properly dissected, the two nerves can be identified and joined with an interpositioned nerve graft by use of microtechnique. Encouraging results in this approach have been reported by Narakas[3] and Millesi.[2] The operation is frequently a long and tedious one and involves multiple roots and multiple nerve grafts.

It is my philosophy in such an injury that one should set about a goal prior to the operation. The surgeon should decide that he should concentrate on elbow flexion and extrinsic muscle power to the hand. One should not be enthusiastic enough to believe that intrinsic power could be restored to the hand. With such a goal, one could concentrate then on the musculocutaneous, median, and radial nerves. The shoulder is controlled by so many muscles that an arthrodesis probably would be more beneficial. With this goal-oriented approach, nerve grafting to specific nerves from roots can be useful.

More distally in the plexus in the cord region or beneath the clavicle, we see mixed lesions involving several nerves. Again, here isolated nerve grafting with strict goals in mind can be useful. If nerve grafts are used over 10 to 12 cm in length, one must be prepared to resect the distal suture site if scarring prevents axonal growth across the suture site.

INDIRECT NERVE TRANSFER

Use of intercostal nerves 2 to 7 to provide axonal regrowth to the plexus has been reported by Seddon,[4] Millesi,[2] and others. I believe that this technique shows promise. It is my strong recommendation that again this technique be used for specific goals in these complex problems. Such limited goals can be intercostal nerve transfer prolonged by nerve graft to musculocutaneous or radial nerve to provide elbow function. We have used this technique and found it helpful in several patients. The recipient nerve is dissected from the brachial plexus. The intercostal nerve is exposed in the midaxillary line and usually two intercostal nerves are used for the musculocutaneous nerve. Intercostal nerves two and three are taken from the midaxillary line with sufficient motor fibers still left to preserve function. They are prolonged by a sural nerve graft, which is approximately the same size as the intercostal nerve. The use of a 7 to 10 cm sural nerve graft is mandatory because there will be too much tension in between the intercostal nerve and direct brachial plexus. The nerve graft is sutured under standard microsurgical technique. Usually this is done with 4.5- or 6-power surgical telescopes using one or two sutures of 8 or 10-0 nylon. The nerve grafts are then brought to the recipient nerve and sutured into place.

Tinel's sign can be followed, and the distal suture site must be treated surgically if Tinel's sign stays at that level. The time interval between surgery and reinnervation of upper arm muscle through this approach is rather lengthy, approaching 1 year. The patients need very little education and have been able to transfer the function of the intercostal nerve to the recipient nerve. I believe this operation should be reserved for young patients. The technique of this operation is illustrated in Fig. 15-2.

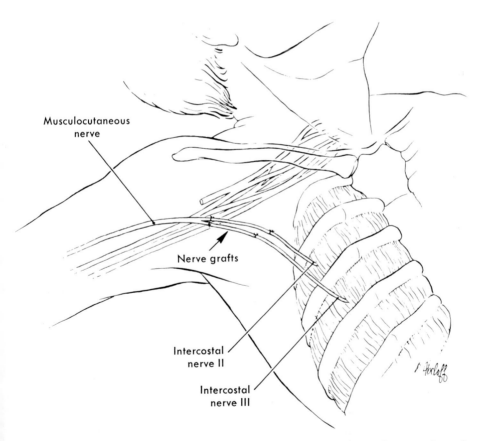

Fig. 15-2. Technique of intercostal nerve transfer to provide axonal regrowth to the plexus.

In summary, we have attempted to show that the development of micro-surgical techniques offers some new possibilities to the surgical approach to the brachial plexus. Microsurgical nerve grafting has enabled the surgeon to bridge the defects in this difficult anatomic region. The transfer of another nerve has been used successfully to reinnervate the innervated portions of the brachial plexus where repair is impossible because of root avulsion. These operations are being performed in a few centers, and it is hoped that in several years the results will prove to be better than that from previous surgical attempts.

REFERENCES

1. Leffert, R. D.: Brachial plexus injuries, Orthop. Clin. North Am. **1:**399-417, Nov. 1970.
2. Mellesi, H.: Surgical management of brachial plexus injuries, J. Hand Surg. **2:**367-379, Sept. 1977.
3. Narakas, A.: Plexo braquial, Revista de Ortopedia y Traumatología **16:**855-920, 1972.
4. Seddon, H.: Surgical disorders of the peripheral nerves, Baltimore, 1972, The Williams & Wilkins Co.

GENERAL DISCUSSION

Dr. Tupper: What are the present feelings about timing of tendon transfers for peripheral nerve laceration above the elbow? Will transfers ever be done at the same sitting as nerve repair?

Dr. Urbaniak: The radial nerve, I guess, would be the easiest one to discuss first. A lot of surgeons emphasized doing the radial nerve and some type of transfer to give finger and thumb extension at the same time. They believe the distal extensors may not return. My belief, even in the delayed repair of 8 to 10 months, would be to just repair the nerve. In our radial nerve repairs, we anticipate getting return of finger and thumb extension as well as wrist extension.

Generally, we don't do the transfers at the same time. We anticipate better nerve recovery than we did in the past. In median and ulnar nerve lacera-tions above the elbow in adults, especially ones that have been severed for more than a year, I would consider simultaneous transfers. For example, I would consider doing an opponens transfer at the same time as an above-elbow median nerve repair. I haven't done any intrinsic transfers at the same time as an ulnar nerve repair.

Dr. Wilgis: I believe that there is a place for some transfers; I believe you should consider anything you do, simultaneously with a nerve repair, as merely an internal splint. You must not do a transfer that will cause prob-lems if the nerve recovers. I have seen a radial nerve in which somebody had transfers and then the radial nerve recovered and they had a constant extension deformity. I think this is a bad approach. As an internal splint, the pronator teres to extensor carpi radialis brevis is a suitable transfer for the radial nerve. As far as the median nerve is concerned, there's probably some indication to do an opponens transfer with a high median nerve lesion. I say this for two reasons: (1) the chances of getting back all opponens function are not terribly good and (2) in sensory reeducation, we found that an individual with normal motor power will get improved sensory recovery. As far as the ulnar nerve is concerned, I think a Zancoli capsulodesis or capsulorrhaphy as an internal splint is a suitable operation to perform in an above-elbow ulnar nerve lesion.

Dr. Tupper: Of all those procedures, the pronator teres to the extensor carpi radialis brevis is a great one because you still retain pronation from it and the patient doesn't have to wear that splint around for so long. The Zancoli is another one in which you don't lose anything. You haven't really stolen any tendons and lost them.

Dr. Urbaniak: The problem with doing the pronator transfer is you can't tell how good your results are. That's why you get good results, Jack. We want to see whether our nerve repair is going to work or not.

Dr. Tupper: Dr. Wilgis, do you do internal neurolysis only with clinical findings or do you do it on the basis of electrical abnormalities?

Dr. Wilgis: Well, I won't do internal neurolysis on the basis of electrical abnormalities. I think I have to say that of all of the median nerve decompressions that we do, probably 15% have preoperative electrical studies; the clinical examination is the one that I rely on. You have to remember that on the electrical study, you can be studying one normal fascicle and all the rest of them can be abnormal. So, I really don't base my indication for intraneurolysis on the electrical study.

Dr. Tupper: Jim, when do you decide to decompress the median nerve after a Colles' fracture at the wrist?

Dr. Urbaniak: In the acute stage, that depends on your clinical evaluation. If the patient has numbness, tingling, and no pain in the hand, I would watch it for a period of 12 to 24 hours. Many times they will improve. If there are no signs of improvement, I would still watch the patient every 3 to 4 hours, and if he showed signs of pain or progression, I certainly would decompress the nerve within the next day. In the old ladies with Colles' fractures, it is not uncommon to have this persistent numbness for a while, but we don't go in and decompress them immediately. It depends a lot on the pain associated with it. Any evidence of severe compression merits immediate decompression. I have followed patients closely, and one or two times I have wished I had decompressed them earlier because I had to decompress them 2 weeks later. I think it is difficult to say.

Dr. Tupper: Do you agree with that, Shaw?

Dr. Wilgis: I don't treat any acute Colles' fractures. The only ones I see are the ones that are in trouble, but we don't hesitate to decompress the median nerve if we believe there's a problem. Frequently there is hemorrhage within the neural sheath and the orthopaedists do follow many along that we eventually decompress some 6 months to a year later. I believe if there is any question, however, a decompression is a very useful procedure. It might avoid that terrible reflex sympathetic dystrophy, which you may see 6 months down the road.

Dr. Tupper: We've always believed that it's important to know from the time you first see the patient with an acute fracture whether or not there is median nerve involvement. It's terribly important to have this documented on the chart, whether or not there is median loss at the time you first see them. Many median nerves are contused at the time of the Colles' fracture, and my feeling is that they don't really require carpal tunnel release. On the other hand, if the numbness develops 2 days later and there was none to begin with, then you have an acute carpal tunnel syndrome that requires mandatory decompression. We've had hundreds of suits in our area, but we've had several involving just this thing. Nobody mentioned whether or not the median nerve was numb at the time of the fracture, and there was just nothing you could do. You can't go back. The patient of course has been well instructed by his attorney by that time.

Dr. Wilgis: I think that if one requires more than one manipulation, in my experience these have had to be opened and decompressed if median nerve symptoms are present.

Dr. Tupper: Dr. Urbaniak, when do you like to repair fresh nerve lacerations—the day of the injury, the night of the injury, or when? And considering repair of the nerve, do you have some comments on delayed primary versus primary and even versus secondary? When do you decide when to do it?

Dr. Urbaniak: Since we've been involved in the replantations, I have changed my philosophy some. I used to do most of my nerve repairs in the first 3 weeks. I would tell the referring physician to close the wound and send them to us. If we saw them in the emergency room, we wouldn't hesitate about cleaning up the wound, either leaving it open or closed, depending on the type and extent of injury. Since we've been involved with so many nerve repairs in replantations, I personally elect to go ahead and take the patient to the operating room immediately and repair the nerve, particularly if there is an associated vascular problem. I'm not talking about a replant or any partial amputation, but about a nerve injury in which there may be an associated vessel involved. Most of my nerve repairs are performed on the day of injury for a lot of reasons. One is for the ease of getting them on the operative schedule, and we believe we can now do them quicker and perhaps better than delayed repair. The results are no different if they're done today, tonight, or 3 weeks later. I really don't think anybody has any evidence. I'm familiar with the work of Dr. Drucker who stated that they do better if they are repaired somewhere between 9 and 21 days because of axon flow or cell body changes or whatever is going on and this may be so. But, I really think the results are no different. So this depends on your particular situation, the condition of the patient and wound and the availability of the operating room.

Dr. Wilgis: Certainly it is a much easier operation if you do it immediately after the laceration, and I think this is something to be considered.

Dr. Tupper: Do you transfer all your ulnar nerves beneath the flexor muscle mass or only those that have an internal neurolysis? Do you ever do a medial epicondylectomy?

Dr. Wilgis: No, I don't do a medial epicondylectomy. I never have. I am aware of the people that do, but we never have. There are two operations we do on the ulnar nerve at the elbow. The first is for the transient ulnar neuritis without motor deficit but with aggravating sensory complaints in essentially a normal elbow. I believe the major problem here is Osborn's fascia, which is a fascial compartment stretching from the two heads of the flexor carpi ulnaris muscle. We release Osborn's fascia and divide the two heads of the flexor carpi ulnaris muscle, which is really distal to the elbow. If you look, you'll find many of these problems do originate right there. Many times it's an individual who has a flexor carpi ulnaris that doesn't divide at all and comes off as almost a common origin. Now for the individual with motor weakness, we do do an internal neurolysis and there we transpose beneath the flexor muscle mass. I have not done a subcutaneous anterior transposition in 5 years. I'm sure that will stimulate some argument.

16. Electrophysiology of nerves

Donald S. Bright
Roni Sehayik

This chapter contains a brief outline of peripheral nerve anatomy and electrophysiology. Some well-established as well as some new concepts in determining the timing and type of nerve repair after peripheral nerve injury are included. This field is difficult and there are rapidly evolving concepts that will improve our ability to assist patients with nerve injuries in the future.

ANATOMY

Important elements of the nerve include the epineurium or outer investing sheath of the nerve and the funiculus (fasciculus), which is surrounded by the perineurium and contains endoneurium. The epineurium and the perineurium are derived from mesodermal tissues, whereas the endoneurium is derived from ectodermal tissues. The epineurium and perineurium contain larger fibers of collagen. Vessels within the perineurium are no larger than a capillary.

Within the funiculus the finer collagen of the endoneurium forms sheaths or endoneurial tubes. Within these sheaths lie the Schwann cells and axons.

There are from 20,000 to 30,000 axons in the median and ulnar nerves at the elbow. The number of funiculi varies from one to 36 in the median, ulnar, and radial nerves and from 30 to 150 in the sciatic nerve.

One anatomic feature that presents particular problems to the operating surgeon is the continual variations throughout the length of the nerve. These include variation in the number of funiculi within the nerve, the funicular pattern within a cross section along the length of the nerve, the axonal composition of each funiculus (sensory, motor, proprioceptive).[27] Thus the percentage of conducting tissue within the cross section of the nerve varies along the length of a nerve.

As the funiculi travel distally in the nerve, they vary in size in a continual pattern because of cross connections between funiculi. More proximally in a nerve each funiculus contain both sensory and motor axons, whereas distally,

200

where the sensory and motor branches leave the main trunk of the nerve, the funiculi are more consistently sensory or motor.

In the cross-sectional area of the nerve, 30% to 90% contains epineurial (nonconducting) tissue. The sciatic nerve at the notch contains over 80% nonconducting tissue acting primarily as a cushion. In the median nerve at the wrist, there is relatively little epineurial tissue and the funiculi are closely packed together.[28]

Throughout the course of the nerve there is a continual pattern of undulations or waves. The axons undulate within the funiculi, and the funiculi undulate within the epineurium. This undulation allows a certain amount of stretch without damage.

FUNCTION

The motor axons originate in the cell body in the anterior horn. They travel within the nerve and are myelinated. They terminate on the motor end plate of muscles where the basal lamina of the muscle has a fold and receptors are present. The end plate is protected by Schwann cells. Transmitter substance is deactivated by cholinesterase after it reaches the receptor.[8] In traveling down the myelinated fiber, the current travels proximal to distal and propagates from one node of Ranvier to another.[13] In myelinated fibers the velocity of the current is related in a positive manner to fiber size, with the slope being approximately 4 to 6.

Sensory axons are technically dendrites or projections of the cell body with the actual axons communicating with the spinal cord. Functionally, however, these dendrites behave exactly like axons. They are referred to as axons in the peripheral nerve. The sensory and pseudomotor axons travel in the peripheral and cutaneous sensory nerves to the various end organs.[21] They are both myelinated and nonmyelinated, with the nonmyelinated fibers having much lower conduction along the axon. Also in the nonmyelinated fibers, conduction velocity is related to fiber size, but with a lower slope than that in myelinated fibers. Skin receptors have properties that transduce mechanical stimuli into patterns of responses rather than modality specific information.[19]

Electrically the nerves have a safety factor with the current available for stimulation along the nerve being approximately four to six times what is normally required to activate the axon distally. In nerve injury when this safety factor fails, there is first a conduction block and then a complete block.

The axon is an extension of the cell body in the spinal cord or in the sensory ganglion and as such is far from its normal nourishment. For continued nerve growth, trophic substances are essential. The Schwann cell plays an important part in nourishing the axon; its trophic influence may be related to nerve growth factor.

Nerve growth factor is believed to affect adrenergic and sensory neuron development, but not motor or parasympathetic neuron development. It is probably a protein, and recently investigators have found that experimentally it prevents the detachment of the synapse from the spinal cord after rhizotomy. The Schwann cell can substitute for nerve growth factor in nerve growth factor—sensitive cells; a sensory neuron can grow in a Schwann cell bed without the addition of nerve growth factor.[3]

Also, axoplasmic transport probably has much to do with the nourishment and function of the axon. Tagged leucine (tritiated), which is a polypeptide, moves down about 410 mm of a nerve a day, a rate that approximates that in the spinal cord. This movement is apparently independent of species, fiber type, and diameter. The rate does not change after distal neurotomy and is independent of the cell body. It depends on oxidative metabolism and is decreased in the devascularized nerve and stopped by 300 mm Hg of tourniquet pressure.[23]

Functionally the perineurium is important. The perineurial sheath provides the tensile strength for the nerve while also acting as a diffusion barrier, resisting infection and maintaining interfunicular pressure. In the cat, nerve conduction is decreased when the perineurial sheath is removed.[23]

NERVE INJURY AND RESPONSE: NEUROTMESIS, STRETCH INJURY, NEURAPRAXIA, CONDUCTION BLOCK

Nerve injuries can be classified as (1) neurotmesis (disruption of the whole nerve), (2) axonotmesis (disruption of the axon within the nerve while the nerve as a whole remains anatomically continuous) and (3) neurapraxia (failure of function without physical disruption of the axon, tube, or nerve trunk). A newer class of nerve injury is that of conduction delay.

Neurotmesis

After division of a nerve trunk, changes take place proximally and distally. Proximally, 10% to 80% of the cell bodies will degenerate and be permanently lost.[26] The percentage of cell bodies that die is believed to be related to the severity of the injury: an avulsion injury would lead to more cell bodies dying than a simple clean laceration. Wallerian degeneration of the nerve takes place distal to the cut nerve.[24] There is a decrease in the size of the funiculus and atrophy of the muscle, with no change in epineurial tissue. The Schwann cell remains present but shrinks in size. The decrease in size of funiculus, muscle atrophy, and decrease in tubule size are roughly parallel.[27]

In the reparative process in neurotmesis, during the first 10 to 20 days, there is central hypertrophy of the cell body.[5] This chromatolysis may be secondary to increased activity of the cell body in aiding regeneration, or to loss of the peripheral trophic factor.

At the site of the nerve interruption axons sprout. Each axon sprouts many times so that there may be more axons distally to the interruption than proxi-

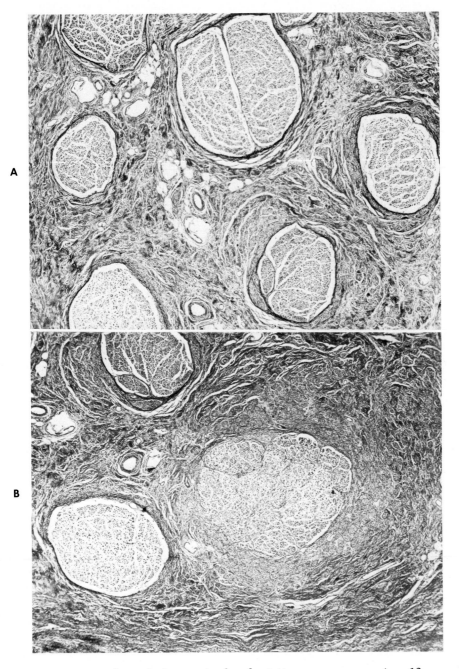

Fig. 16-1. Sections through the proximal and sciatic nerve neuroma in a 12-year-old after a shotgun blast to the knee. **A,** Proximal in the neuroma the funiculi are fairly well defined with some increase in epineurial collagen and scar formation. **B,** There is some disorientation of a clear funicular pattern. In the center are sprouting axons outside of the normal funicular border of the perineurium. An adjacent funiculus remains fairly well defined. **C,** More distal in the neuroma there is general disorientation of the funicular pattern. Axons are traveling in longitudinal, horizontal, and oblique directions with extensive scar formation both intraperineurially and extraperineurially. Clinical, anatomic, microscopic, and electrophysiologic means are needed to determine in the clinical setting where the function and anatomy of the nerve are acceptable for repair and where the disorganization makes repair impossible.

Continued.

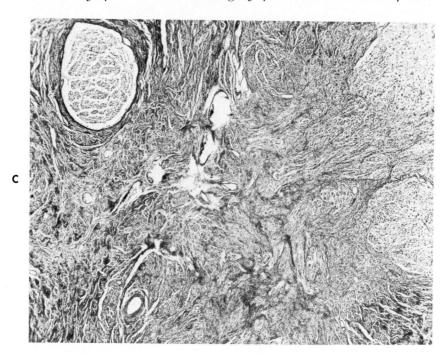

Fig. 16-1, cont'd. For legend see p. 203.

mally (Fig. 16-1). If these axons travel down endoneurial tubes, the Schwann cells and endoneurial tubes hypertrophy and remyelinate the axons. When the motor and sensory end plates are reached, if the nerves and end plates are functionally related, the nerve resumes its function, but at a decreased level.

Axonotmesis

In peripheral nerve stretch, the elastic limit is about 10% to 15% stretch and the mechanical limit is 15% to 23% stretch (7.5 cm/min).[27] During such injury the nerve trunk elongates, the wavy pattern of the funiculus straightens out, the axon fiber breaks, and then there is disruption of the funiculus. This is followed by separation of the nerve. In severe stretch there is interruption of axons at different levels. At each individual level, regeneration proceeds as with neurotmesis.

Neurapraxia

In neurapraxia, because of localized crush or pressure or temporary devascularization, there is loss of nerve function. In minor injuries, the loss of function may be transient; in more prolonged or severe injuries, the axons may undergo wallerian degeneration distal to the site of injury. Because the endoneurial tubes are not disrupted, the regenerating axons have a smooth path to the same end organ as before the injury. Largely because of this fact, recovery after neurapraxia is good.

Conduction delays

Certain injury phenomena of nerves result from conduction delays. When there is prolonged compression as on the median nerve in a carpal tunnel syndrome, or with perineurial fibrosis from callous or scar formation, there is *impaired* but not absent nerve function.

In one type of conduction delay there can be a decrease in the action potential height in traversing the injured area because of impaired function or structure of the myelin.[24] An alternate block occurs with a change in the refractory period of the nerve and an increasing stimulus rate. In this condition, fewer impulses traverse the injured area because of the relative increase in the refractory period of each individual fiber.[29] Franz and Iggo[6] showed that with increased cooling as the stimulus frequency was increased, the nerve only responded to a certain percentage of the stimuli. In the trains block, only the first impulse gets through; the remaining impulses are blocked at the injured area. This is more impaired conduction than alternate block.

Absence of any conduction is considered complete block.

Conduction blocks or delays can explain some of the features of neurapraxial nerve-compression syndromes. They also can explain the observation that the function of a nerve can change acutely after decompression, presumably because of a reversal of conduction blocks. These conduction blocks can be considered as type ½ in Sunderland's classification. They generally affect motor more than sensory or autonomic nerves.

In peripheral nerve compression syndromes there is relative anoxia from pressure. The larger caliber fibers are affected initially, and with continued pressure there are endothelial changes with increases in pressure, edema, and fibrosis within the funiculus. Conduction abnormalities ensue, followed by complete dysfunction of the axon. Such damage can be partially or completely reversed depending on the time factor of release. Early after release the conduction abnormalities may correct, but some axons will have to completely regenerate distally and may take up to several years to recover their function. Ochoa has shown that in acute and chronic nerve compression lesions caused by mechanical compression, axoplasm is pushed away from the increased pressure area. The Schwann cell and myelin are invaginated. In the chronic lesion this appears much like tadpoles lined up.[22] The bulbous end contains excess myelin including the inner and outer lamellae. This histologic finding has been verified in man with compression lesions in nerves.

Neuroma pain

The pain of neuromas has both intrinsic and extrinsic causes. Extrinsic pressure from fracture fragments, callous formation, or dense scar can in many instances cause continual pain or pain with joint motion. Intrinsic factors such as intraneural collagenization and disorganization also can play a role. Several additional theories such as the fiber-dissociation theory, which postulates a selective loss of large fiber myelin; or cross excitation from one fiber to another; or spontaneous pacemaker activity of the regenerating nerve, are all possible contributing factors to the pain of a neuroma.

NERVE REPAIR
Essential principles

The amount of local injury to the nerve must be known. In some crushing, stretch, or avulsion injuries it will take several days to weeks before the full extent of axonal damage can be determined. In these instances, delayed nerve repair is often preferable since the surrounding tissue may also be severely injured and may have to be excised either shortly after the injury or at a later time. In cleanly severed nerves acute repair may be preferable.

Orientation is important in nerve repairs because functionally related axons must be opposed to each other.[9] This is especially true distally where there is clear differentiation between motor and sensory areas of the nerve. Orientation is usually not difficult in acute, clean lacerations when minimal nerve is resected. It becomes more difficult with segmental loss of nerve tissue or proximal lesions, delayed repair, or where there is a larger proportion of connective tissue than conducting tissue. Other important factors include the differences in the size, number, and rotation of funiculi.

Magnification either by loupes or microscope aids in determining the funicular pattern and in ensuring opposition of the funiculi.

The suture material should be nonreactive and not constrict the funiculi (Fig. 16-2).

Increased tension is detrimental to a good nerve repair.[10,20] Proximal and distal dissection and positioning of the extremity can relieve some tension at the time of repair. In a study of interfascicular nerve grafting in primates, Hudson[12] found that scar formation was detrimental. Millesi[20] concluded that when tension is present grafting should be performed; in most cases a bundle graft is more appropriate than individual fascicular grafting.

In an experimental study carried out at Letterman Hospital McCarrol found that nerve grafts and increased tension decreased function whereas epineurial versus perineurial sutures showed no difference.[18] Orgel studied sciatic nerve repair in rabbits by electrophysiologic methods and found no difference in epineurial versus fascicular repair.[25]

Adaptation

In composite tissue toe-to-hand transfers in which the nerve is transferred along with tissue, the measured function in the hand is occasionally better than it was when the tissue was on the foot. This phenomenon is referred to

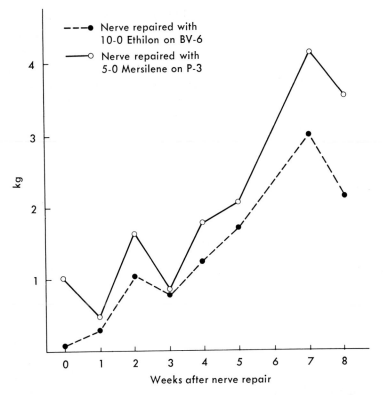

Fig. 16-2. Repaired nerve strength in experimental animal. Comparison between perineurial suture with 10-0 monofilament and epineurial suture with 5-0 Mersilene. During the first week the epineurial suture is clearly stronger. After 7 days the suture strengths approximate each other and there is an increase in strength in both epineurial and perineurial repair.

as adaptation. That adaptation takes place is fairly well agreed upon, but whether it takes place in the mechanosensory receptors or in the cortex is not clear.

ELECTRICAL AND CLINICAL PROPERTIES OF THE INJURED AND REPAIRED NERVE
Electrical properties

Neural tissue has electrical properties that change during propagation of an impulse, exhibiting a decrease in resting potential across the axolemma and an associated flow of sodium, potassium, and other ions across its membrane. This is called an action potential. The summation of the action potentials of many neural fibers in a nerve trunk is referred to as the compound action potential. It is characterized by a very rapid depolarization and slower repolarization to its resting state.

The minimum intensity of the stimulus required to evoke an action potential is called the "threshold stimulus." Evoked action potential in a nerve may be initiated by an electrical stimulus that differs in pattern from a natural stimulus since an electrical stimulus bypasses the receptors and activates fibers on the basis of their diameter. The ability of the nerve to propagate an action potential once the threshold has been bypassed, without a change in wave pattern, is called the all-or-none response.[24]

In the early stage of an action potential, the neural tissue will not respond to another stimulus; this is called the absolute refractory period. After this, it will respond to a strong stimulus, or with less response to the same stimulus; this is called the relative refractory period.[2]

Nerve conduction velocity is related not only to nerve size but also to the differences between myelinated and unmyelinated nerve fibers. The greater velocity in myelinated fibers is secondary to the ability to confine ionic changes to the nodes of Ranvier; unmyelinated fibers require the progression of local circuit flow along the length of the fiber. Injured nerves with decreased myelin and regenerating axons exhibit decreased conduction velocity; a typical example is the carpal tunnel syndrome. In addition, the number of ions moved by the action potential is proportional to the axon surface area and the amount contributed by larger fibers is greater than smaller fibers.

Compound action potential of a nerve trunk thus has been used to yield great diagnostic information through interpretation of its shape, size, latency, presence or absence, and frequency of occurrence.[14] The smooth pattern of a compound action potential is characteristic of normal nerve. One that is broad with several peaks is caused by dispersion of many single action potentials, depending on the number of fibers and size of nerve trunk.

Clinical evaluation

Preoperative and postoperative study. Clinical examination begins with a motor examination. This includes muscle rating, and bulk. Lidocaine blocks at and above the lesion of the involved nerve and the nerve that could exhibit cross-over innervation are given. For the median nerve at the wrist, for example, the ulnar nerve is blocked at the wrist and at the elbow.

The sensory examination should record responses to deep pain, protective sensation such as sharp and dull, hot and cold, two-point discrimination, static as well as moving, and pseudomotor function as evidenced by the sweat test.[21] Vibratory sense can also be tested.

A histamine test can be used to differentiate peripheral versus preganglionic sensory injury, and in brachial plexus lesions a myelogram can determine whether there has been nerve root avulsion from the spinal cord.

Cold intolerance can be subjectively and objectively measured and is present in nerve injuries, vascular injuries, and a combination of nerve and vascular injuries. Subjectively, cold intolerance is evidenced by pain and coldness of the digit when subjected to either cold water or cold environment. Objectively, a cold pressor test can be used, by immersion of the hand in ice water and determination of the warm-up time in comparison with the opposite normal digit. Abnormal cold intolerance will usually be evidenced by an extremity that cools to a lower temperature and has a slower warm-up time than the normal digit.

Electromyography and sensory and motor conduction velocities can be performed routinely and are helpful in determining the state of regeneration and documenting advances in regenerating nerve.[1] Electromyography is probably most useful in complete nerve lesions where fibrillations in the absence of action potentials are demonstrated as early as 3 weeks after the initial lesion. As regeneration takes place, there will be a decrease in the fibrillations, and some voluntary motor action potentials will appear several months prior to any clinical evidence of motor regeneration.[11] This can be helpful in determining those cases in which it is difficult to determine whether a nerve needs to be resutured or not.[1]

Sensory conduction velocities are more difficult to obtain but may be an earlier or more sensitive way of determining compression lesions or lesions high in the axilla.

Motor conduction times are, of course, relatively simple to obtain and can accurately help in assessing nerve-compression syndromes.[7]

Intraoperative study. In the operating room the use of electrophysiology has been advanced by some of the fine work of Terzis, Williams, Kline, and Hakstian[9,14-16,30,31] (Fig. 16-3). Elegant and comprehensive electrical equipment can be used in conjunction with microsurgical techniques so that one may dissect out individual funiculi and obtain recordings from them to determine presence of electrical continuity in certain nerve lesions. These advances are certainly useful in some cases where the technical personnel and specialized equipment are available.

The patient, however, can be used as his or her own electrophysiologist if the procedure is done under local anesthesia and a small stimulator is used on individual fasciculi. If there is an untidy wound, the nerve can be trimmed back and with the patient awake the fascicular groupings can be determined. Local nerve stimulation with a small-tipped stimulator of 2 to 3 volts or several milliamperes is most appropriate. The nerve can be mapped proximally with the sensory funiculi mapped.

At the distal end several methods can be used to determine the orientation of the nerve. If the wound is explored within 72 hours after injury, the motor funiculi can be determined by stimulation of the cut distal end, to which the appropriate muscle mass will contract[17] (Fig. 16-4). Alternately the nerve can be dissected distally with the funicular pattern determined by anatomic means. This method of orientation can be used in conjunction with (1) match-

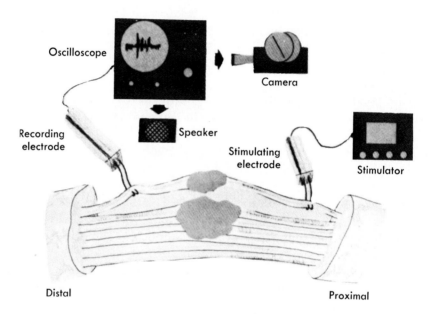

Fig. 16-3. Record above and below the lesion in conjunction with the careful preoperative clinical evaluation and the intraoperative stimulation at this point probably provides the most advantageous way of determining nerve function in partial lesions. (From Terzis, J. K., Dykes, K. W., and Hakstian, R. W.: J. Hand Surg. **1:**52-66, 1976.)

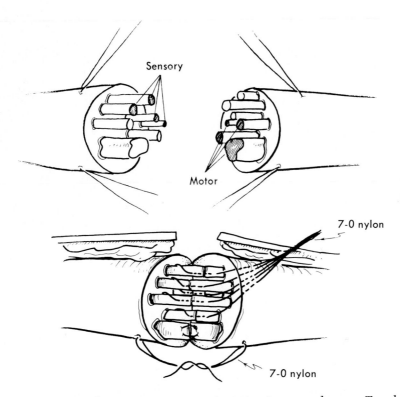

Fig. 16-4. Schematic of attempts at proper orientation in severed nerve. *Top drawing,* Sensory fascicles can be determined with mapping with the patient awake. The motor fascicles can be determined by anatomic dissection, or, within 72 hours of injury, stimulation of the distal motor fascicles will produce contraction of the innervated muscles. *Bottom drawing,* Orientation of perineurial sutures for correct alignment of the fascicles with an epineurial suture for strength.

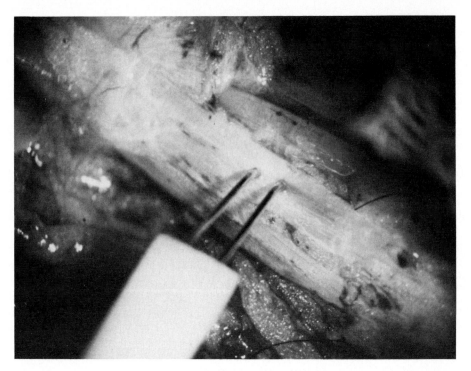

Fig. 16-5. View through microscope of stimulation of a 2 mm nerve with bipolar electrode.

ing cut ends of vessels found in the epineurium, (2) matching cut edges, and (3) using the methylene blue test to contrast connective tissue from neural tissue.

In neuromas in continuity or in partial lesions, dissection above and below the lesion can be carried out under local anesthesia and stimulation of motor fascicles proximal to the lesion or sensory fascicles distal to the lesion can determine which portions of the nerve are functionally intact (Fig. 16-5).

The electrical properties of nerves also determine intraoperative topography of the nerve in our nerve implants. For example, in placing the sensory feedback prosthesis or in percutaneous nerve implantation for pain problems, the nerve can be explored under local anesthesia and the electrodes placed on the appropriate fascicles after mapping.

Daniel and Terzis have also shown that the intraoperative determination of the electrical properties of the nerve is useful in converting an injury with a large skin defect and no sensibility to one with coverage and sensibility.[4] This has been useful in using an intercostal fiber to cover the buttocks of paraplegics.

CONCLUSION

A knowledge of the basics of neural physiology coupled with a thorough preoperative examination and the use of various intraoperative devices often readily available to the operating surgeon can aid in obtaining a better result after injury of peripheral nerves.

ACKNOWLEDGMENT

Work in this chapter was partially supported by NIH Grant no. 1 RO1 GM25666.

REFERENCES

1. Ballantyne, J. P., and Campbell, M. J.: Electrophysiological study after surgical repair of sectioned human peripheral nerves, J. Neurol. Neurosurg. Psychiatry **36**:797, 1973.
2. Brindley, F. J.: Excitation and conduction in nerve fibers, In Mountcastle, V. B., editor: Medical Physiology, St. Louis, 1974, The C. V. Mosby Co., vol. 1, pp. 34-76.
3. Bunge, R.P.: Some observations on the role of the Schwann cell in peripheral nerve regeneration. In Jewett, D. L., and McCarroll, H. R., Jr., editors: Nerve repair and regeneration: its clinical and experimental basis, St. Louis, 1979, The C. V. Mosby Co.
4. Daniel, R. K., Terzis, J., and Midgley, R.: Restoration of sensation to an anesthetic hand by a free neurovascular flap from the foot, Plast. Reconstr. Surg. **57**:275, 1976.
5. Ducker, T. B.: Metabolic factors in surgery of peripheral nerves, Surg. Clin. North Am. **52**:1109, 1972.
6. Franz, D. N., and Iggo, A.: Conduction failure in myelinated and non-myelinated axons at low temperatures, J. Physiol. **199**:319, 1968.
7. Gilliatt, R. W.: Recent advances in the pathophysiology of nerve conduction. In Desmedt, J. E., editor: New developments in electromyography and clinical neurophysiology, Basel, 1973, S. Karger, AG., pp. 2-18.
8. Guth, L.: Trophic influences of nerve on muscle, Physiol. Rev. **48**:645, 1968.
9. Hakstian, R. W.: Funicular orientation by direct stimulation. An aid to peripheral nerve repair, J. Bone Joint Surg. **50-A**:1178, 1968.
10. Highet, W. B., and Sanders, F. K.: The effects of stretching nerves after suture, Br. J. Surg. **30**:355, April 1943.
11. Howard, F. M.: The electromyogram and conduction velocity studies in peripheral nerve trauma, Clin. Neurosurg. **17**:63-76, 1970.
12. Hudson, A., Kline, D., Bratton, B., and Hunter, D.: Axonal growth at the suture line. In Jewett, D. L., and McCarroll, H. R., Jr., editors: Nerve repair and regeneration: its clinical and experimental basis, St. Louis, 1979, The C. V. Mosby Co.
13. Huxley, A. F., and Stämpfli, R.: Evidence for saltatory conduction in peripheral myelinated nerve fibers, J. Physiol. **108**:315, 1949.
14. Kline, D. G., Hackett, E. R., and May, P. R.: Evaluation of nerve injuries by evoked potentials and electromyography, J. Neurosurg. **31**:128, 1969.
15. Kline, D. G., and Nulsen, F. E.: The neuroma in continuity: its preoperative and operative management, Surg. Clin. North Am. **52**:1189, 1972.
16. Kline, D. G., and Hackett, E. R.: Value of electrophysiology tests for peripheral nerve neuromas, J. Surg. Oncol. **2**:299, 1970.

17. Landau, W. M.: The duration of neuro-muscular function after nerve section in man, J. Neurosurg. **10:**64, 1953.
18. McCarroll, H. R., Jr., Rodkey, W. G., and Cabaud, H. E.: Results of suture of cat ulnar nerves: a comparison of surgical techniques. In Jewett, D. L., and McCarroll, H. R., Jr., editors: Nerve repair and regeneration: its clinical and experimental basis, St. Louis, 1979, The C. V. Mosby Co.
19. Melzack, R., and Wall, P. D.: On the nature of cutaneous sensory mechanisms, Brain **85:**331, 1962.
20. Millesi, H.: Further experience with interfascicular grafting of the median, ulnar and radial nerves, J. Bone Joint Surg. **58-A:**209, 1976.
21. Mountcastle, V. B.: Sensory receptors and neural encoding: introduction to sensory processes. In Medical physiology, St. Louis, 1974, The C. V. Mosby Co., vol. 1, pp. 285-306.
22. Ochoa, J.: Histopathology of common mononeuropathies. In Jewett, D. L., and McCarroll, H. R., Jr., editors: Nerve repair and regeneration: its clinical and experimental basis, St. Louis, 1979, The C. V. Mosby Co.
23. Ochs, S.: Calcium requirement for axoplasmic transport and the role of the perineurial sheath. In Jewett, D. L., and McCarroll, H. R., Jr., editors: Nerve repair and regeneration: its clinical and experimental basis, St. Louis, 1979, The C. V. Mosby Co.
24. Ochs, S.: Elements of neurophysiology, New York, 1965, John Wiley & Sons, Inc.
25. Orgel, M. G.: A critical review of histologic methods used in the study of nerve regeneration. In Jewett, D. L., and McCarroll, H. R., Jr., editors: Nerve repair and regeneration: its clinical and experimental basis, St. Louis, 1979, The C. V. Mosby Co.
26. Stein, R., Hoffer, J. A., Gordon, T., et al.: Long-term recordings from cat peripheral nerves during degeneration and regeneration. In Jewett, D. L., and McCarroll, H. R., Jr., editors: Nerve repair and regeneration: its clinical and experimental basis, St. Louis, 1979, The C. V. Mosby Co.
27. Sunderland, S.: Nerves and nerve injuries, Baltimore, 1968, The Williams & Wilkins Co.
28. Sunderland, S.: The anatomical basis of nerve repair. In Jewett, D. L., and McCarroll, H. R., Jr., editors: Nerve repair and regeneration: its clinical and experimental basis, St. Louis, 1979, The C. V. Mosby Co.
29. Tasaki, I.: Nerve excitation, a macromolecular approach, Springfield, Ill., 1968, Charles C Thomas, Publisher.
30. Terzis, J.: Sensory mapping. In Entin, M., editor: Clinics in plastic surgery, Philadelphia, 1976, W. B. Saunders Co.
31. Williams, H. B., and Terzis, J. K.: Single fascicular recordings: an intraoperative diagnostic tool for the management of peripheral nerve lesions, Plast. Reconstr. Surg. **57:**562, 1976.

17. Fascicular nerve repair

Jack W. Tupper

Within a peripheral nerve, the nerve fiber (axon and its sheath) is the smallest functional unit. Bundles of these fibers contained by specialized tubular membrane, the perineurium, form the smallest surgical unit, the funiculus (or fasciculus). This may vary from less than 0.1 mm to several millimeters in diameter. The funicular contents are under axoplasmic pressure and are therefore always round in cross section (Fig. 17-1). In contradistinction to the epineurium, the perineurium forms not only a physical but a physiologic barrier as well, allowing preferential passage of some materials. Capillaries form the only true intrafunicular vessels.

Funiculi may pass singly along the nerve or may be arranged in groups. Surrounding funiculi and funicular groups, binding all together, is a loose areolar tissue, the intraneural epineurium (Figs. 17-2 and 17-3). In this tissue are the blood and lymph vessels. Surrounding all of this to form the outer layer of the peripheral nerve is a more or less tubular membrane, the circumferential epineurium (Fig. 17-4).

From an anatomic standpoint, nerve repairs may be of several types:
1. Epineurial—sutures through the circumferential epineurium only.
2. Epineurial plus a few sutures in corresponding bundles (in large nerves).
3. Large bundle repair—removal of circumferential epineurium and suturing of large bundles (in large nerves).
4. Perineurial (funicular, fascicular)—both circumferential and intraneural epineurium are discarded at the repair site; funiculi are repaired with sutures in the perineurium only; even in this type, bundles of very small funiculi (less than 0.2 mm) are usually sutured as a unit.

There are approximately 25 funiculi in the median nerve at the wrist (Figs. 17-10 to 17-12) and four to five in a proper digital nerve (Figs. 17-8, 17-13, and 17-14).

If an epineurial repair is done, there is a gross orientation of the nerve ends but poor funicular coaptation. A tight closure inhibits escape of budding axons but may make intraneural hematoma more likely. Since a peripheral nerve is

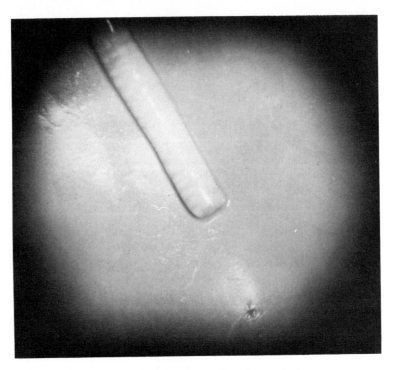

Fig. 17-1. Single funiculus (fasciculus).

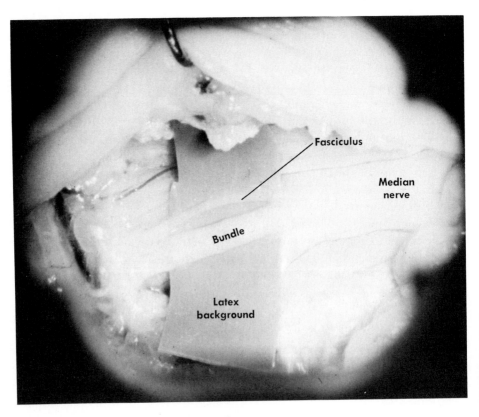

Fig. 17-2. Median nerve in wrist.

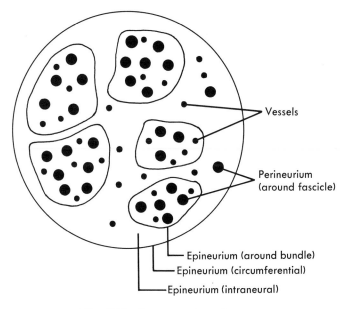

Fig. 17-3. Cross section of nerve.

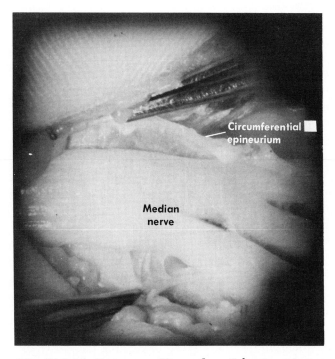

Fig. 17-4. Median nerve. Circumferential epineurium.

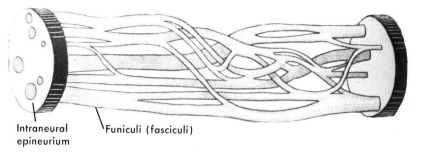

Intraneural
epineurium

Funiculi (fasciculi)

Fig. 17-5. Nerve trunk shows proportion of funicular to nonfunicular material. (From Sunderland, S.: Nerve and nerve injuries, Edinburgh, 1972, Churchill Livingstone.)

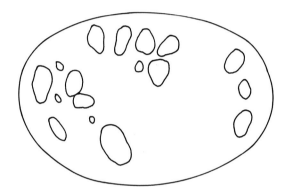

Fig. 17-6. Cross section of nerve showing proportion of funiculi to nonfunicular tissue.

often 50% interfunicular tissue (Fig. 17-5 and 17-6), it would follow that regenerating axons would have approximately that percentage of growing down a distal perineurial tube rather than into the tissue between. A specific funicular juncture, if motor and sensory can be sorted, theoretically would give a better percentage.

Accurate funicular matching can be done only in primary repair of sharply divided nerves. At the wrist level, the motor funiculus is separate and can usually be identified, but proximally funiculi will be mixed in their sensorimotor content (Fig. 17-5).

If a graft is to be used, the repair may be either epineurial or perineurial. The sural is the usual donor nerve. If a funicular graft is to be carried out, the epineurium must be removed and the funiculi dissected into lengths determined initially by the distance between branching funiculi, so that the length of funicular graft is essentially one fairly homogeneous strand. Not all funicular material within a nerve is useful, many being too small in size. These funicular grafts may then be sutured to bridge the gap between proximal and distal funiculi in the injured nerve.

TECHNIQUE OF FUNICULAR REPAIR

A piece of light blue ordinary latex balloon serves nicely as a background. It is readily available, cheap, and does not give a light reflection. Frequent flushing using a plastic BSS bottle* with a blunt needle allows easier identification of tissues to be discarded. The irrigant solution is heparinized saline solution, which keeps the fine suture materials from sticking to the wound surface. My preference in suture material is the S & T 50-micron (5-V) *short* (3 mm) straight needle swaged onto 18-micron nylon.† It is difficult to carry out accurate perineurial sutures with larger needles.

Dissect away the circumferential epineurium from the end of the nerve for a distance approximately equal to the diameter of the nerve.

If dealing with a large nerve, identify funicular bundles and dissect them initially as bundle units, proximally and distally. Match them with what appear to be corresponding units and temporarily loosely suture them together. Then, one bundle at a time, dissect all funiculi from each other, removing all the intraneural epineurium. Frequent flooding of the field will aid in cleanly preparing the funiculi. Each funiculus shows a spiral pattern in the perineurium (Fig. 17-1). These are pleats that disappear on axial stretch and reappear when tension is relaxed. The funiculi from the two paired bundles are arranged in a fan-shaped pattern on a flat surface facing each other (Fig. 17-9). These are then matched one to another by size. Protruding from the perineurial cuff are the gelatinous intrafunicular contents (Fig. 17-7). This is trimmed flush with the perineurium (Fig. 17-1), and two sutures are then placed at 180 degrees from each other (Fig. 17-8). Axoplasmic leak will then usually cease. If only one suture is used, there is a possibility of torsion of the funiculus with loss of contact (Fig. 17-9). The rest of the funiculi in the bundle are then matched and sutured in like manner. Then the next bundle is dealt with in similar fashion until repair is complete (Figs. 17-10 to 17-12).

In the smaller nerves such as the digital, the funiculi number 3 to 5 and are not formed into bundles but pass singly through the nerve (Figs. 17-13 and 17-14).

A delay of only a few days will result in shrinkage of the distal perineurial tubes and make repair slightly more difficult.

A secondary repair after scar and neuroma formation have occurred requires a resection of the scar regardless of whether the repair is to be perineurial or epineurial. If a funicular juncture is to be used, the multiple new funicular sprouts must be removed until a normal funicular anatomy is reached. This may leave a sufficient gap so that a graft is required.

Text continued on p. 224.

---

*Alcon Co., P. O. Box 2664, Fort Worth, Texas 76101.
†S & T Chirurgische Nadeln, 7893 Jestetten/GRD, Postfach 93, West Germany. Also Ethicon, Inc., 3640 Allendale Drive, Somerville, N.J. 08876.

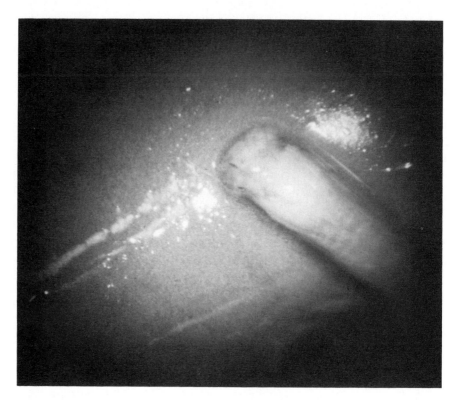

Fig. 17-7. Intrafunicular contents protruding beyond perineurium.

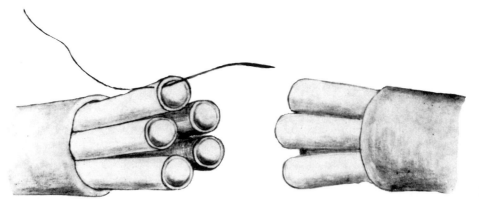

Fig. 17-8. Funicular repair. Digital nerve using perineural sutures.

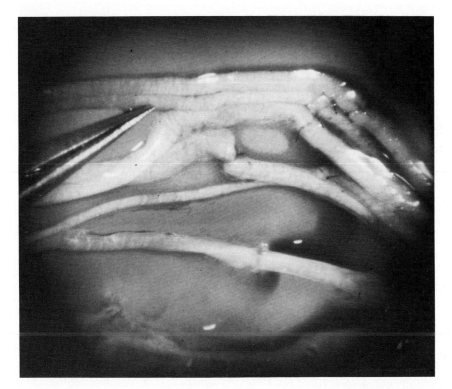

Fig. 17-9. Funicular grafting. Note torsion of one funiculus after only one suture.

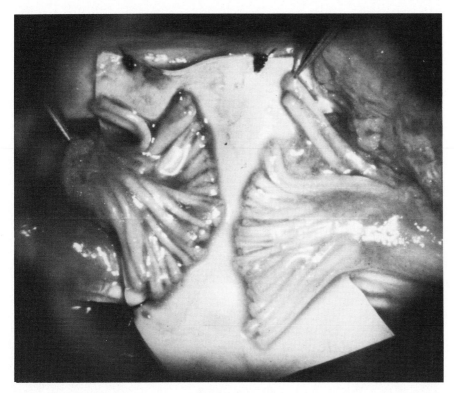

Fig. 17-10. Median nerve funicular dissection prior to repair. Uppermost funiculus is motor in function. Approximate number of funiculi, 25.

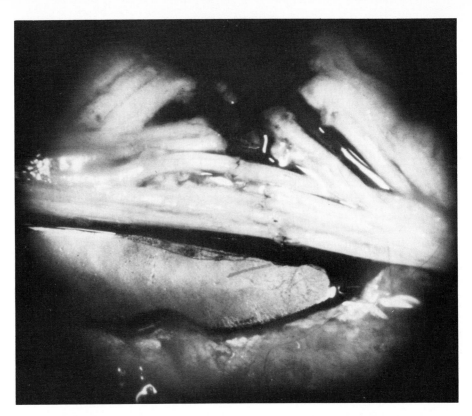

Fig. 17-11. Median nerve funicular repair partly completed.

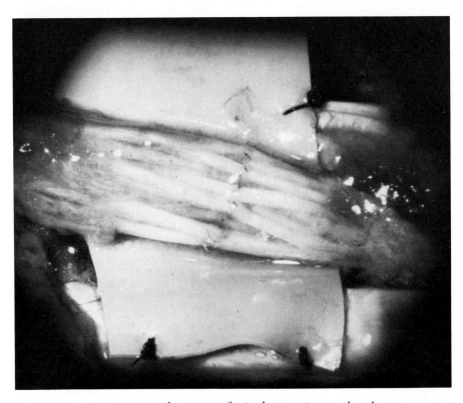

Fig. 17-12. Median nerve funicular repair completed.

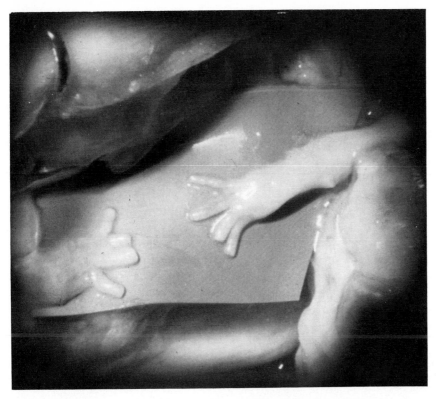

Fig. 17-13. Digital nerve prepared for funicular repair.

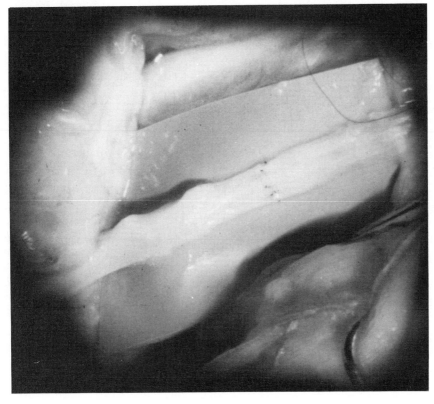

Fig. 17-14. Digital nerve funicular repair completed.

FUNICULAR GRAFT TECHNIQUE

The sural is the best donor nerve. It may be removed while the patient is supine, but this is carried out more easily in the prone position particularly if both sural nerves are to be removed. Frequently, the grafts are removed and prepared the day prior to insertion if the necessity for grafting is known. These may then be stored at 4° C overnight. Blood-storage refrigerators are kept at this temperature.

Working on a moist plastic surface, each funiculus is dissected free from the others. The funiculus is kept as a unit until branching occurs where it is transsected. Usually the larger funiculi in the nerve are the ones most suitable. These funicular lengths are then stored in a sealed jar with a slightly moist sponge overnight. Then, after preparation of the proximal and distal nerve stumps in the manner described above, these funiculi are trimmed to the necessary length and suturing carried out (Figs. 17-9 and 17-15). The original proximodistal orientation of the graft funiculi is believed to be not important. The proximal nerve stump will usually have more funiculi than the distal and

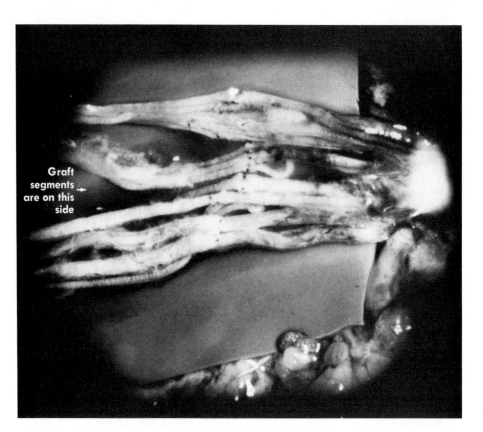

Graft segments are on this side

Fig. 17-15. Funicular nerve graft.

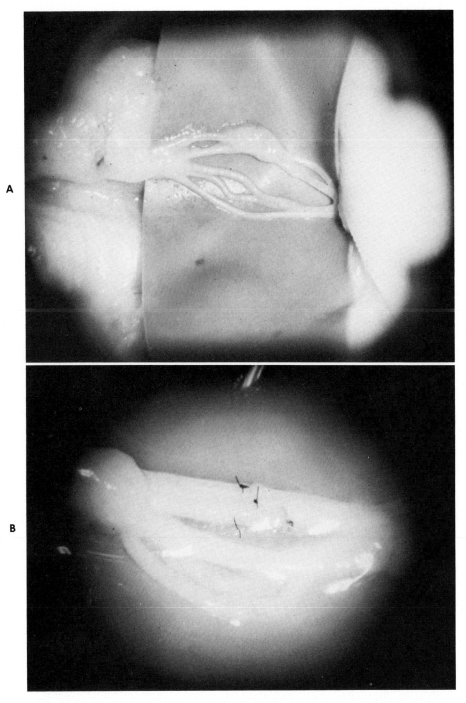

Fig. 17-16. Digital nerve. Old partial section showing painful neuroma. Some sensibility remained. **A,** Two funiculi had been cut. **B,** Neuroma resected and severed funiculi repaired. No surgical damage was done to the three unsevered funiculi.

therefore all distal junctures are made first. These are then covered with a piece of plastic to prevent sticking to gloves, gowns, and so forth, and then the proximal junctures are carried out. An attempt is made to place grafted material in a vascular bed of muscle, fat, or areolar tissue.

It is not yet possible to define the usefulness of fascicular repair because insufficient nerves have been repaired and followed at the present time. Preliminary results are as follows: In digital nerve repairs on a funicular basis, there were 14 cases, with an age over 21 years, followed for 1 year or more. In the cases, the von Frey tests were 2.57 compared with a normal of 1.65. Two-point discrimination was 9.82 if all patients with no two-point discrimination at all were measured as 15 for purposes of obtaining an average.

There were 27 patients with epineurial repairs with the same qualifications. In these, von Frey tests equaled 2.55 and two-point discrimination 7.63. This indicates that there is approximately the same results from each.

In nerve grafts with the same qualifications, there were two cases that had epineurial grafts, and these both had a von Frey test of 1.65 and a two-point discrimination of 15 (no two-point discrimination at all).

There were six funicular nerve grafts done on digital nerves. These had a von Frey test of 1.9 and a two-point discrimination of 9.5.

There have been insufficient numbers of median and ulnar nerves above the wrist to draw general conclusions. Individual cases would indicate that dissecting the funiculi from a sural nerve does not do any particular harm. In general, one may say that for repair or for grafting completely severed nerves, there is no indication at the moment that funicular repair is either better or worse than epineurial.

It would seem that the ideal indication for funicular dissection and repair or grafting would be in the partially divided nerve (Fig. 17-16), for the uninjured funiculi could be dissected free from the severed ones and a specific repair could be carried out. This would prevent additional surgical damage to the uninjured funiculi, reduce the chance of neuromatous pain, and encourage restoration of some sensation.

READINGS

Bora, F. W.: Peripheral nerve repair in cats: the fascicular stitch, J. Bone Joint Surg. **49-A:**659, 1967.

Sunderland, S.: Nerves and nerve injury, Baltimore, 1968, The Williams & Wilkins Co., chapters 7, 8, 29, 30, and 45.

18. Toe-to-hand transfer

Joseph E. Kutz
Cathy B. Thomson
Howard W. Klein

"Just as the neurovascular pedicle method of composite tissue transfer unshackled the older but limited procedures and made possible more accurate planning in substituting for the structural loss, so must the new freedom, afforded the transfer of composite tissue through microvascular surgery, not fail to utilize established structural and functional principles. Nor must the urge to use the free transfer method lure the surgeon from a safer, more predictable procedure."

J. W. Littler*

The toe-to-hand transfer is a microsurgical procedure consisting of a free vascularized graft involving one or multiple toes that is used to restore finger and thumb function in the reconstruction of the severely traumatized hand. The graft is vascularized by anastomosing its original blood supply (the dorsalis pedis artery and branches; the saphenous vein and branches) to a recipient vessel in the hand (radial, ulnar, and metacarpal arteries, cephalic vein, and its branches). The sensitivity so important in normal hand function is restored by anastomosis of the digital nerves of the respective toes to the median, ulnar, radial, and digital nerves of the hand. Joint motion and stability are restored through reattachment of the flexor and extensor tendons, respectively. The patient is therefore given a cosmetically acceptable, mobile, stable, and sensitive digit, which often allows use and function of the injured hand to return to extremely satisfactory levels. Patient satisfaction is of utmost importance as the dissatisfied patient uses his hand poorly postoperatively and may even use it less than preoperatively. Therefore patient selection is critical and a thorough knowledge of the patient's personality profile, socioeconomic status, occupation, and past medical history is essential. A preoperative evaluation by a therapist is used not only to help assess function but also to determine the patient's ability to successfully undertake the vigorous therapy

---

*Littler, J. W.: On making a thumb: one hundred years of surgical effort, J. Hand Surg. 1(1):35, July, 1976.

program needed postoperatively to provide a good functional result. Cosmesis, although usually acceptable to most patients with toe transfers, is not an indication for the procedure and its presence postoperatively does not ensure good function of the hand.

HISTORICAL REVIEW

Toe-to-hand transfers were used by Nicoladoni[7] in 1900 for reconstruction of the hand after thumb loss. In 1969, Cobbett[2] in England reported a successful transfer of a great toe to replace an amputated thumb. Buncke[1] in 1971 and 1973 described the transfer of a great toe by microvascular anastomosis, and since then numerous reports have followed. O'Brien reported on hallus-to-hand transfer in 1975[8] and published three case reports of successful transfer of the second toe based on the dorsal vascular system of the dorsalis pedis artery and saphenous vein in 1978.[9] Our clinical experience with these transfers parallels that of the above authors and will be described below.

PATIENT SELECTION

The patient chosen as a candidate for a free vascularized toe transfer must be carefully selected and must first have been considered for the following methods of reconstruction.[6]

1. *Thumb reconstruction alone*
   a. *Conservative management.* Although the absence of the thumb presents a critical disability with loss of refined pinch and grasp (Littler[5]) not every patient requires surgical correction. An unskilled worker (especially heavy manual laborer) may be, in fact, hindered by such attempts and be rendered unable to ever return to his regular occupation. Therefore the patient and his desires for postoperative function should be carefully considered and outlined so as to choose the procedure best suited to give the most functional result.
   b. *Phalangization of first metacarpal.* This method can be used when there is minimal scarring and a relatively mobile metacarpal. It can be combined with transfer of an adjacent stump, which will contribute to deepening of the thumb web space. It requires that sensible, mobile, and vascularized skin coverage be available for best functional results.
   c. *Construction of a thumb post.* This consists of using a tubed pedicle incorporating a bone graft. The graft can be done as part of the first stage or as a secondary procedure. Next, for restoration of sensibility, a neurovascular island graft is recommended. Postoperative occupational therapy has proved helpful in the sensory reeducation of these patients. Heavy manual laborers with subtotal amputations of the thumb have proved to be good candidates because an intact finger is not sacrificed and the procedure does not risk narrowing the thumb web space of the palm.

d. *Digital transposition (pollicization).* This procedure is well used in reconstruction of congenital absence of the thumb. It can give excellent cosmesis and restore digital length, sensibility, and a quite functional range of motion. Unfortunately, in posttraumatic situations there is usually multiple digital amputations and associated digital injury so that pollicization is not possible. However, when this procedure is feasible and the patient accepts its recommendation, the functional result obtained can be anticipated to be extremely satisfactory. It is well suited in the thumb after total or subtotal ray amputation. The appropriate length for good cosmesis and function can be chosen at the time of surgery and the digital transfer performed as outlined for congenital cases. As a one-stage procedure, it offers the advantage in providing an alternative to the patient who desires more than conservative management but who is not physiologically or psychologically suited for multiple-staged procedures as described under methods (c) or (e).

e. *Digital transfer.* After all the above treatment methods have been considered, free vascularized transfer of the great toe or second toe is an additional approach that might be selected. The following criteria are important prerequisites:
   (1) When there is an amputation with base and thenar muscles intact.
   (2) When sensory return is important.
   (3) When the index finger is essential for normal daily activities or occupational skills requiring fine work and is therefore unsuitable for pollicization.
   (4) When the patient refuses pollicization but desires more than conservative management and less than a two- or three-staged reconstructive procedure.
   (5) When a patient is extremely well motivated and will sacrifice some cosmesis for a satisfying functional result.
   (6) When a thorough physical examination and review of past medical history does not indicate a predisposing factor, such as collagen vascular disease, advanced arteriosclerosis, osteoporosis, peripheral neuropathies, and bleeding dyscrasias, which might compromise the vascular anastomosis, nerve regeneration, or wound bone healing processes.

2. *Digital reconstruction alone.* When the thumb is not involved in the injury and remains mobile with intact sensibility, many methods of conservative management can be employed to treat the digital loss. Patients can learn to bypass the involved digit or modify hand function to accommodate it. However, if there is enough shortening to prevent pinch activities, an "on-top plasty" described by Kelleher[3] or phalangization of adjacent short digits is possible. If there is no available sensitive skin locally to be used for reconstruction, a neurovascular island pedicle may be used. Frequently multiple

digits involved are reconstructed with insensitive flaps (such as the groin flap) and the area that is denervated is too large to reinervate. In this situation, digital transfer of one or two toes is indicated.

3. *Thumb and digital reconstruction.* In clinical situations where multiple digits and the thumb are involved, satisfactory hand function frequently is dependent on reconstruction of both deficits. A digit used for pollicization or phalangization in thumb reconstruction can be replaced by digital transfers. Multiple transfers can be fashioned at surgery to the appropriate lengths to function effectively with the reconstructed thumb. Patient selection is especially critical with this procedure because it entails more surgery and a more intensive postoperative therapy program.

A combination of the methods described above may be appropriate but require multiple-staged procedures, and the digital transfer can be accomplished at one stage. A thorough preoperative evaluation is needed for careful selection of the best procedure for this challenging clinical situation.

PREOPERATIVE ASSESSMENT

The patient selected for digital transfer needs a comprehensive evaluation, which includes a detailed history of the injury and its mechanism. The degloving and crush type of injuries will most likely have more severe tissue damage and involvement compared to the sharp, tidy injuries. An exact knowledge of the acute treatment rendered will be valuable in identification of vital structures at the time of transfer. A complete knowledge of the past medical history and findings on physical examination is essential for determination of any predisposing factors that might put the transfer at risk. The evaluation of a therapist is used to record parameters of hand function and outline the postoperative program to be followed. Several patient visits are required to establish the personality profile, occupational skills, and socioeconomic status, which will help ensure a satisfied patient result. A preoperative arteriogram of the involved upper extremity and lower extremity to be used is obtained. The patient is considered a candidate when the above evaluation is completed.

TECHNIQUE

The operation itself requires two teams, one preparing the hand and the other mobilizing the toe. The hand may be prepared first, and no definitive moves should be made by the other team until this is accomplished. This might save a needless amputation in the event that the vasculature of the thumb site created a problem or other unforeseen difficulties arose. For the more experienced microsurgical teams, both sites can be prepared simultaneously.

1. *Preparation of hand site*
   a. Appropriate skin flaps are incised to expose the veins on the dorsum of the hand. The veins are isolated and clamped with micro-occlusion clips.

b. The radial artery (or branches) is dissected out and prepared for anastomosis. The length of this mobilization will vary according to each patient.

c. The flexor and extensor pollicis longus are located and transfixed with Keith needles. The recipient bone at the base of the thumb is prepared for the toe.

d. The nerves to the thumb are dissected out with adequate length for suturing without tension.

2. *Mobilization of toe*

a. The toe is circumscribed with a racquet-shaped incision, and the veins are isolated through the dorsal aspect and clamped with micro-occlusion clips (Fig. 18-19, *A*).

b. The extensor tendon is dissected proximally and transsected over the base of the metatarsal.

c. The dorsalis pedis artery is dissected to the digital vessels with ligation of all branches of that vessel to prepare for the anastomosis.

d. On the plantar surface, the digital nerves and flexor tendons are transsected at levels of adequate length for anastomosis.

e. The toe is transsected at the level previously determined for adequate length of the thumb (Fig. 18-19, *B*).

f. The patient is placed on an anticoagulation regime during the anastomosis procedures.

POSTOPERATIVE MANAGEMENT

An anticoagulation regime consisting of 1 unit of low molecular weight dextran per day for 7 days and aspirin has been employed. The use of heparin has been discontinued. Prophylactic antibiotics are used for 5 to 7 days if not contraindicated. Bed rest is observed with elevation of both hand and foot until swelling resolves. No weight bearing is suggested until complete wound healing occurs. Gentle range of motion is begun at 3 weeks and postoperative dynamic splinting is used if necessary. Internal fixation is discontinued when bony union is seen on the radiograph or at 4 to 6 weeks when the soft-tissue supporting structures are strong and intact.

COMPLICATIONS AND SECONDARY PROCEDURES

Although there are few reported complications in the literature except for those of a vascular nature, clinical experience with long-term results has revealed some additions. With greater attention to meticulous microsurgical technique, failure as a result of thrombosis is more likely the exception rather than the rule. In the presence of a thrombosis or threatened thrombosis, the patient is returned to the operating room immediately and reexplored. Acute as well as subacute (3 weeks) vascular occlusion has been observed. There has been one incidence of delayed bony union requiring bone grafting as a secondary procedure. Tendolysis, capsulectomy, and neurolysis were necessary

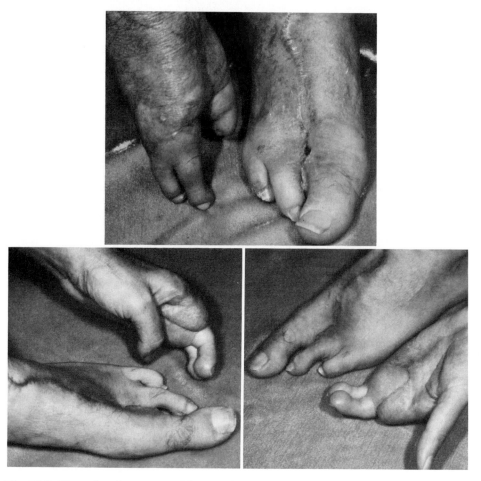

Fig. 18-1. There has been no problem with gait noted postoperatively in toe transfers in patients like this.

in one patient. Web-space deepening has been employed to treat long-standing contractures and to improve range of motion. One patient sustained a fracture of his toe transfer (Fig. 18-11, *B*), which healed spontaneously with conservative management. Hypersensitivity in the area of digital nerve anastomosis was successfully treated in one incidence by transcutaneous nerve stimulation. There have been no difficulties with gait noted in either great toe or multiple toe transfers (Fig. 18-1). Wound healing is extremely important, and skin grafting has sometimes been employed to decrease skin tension at the time of closure. Some patients may note hypertrophic scarring or areas of numbness across the dorsum, but this has had no effect on foot function. No wound infections have been observed although delayed wound healing necessitated skin grafting in one patient.

CASE PRESENTATIONS

The following patients were selected to illustrate indications, postoperative functional results, and complications of the free vascularized toe transfer.

Multiple-digit amputations with intact thumb. W.G. is a 32-year-old right-handed male who sustained a bilateral degloving injury at work after both hands were caught in a printing roller machine in July 1975. He underwent initial débridement including amputation of the right index finger and amputation of the distal phalanx of the right thumb with application of a groin pedicle flap. His left hand was more severely involved. Débridement included amputation at the bases of the proximal phalanges of the left index, middle, ring, and little fingers. Thirteen days later he had a groin pedicle flap applied to the left hand. The groin flaps were divided and reconstruction of both hands was begun. In March 1976 a neurovascular island flap from the right ring finger to the right thumb was performed. A free vascularized transfer of the left second and third toes to the left hand was performed in June 1976. Preoperatively, the left thumb was stated to have normal range of motion and sensation. The procedure was performed by two operative teams. A V incision was made on the dorsum of the left foot. With careful meticulous dissection, the dorsalis pedis artery was identified along with one volar artery. The metatarsals were divided distally along with the plantar and dorsal tendons. The wound was closed primarily after further partial excision of the second metatarsal. Simultaneously a team had identified multiple veins, the radial and ulnar arteries, and the extensor tendons in the left hand. The heads of the third and fourth metacarpals were excised and slots were fashioned in the medullary canals for the metatarsals. Kirschner wire fixation was employed to secure adequate fixation. The tendons were repaired by primary anastomosis of the extensors and flexors of the second toe. A palmaris longus tendon graft was used for repair of the third toe flexor. The venous anastomosis was performed with use of five veins. The arterial anastomosis consisted of two repairs with use of the radial and dorsalis pedis arteries in addition to a metacarpal and volar artery, which required a vein graft. The nerve repair consisted of a dorsal nerve from the toes to the radial nerve of the hand. Postoperatively there was excellent vascularization of the transfer with good capillary refill. Both hand and foot were immobilized with plaster splints until adequate wound healing occurred. Weight bearing was initiated at 3 postoperative weeks. In December 1976 the patient was returned to the operating room for defatting of the flap, tendolysis of the flexor tendons, and ray excision of the second metatarsal to increase the thumb web space. On examination in April 1978, two-point discrimination of the radial toe was recorded at 9 mm and the ulnar toe at 11 mm. There was active flexion and extension at all joints, and the patient was using his hand without difficulty to pick up and support objects (Figs. 18-2 to 18-6).

Multiple-digit amputations with absent thumb. J. P., a 19-year-old white

Text continued on p. 238.

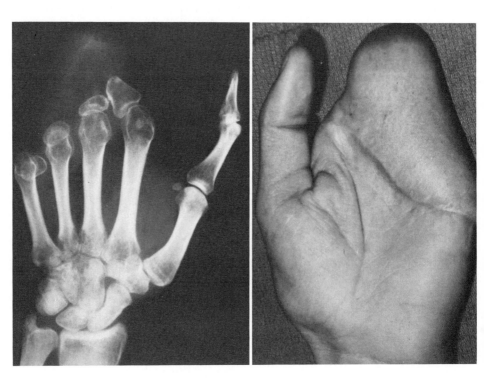

Fig. 18-2. Preoperative photo and radiograph showing intact thumb and multiple digit amputations. (W.G.)

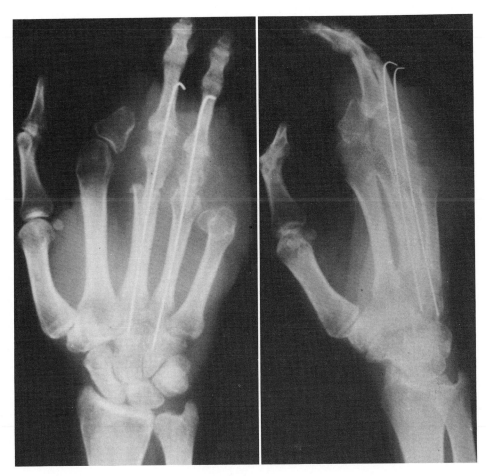

Fig. 18-3. Anteroposterior and lateral radiographs of the hand showing fixation and position of the second and third metatarsals after transfer. (W.G.)

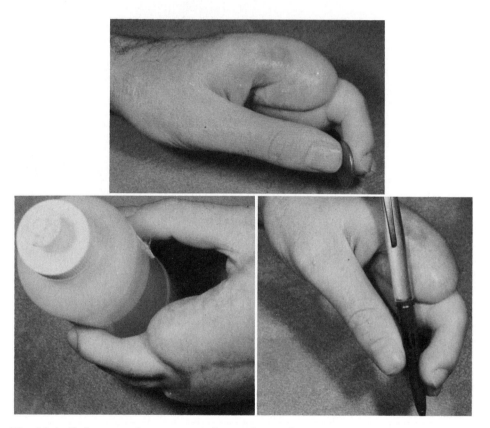

Fig. 18-4. Ability to pick up coins and grasp large objects shown 6 months postoperatively. (W.G.)

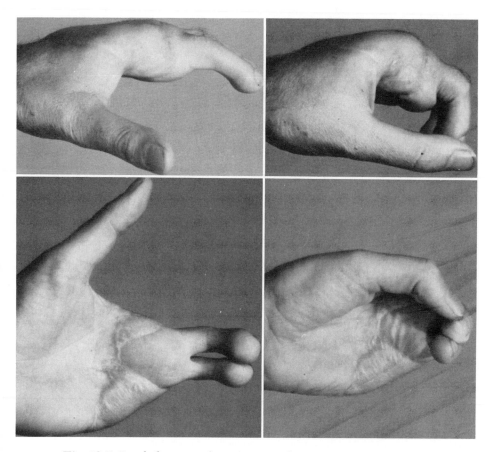

Fig. 18-5. Pinch function shown 16 months postoperatively. (W.G.)

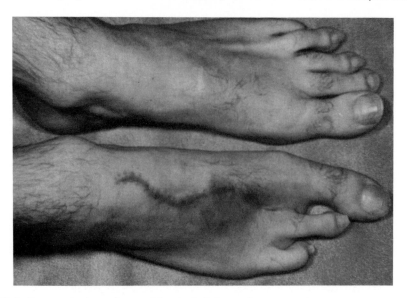

Fig. 18-6. Postoperative photo of healed defect after multiple toe transfer. No gait problems noted. (W.G.)

male, was flown to Louisville from Michigan after amputation of the left hand by a power saw at the mid to distal metacarpal level on July 25, 1974. On initial admission he had total replantation of the thumb, index, long, and ring fingers. Postoperative course showed progressive necrosis of the fingers and thumb. The necrotic hand was debrided 2 weeks later and a groin flap raised to cover the defect. Five months after the injury, the left second toe was transferred to the left hand with revision of the pedicle flap and construction of an opposable thumb post with a bone graft from the second metacarpal to the fifth meta-carpal. At that time his grasp was 10 p.s.i., and he was able to hold the weight of an ophthalmoscope. Six months later the metacarpal post was lengthened and the previous flap thinned to deepen his web space. Eight months after the accident, the patient returned to his previous occupation working as a packer and using his left hand. He has had return of hot and cold sensation. In November 1975 his two-point discrimination on his thumb was 9 mm on the radial side, 1 cm on the ulnar side and 6 mm on the dorsum. In May 1977, while using his hand, he stated that he had sudden onset of pain and swelling in the thumb after a traumatic episode. Radiographs obtained showed a non-displaced fracture of the metacarpal-metatarsal junction, which healed un-eventfully with simple splinting. He continues to have excellent function and participates in bowling and basketball on a limited basis (Figs. 18-7 to 18-11).

Multiple-digit amputations with partial thumb loss (pollicization or phal-angization possible). W.B. is a 59-year-old male who sustained a degloving injury to his dominant right hand in January 1975. He caught his hand in a grain elevator resulting in a dislocated wrist, avulsion injury to both phalanges

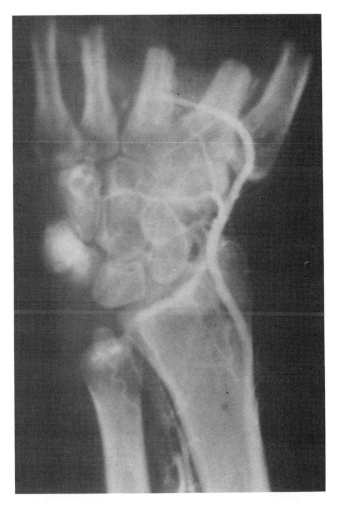

Fig. 18-7. J.P.'s preoperative arteriogram showing position of radial artery and branches suitable for anastomosis.

of the thumb, amputation through the proximal interphalangeal joint of the index finger, amputation through the metacarpals of the middle and ring fingers, and amputation through the metacarpal joint of the little finger. He was treated primarily with débridement and primary closure. He was referred for evaluation in November 1976. The index finger was noted to have zero to 40 degrees of motion at the metacarpophalangeal joint and a two-point discrimination of 1 cm of the stump. After preoperative angiography of the right arm and left leg, the patient underwent free vascularized transfer of the second and third toes to the second and fifth metacarpals (Fig. 18-14). The proximal phalanx of the index finger was then phalangized to the first metacarpal. He underwent bone grafting to the transferred toes for delayed union of the metacarpals and tendolysis of the flexor and extensor tendons at 4 postopera-

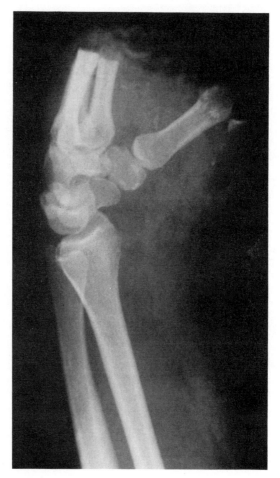

Fig. 18-8. Preoperative lateral radiogram of J.P. in December 1974 showing multiple digit amputation with absent thumb.

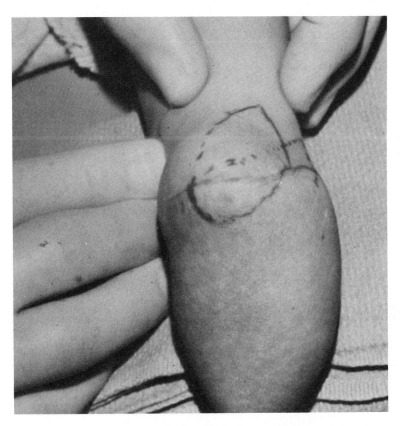

Fig. 18-9. At surgery, incision is marked on thumb-recipient site. The skin coverage provided by the previous groin flap is illustrated. (J.P., May 1974)

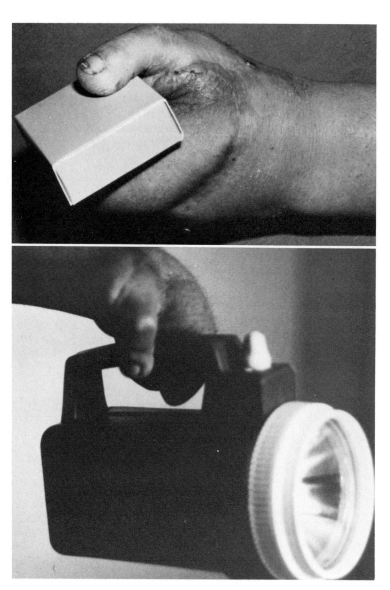

Fig. 18-10. J.P. at 8 months postoperatively is able to grasp large objects and has a two-point discrimination radially of 9 mm and ulnarly of 1 cm.

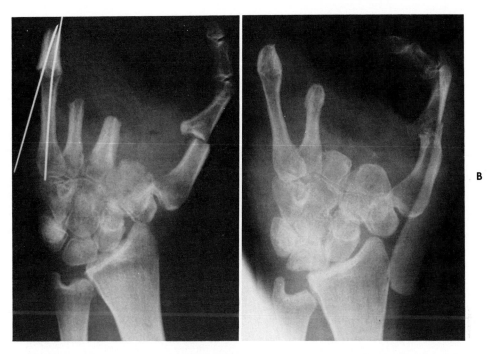

B

Fig. 18-11. A, J.P. at 2 months postoperatively. Anteroposterior radiograph of position of toe transfer and metacarpal bone graft with fixation. **B,** Nondisplaced fracture of thumb sustained 30 months postoperatively is shown splinted. Fracture healed uneventfully with conservative management.

tive months. On examination in June 1978, he was noted to have protective sensation and was using his hand at work. The only complaint was some degree of cold intolerance with weather changes (Figs. 18-12 to 18-17).

Multiple-digit amputations with partial thumb loss (pollicization or phalangization not possible). S.G. is an 11-year-old right-handed female who sustained an electrical burn to her left hand at age 4. Her thumb was amputated at the metacarpophalangeal joint and the index and middle fingers were deeply burned. She was initially treated with multiple skin grafts. In August 1976 she presented with a contracture of the first web space and a contracted nonfunctional index finger unsuited for pollicization. The middle finger was also scarred and contracted from previous grafting. A transfer of the right second toe to the thumb metacarpal along with a ray amputation of the nonfunctional index finger was performed. One postoperative year later she had a two-point discrimination of 5 mm and good range of motion with ability to oppose, abduct, and extend the thumb. Postoperative night splinting was used for prevention of a web-space contracture (Figs. 18-18 to 18-20).

H.D., a 29-year-old white female, was initially seen in the emergency room in April 1974 with a crush injury of the left hand with complete amputation of the left ring finger at the carpometacarpal area, comminuted fracture of the

Text continued on p. 253.

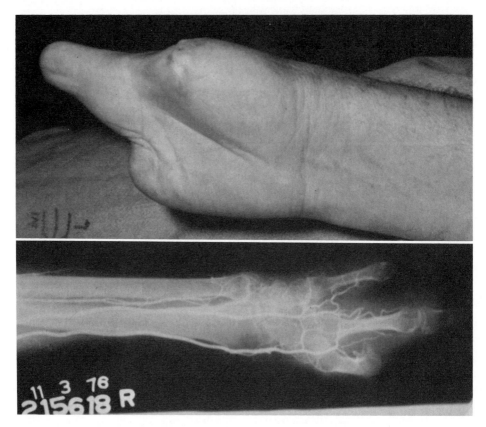

Fig. 18-12. W.B.'s preoperative condition and arteriogram showing multiple digit amputations with partial thumb loss. Index finger used for phalangization.

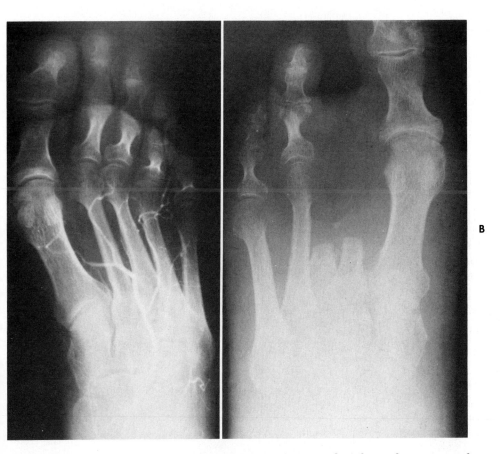

B

Fig. 18-13. A, Preoperative arteriogram of W.B. showing dorsalis pedis artery and branches. **B,** Postoperative anteroposterior radiograph showing level of metatarsal resection.

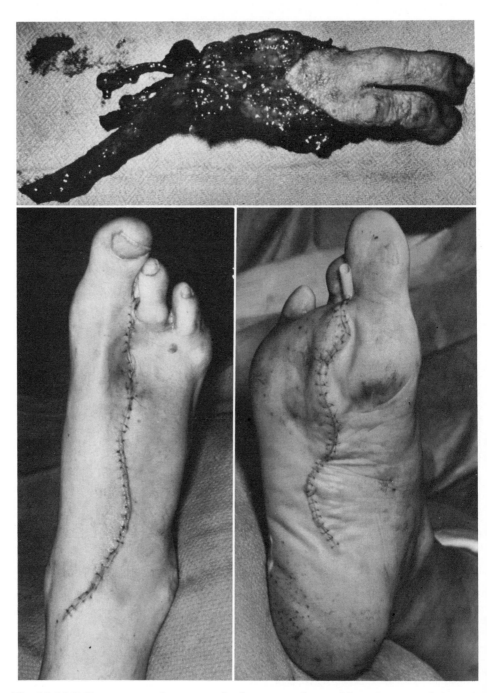

Fig. 18-14. W.B. at surgery showing multiple toe transfers and foot after wound closure.

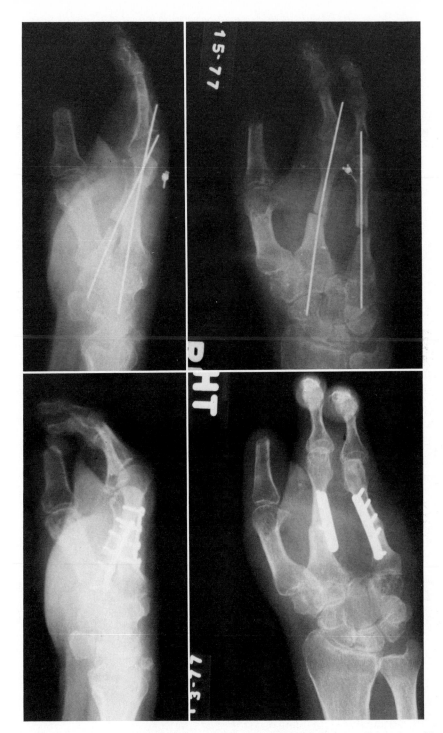

Fig. 18-15. Postoperative radiographs showing initial Kirschner wire fixation and bone grafting done 4 months later on toe transfers. Pollicized index finger is also shown. (W.B.)

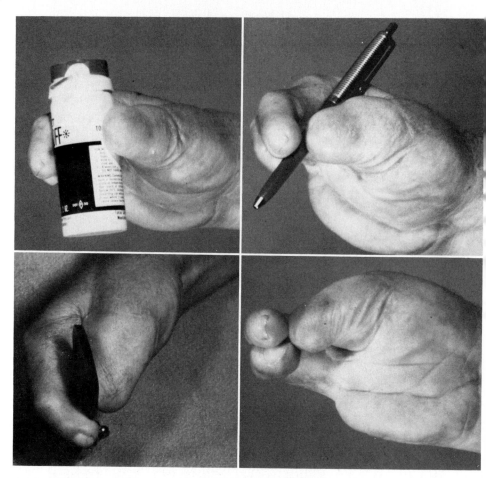

Fig. 18-16. W.B. 17 months postoperatively can grasp large objects, support a pen, and pinch small objects.

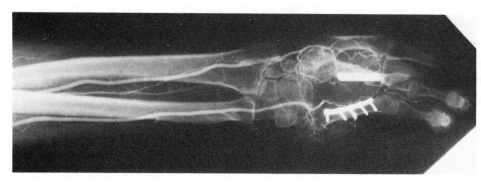

Fig. 18-17. Postoperatively at 16 months, arteriogram shows digital blood supply to transferred digits.

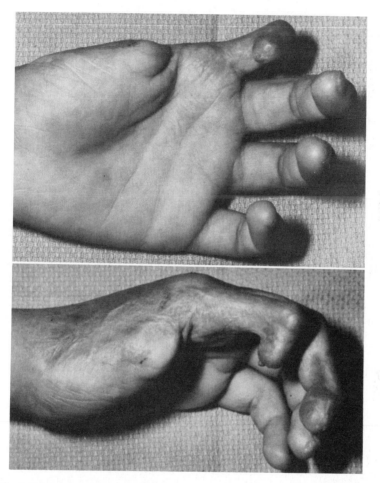

Fig. 18-18. S.G.'s preoperative contractures of index and middle finger with partial thumb loss. (Pollicization not possible.)

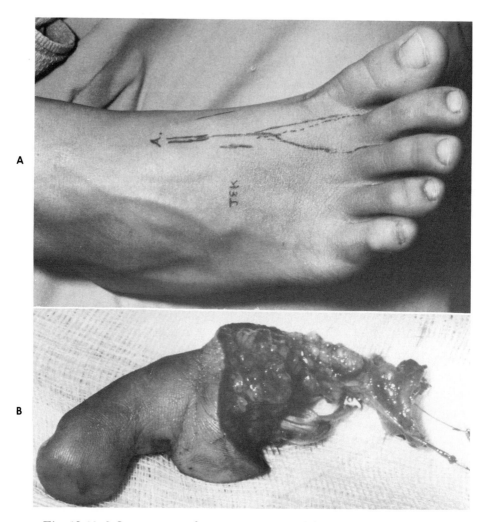

Fig. 18-19. S.G. at surgery showing incision and free vascularized toe graft.

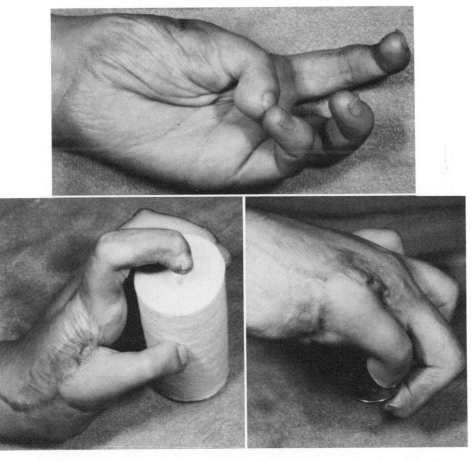

Fig. 18-20. S.G. at 4 months postoperatively is shown opposing thumb to little finger, and grasp-pinch function is present.

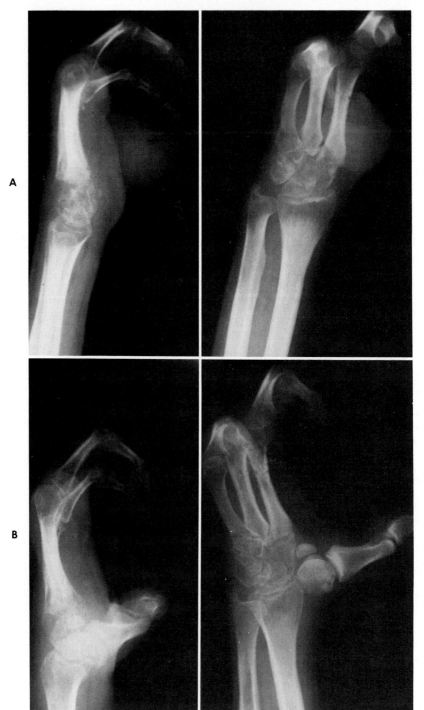

Fig. 18-21. A, H.D.'s preoperative radiographs after punch-press injury and failed replantation attempt. **B,** Postoperative radiograph of her great-toe transfer.

fourth metacarpal, dislocation of the second, third, and fifth metacarpals from the distal carpal row and amputation of the thumb with destruction of the flexor tendons of all fingers. She initially underwent exploration and débridement of the wounds, immobilization of the fractures, repair of the flexor tendons of the thumb, index, and long fingers, arterial repair of the index and long fingers and radial artery to the thumb. She was followed in the office and was found to have nonviability of the thumb, thenar eminence, and volar aspect of the little finger. She was readmitted to the hospital for amputation and groin pedicle flap coverage. Eight months after her initial injury, she underwent transfer of the left great toe to the left hand. She was discharged approximately 2 weeks after the transfer and was doing well. However, she returned to the hospital 5 days later complaining of coldness and pallor of the toe transplant. She was taken to surgery where an exploration of the vascular anastomosis revealed complete thrombosis of the artery. A saphenous vein graft was then used to replace the thrombosed vessel. Postoperatively, the vein graft was occluded, and subsequent thrombectomy and arteriotomy were performed. Skin necrosis developed in several areas of the transferred digit. However, it continued to survive. One month after the transfer, the necrotic tip of the thumb and the web space of the digit transfer required a split-thickness skin graft. She was discharged from the hospital 1 week later. No further vascular complications were noted, and the toe remained viable. When last evaluated 2½ years postoperatively, she was using her left hand as an assist (Fig. 18-21).

REFERENCES

1. Buncke, H. J., McLean, D. H., George, P. T., et al.: Thumb replacement. Great toe transplantation by microvascular anastomosis, Br. J. Plast. Surg. **26**:194, 1973.
2. Cobbett, J. R.: Free digital transfer. Report of a case of transfer of a great toe to replace an amputated thumb, J. Bone Joint Surg. **51-B**:677, 1969.
3. Kelleher, J. C., Sullivan, J. C., Biabak, G. J., et al.: "On top plasty" for amputated fingers, Plast. Reconstr. Surg. **42**:242-248, 1968.
4. Littler, J. W.: On making a thumb: one hundred years of surgical effort, J. Hand Surg. 1(1):35, 1976.
5. Littler, J. W.: Restoration of the amputated thumb. In Littler, J. W., Cramer, L. M., and Smith, J. W., editors: Symposium on reconstructive hand surgery, St. Louis, 1974, The C. V. Mosby Co., pp. 202-212.
6. Murray, J. F.: The missing thumb. In Littler, J. W., Cramer, L. M., and Smith, J. W., editors: Symposium on reconstructive hand surgery, St. Louis, 1974, The C. V. Mosby Co., pp. 214-221.
7. Nicoladoni, C.: Daumenplastik und organischer Ersatz der Fingerspitze (Anticheiroplastik und Daktyloplastik), Arch. Klin. Chir. **61**:606, 1900.
8. O'Brien, B. M., MacLeod, A. M., Sykes, P. J., et al.: Hallux to hand transfer, Hand 7:128-133, 1975.
9. O'Brien, B. M., MacLeod, A. M., Sykes, P. J., Browning, F. S. C., and Threlfall, G. N.: Microvascular second toe transfer for digital reconstruction, J. Hand Surg. 3(2):123-133, 1978.

19. Free vascularized bone grafts

Joseph E. Kutz
Cathy B. Thomson

Bone grafting has long been a surgically direct method of accomplishing many objectives. These include bridging bony defects caused by bone loss secondary to trauma, defects secondary to fibrous nonunions, defects secondary to bony absorption after disuse or infection, and defects associated with reconstructive surgery. The main purpose of the grafting is related to the clinical situation in which it is employed. However, generally it can be stated that grafting provides the needed bone matrix onto which osteoblasts lay down new osteoid. Gradually the defects fill in with new bone, and in time under the forces of normal stress, a solid bony union is formed. The factors that are now known to promote healing are the use of cancellous graft, rigid fixation of the graft, absence of infection, good neighboring tissue vascularity and viability, and normal, durable skin coverage. Normal sensitivity is not mandatory but has been observed to be associated with long-term acceptable results.

A free vascularized bone graft uses all the above principles and adds the specific advantage of supplying its own vascularized pedicle. The technique (described on p. 256) includes microsurgical dissection, and an arteriovenous anastomosis is performed to guarantee increased vascularity to the recipient area. This is believed to increase incidence and rates of healing allowing the patient to be mobilized earlier. The indications are similar to those described for bone grafting above. However, because of the advantages of a pedicle blood supply, clinical experience has revealed other advantages associated with the procedure. These include bridging large defects such as needed in ablative injuries of the upper and lower limbs, ablative surgery for bone tumors, large segmental nonunions, epiphyseal arrest injuries, and congenital disorders, that is, radial or ulnar clubhand. The possibilities of restoration of a joint surface and preservation of the growing epiphysis adds tremendous application and clinical scope to this procedure.

HISTORICAL REVIEW

Since the report of Strauch, Bloomberg, and Lewin[4] in 1971 who reconstructed the jaw in a dog using a rib graft with its vascular pedicle, few other successful experimental models have been reported. A vascular pedicle was divided and reanastomosed in dogs by McCullough and Fredrickson[2] in 1973. In 1974, Ostrup and Fredrickson[3] reported direct free transfer using microvascular anastomotic techniques of living rib bone grafts to the mandible in dogs. They emphasized the importance of the endosteal (nutrient) blood supply. In 1975 Taylor[5] et al. described the actual technique employed in two patients with ablative injuries to the lower limbs. In 1977 Taylor[6] again summarized the technique and added one additional case. The purpose of this discussion is to present additional clinical experience as well as varied methods of technique that have proved to be successful.

PREOPERATIVE ASSESSMENT

The status of the *recipient site* is evaluated along with length of the defect to be bridged, presence of possible sepsis, viability and vascularity of surrounding soft tissue, and quality of available skin coverage.

Bony defect. A bony defect is measured on routine radiographs and estimated from a clinical exam. The size of the donor graft will vary depending on the recipient defect length and also on the type of fixation chosen. A variety of fixations have been employed and involve both internal and external devices. The choice depends on the recipient site and the experience of the surgeon. One should choose a device that allows the patient to be mobilized as early as possible while still providing rigid fixation of the graft (usually with the addition of plaster of paris).

Vascularity. A preoperative arteriogram of the recipient site is obtained (anteroposterior and lateral views), and an anastomosis site is chosen. Careful dissection is carried out in this area so as not to injure the vessels. Once identified, they are staged with microclips and protected from trauma until the anastomosis is completed.

Viability. The status of the soft tissue is evaluated at the time of surgery. Necrotic areas of tissue are debrided and all viable muscle, fascia, and subcutaneous fat layers are preserved.

Sepsis. A thorough débridement is carried out, and cultures are obtained. Clinical experience has shown that vascularized bone grafting has been successful both in chronic and subacute bone infections if careful attention is given to débridement, rigid fixation, and adequate skin coverage.

Skin coverage. The quality and amount of local skin is carefully assessed preoperatively. Insufficient or poor-quality skin does not necessarily preclude grafting. Local flaps and delayed flaps transplanted from the donor site have been used with success. Flap coverage is superior to skin grafting (either full- or split-thickness) and should be used first.

The status of the *donor area* is also evaluated as to available length, vascularity, presence of an epiphysis, skin coverage, and site.

Donor length. Donor length is determined by measurement on routine radiographs. Lengths of up to 25 cm have been obtained from the fibula without postoperative functional deficits. Multiple grafts involving adjacent rib segments are also available.

Vascularity. A preoperative arteriogram is advised because of the normal anatomic variations present when the fibula is considered. The vessels available include the geniculate arteries surrounding the knee and the peroneal arteries. A knowledge of the normal anatomy and its variations is mandatory both for interpretation of the arteriogram and isolation of the vessels at surgery. The vascularity of the rib graft is less subject to variation, and the anterior and posterior intercostal vessels are identified without difficulty.

Epiphysis. The presence of a growth center depends on the goal of the procedure. The proximal head of the fibula has been used clinically and appears to represent a reasonable donor.

Skin coverage. A large recipient defect can be covered with local flaps as well as skin attached to the donor-graft site. Clinically successful experience has been seen when adjacent rib segments and the surrounding skin from the chest wall are grafted. A delay of 10 to 14 days is required and the graft is transferred with surrounding soft tissue and skin flaps. Other methods of coverage include the standard flaps, such as the groin flap, latissimus dorsi flap, and abdominal pedicle flap, done before the grafting procedure.

Site. The donor site choice depends on the length and type of defect to be covered, the preference of the surgeon, and the general condition of the patient. Rib grafts postoperatively require a chest tub and conscientious pulmonary toilet. Fibula grafts postoperatively require a period of plaster immobilization and non–weight bearing ambulation. No permanent functional loss has been noted after either procedure.

After the preoperative evaluation is finished, the procedure is performed according to the standard technique of rigid bone fixation, microsurgical arteriovenous anastomosis, and skin coverage, as outlined. Heparin has not been used postoperatively but low molecular weight dextran (LMD) and aspirin in routine dosages has been so employed. The fixation devices are maintained until bony union is apparent on radiographs. Weight-bearing where appropriate is encouraged and joint range of motion is emphasized as well as muscle-strengthening exercises. Postoperative fracture through the graft has been seen, but with standard treatment the fracture healed spontaneously. Infections and nonunions have not been noted.

PROCEDURE (TECHNIQUE)

The operation can be performed with one or two teams. The preoperative planning just outlined is a integral part in the determination of the success or failure of the procedure.

Preparation of recipient site

An incision is made to expose the bony defect so that adequate exposure is allowed but no compromise of the skin circulation. Meticulous dissection with use of magnification is needed for identification of the vessels to be used for anastomosis. Minimal trauma to the adjacent soft tissue is imperative to minimize postoperative swelling. The ends of the bony defect are fashioned with a rongeur and curette so that briskly bleeding bone is exposed. The soft tissues are kept moist with irrigating solutions of Ringer's lactate with or without prophylactic antibiotics added. The defect is then remeasured and attention is given to the donor site.

Preparation of donor site

Rib graft. The chest is prepped and draped in the usual manner. A transverse incision is made over the ribs to be transferred. Dissection is directed to isolation of the anterior and posterior intercostal vessels that are tagged for use in the anastomosis. The rib or ribs are divided with a bone cutter and transferred with its periosteal blood supply intact. The defect is then closed primarily after insertion of a chest tube. The rib segments measuring up to 30 cm can be obtained, and multiple segments can be transferred (with or without delaying the pedicle). An articular surface is available and the adjacent muscle, overlying skin and nerve, are transferred with the pedicle. There is no epiphyseal growth center available in contrast to the fibula graft.

Fibula graft. An incision is made over the posterolateral margin of the fibula, and dissection is carried down to the muscular layer surrounding the bone. Care is taken to preserve the "periosteal sleeve" of the segment to be transferred as well as some surrounding soft tissue. This is done to protect the periosteal blood supply. The vessels for anastomosis are identified and include the peroneal arteries or the lateral geniculate arteries. Microsurgical technique is used to prepare the vessels for anastomosis.

Arteriovenous anastomosis and fixation of graft

Primary anastomosis of the artery and vein is carried out, and occasionally a vein graft is employed. It is important that the anastomosis fulfills the basic principles of microsurgical technique. There should be no tension, no opportunity for the vascular stalk to kink on itself, and positive patency tests of both artery and vein (Acland[1]). The fixation device is applied before the anastomosis so that there is no chance of disruption. Devices including external fixation (Hofman, Wagner) and internal fixation (AO compression plates, screws, Steinman pins) are used alone or sometimes in conjunction with each other so that *rigid fixation* is accomplished. If an articular surface is being transferred, a Kirschner wire or Steinman pin is used to immobilize the joint. Hemovac drainage is left in place for 48 to 72 hours. Postoperative management with low molecular weight dextran and aspirin is common, and heparin is not prescribed. The extremity is splinted in a position of function, and plaster immobilization is continued until bony union is seen on routine radiographs.

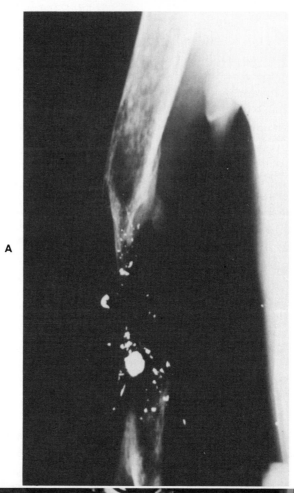

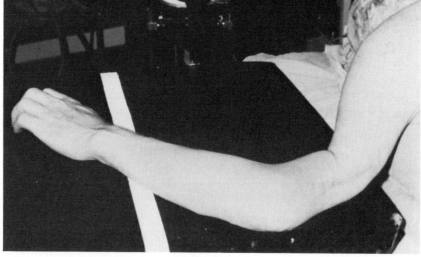

Fig. 19-1. A, Anteroposterior radiograph of R.L. showing large bony defect of midshaft humerus secondary to gunshot wound. **B,** Preoperative view showing flail upper extremity. (**A** and **B** from Weiland, A. J., Kleinert, H. E., Kutz, J. E., and Daniel, R. K.: Vascularized bone grafts in the upper extremity. In Serafin, D., and Buncke, H., editors: Microsurgical composite tissue transplantation, St. Louis, 1979, The C. V. Mosby Co.)

INDICATIONS

Clinical experience has shown the following case illustrations to represent appropriate applications of the technique described.

Ablative injuries of extremities. R.L., a 34-year-old white male, presented with pain in the left arm. He had sustained a gunshot wound that resulted in a large bony defect and flail left arm secondary to radial nerve palsy. He underwent fibular bone graft to the humeral defect and neurolysis of the radial

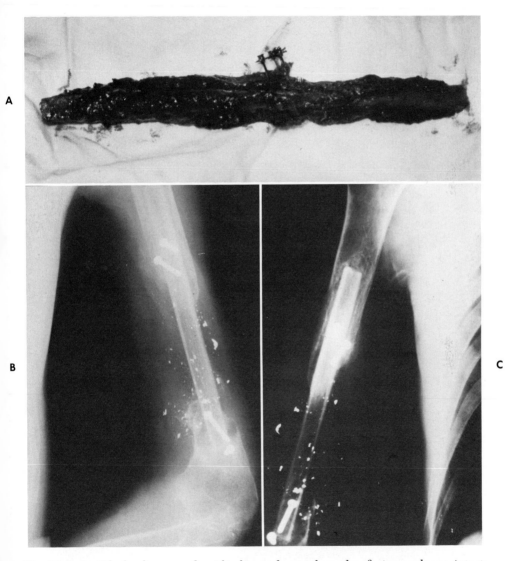

Fig. 19-2. A, Fibular bone graft with clamped vessels and soft-tissue sleeve intact. Measures 17 cm. **B** and **C,** Fibular bone graft respectively 2 and 3 months postoperatively showing callus formation and viability of graft.

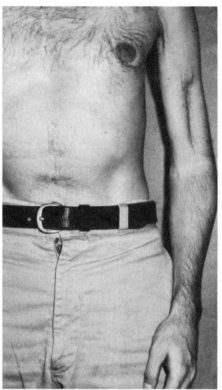

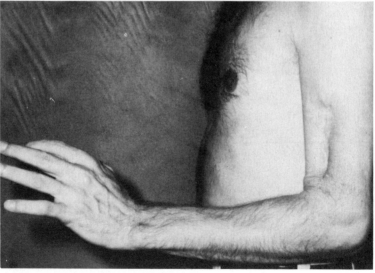

Fig. 19-3. At 13 months postoperatively there is a stable humerus with good alignment. Range of motion of elbow, 15 to 90 degrees.

nerve in December 1976. The graft measured 17 cm and was inserted into the intramedullary canal of the two humeral fragments. The graft was secured with cortical screws. Postoperative radiographs show incorporation of the graft, and the arm is no longer flail. He regained function of his radial nerve. (See Figs. 19-1 to 19-4.)

Ablative surgery for bone tumors. I.C., a 43-year-old white female, was seen because of complaints of pain in the left wrist and forearm. On radiologic examination, she had a large radiolucent defect involving the distal radius with pathologic fracture. Tissue diagnosis of giant cell tumor was confirmed during surgery. An en bloc resection of the tumor was performed, and a fibular graft was obtained. An anastomosis of the radial and inferior lateral geniculate arteries was performed. A compression plate as well as multiple pins was applied. Postoperative radiographs at 4 months showed callus formation at the osteotomy site. (See Figs. 19-5 to 19-10.)

Large segmental nonunions. G.P., a 19-year-old white male, was injured in a motorcycle accident in May 1977. He sustained a severe brachial plexus injury, fractures of the metacarpals of the left hand, and an open comminuted fracture of the left tibia. The tibial fracture received standard treatment but resulted in a large segmental nonunion involving approximately 8 inches of bony defect. There was also an associated skin defect with tibia exposed. This was treated unsuccessfully with multiple skin grafts and débridements. The fibular grafting was done in two procedures. The first procedure involved a delay of the ribs (eighth and ninth) and overlying soft tissue and skin (19 × 31 cm in anteroposterior dimension). A second-stage procedure involved transfer of the free flap graft 14 days later. Internal fixation (K-wire) and external fixation (Tower apparatus) was employed. (See Figs. 19-11 to 19-15.)

Epiphyseal arrest injuries. S.S. was born with a congenital skin defect involving the right forearm. At 3 weeks the ulcer was debrided and closed. At 1 month a second débridement was necessary for ulceration and necrosis. She

Text continued on p. 273.

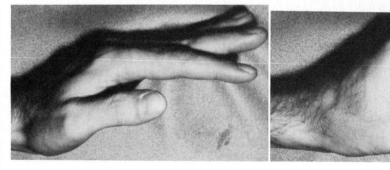

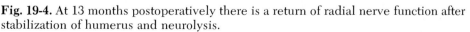

Fig. 19-4. At 13 months postoperatively there is a return of radial nerve function after stabilization of humerus and neurolysis.

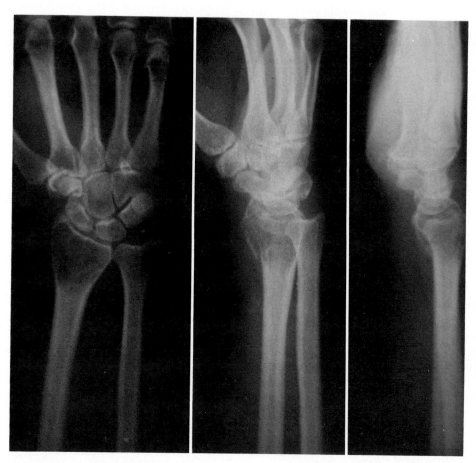

Fig. 19-5. I.C. presented with painful wrist and pathologic fracture of distal radius.

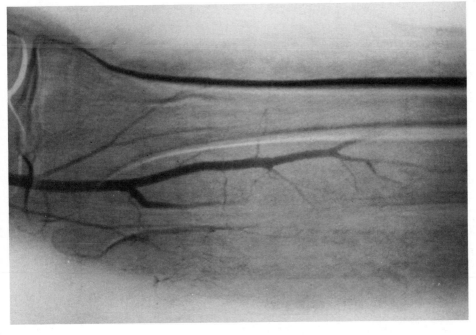

Fig. 19-6. Preoperative arteriogram shows position of geniculate and peroneal vessels in donor site.

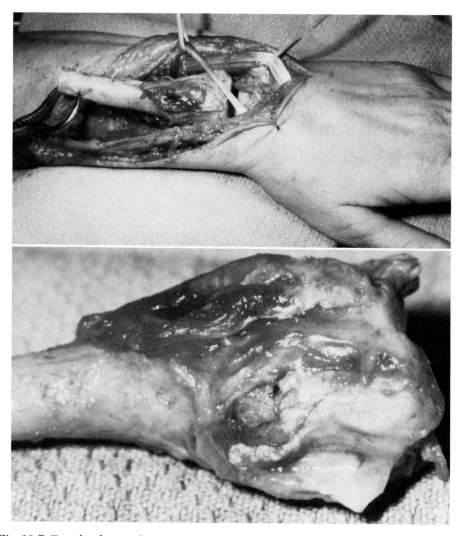

Fig. 19-7. Distal radius is shown at surgery. Pathologic specimen was giant cell tumor.

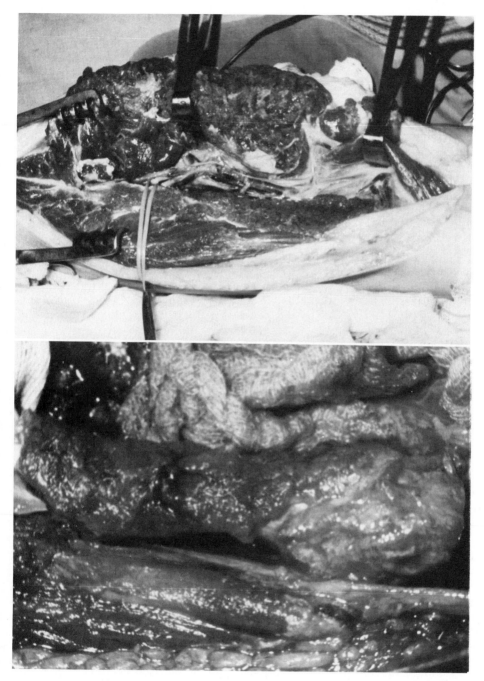

Fig. 19-8. Approach to fibula at surgery with arteriovenous supply marked. Graft is taken with soft-tissue (and endosteal) sleeve intact.

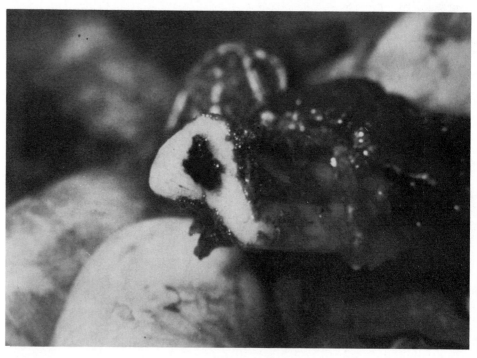

Fig. 19-9. Graft end at surgery illustrating endosteal blood supply and tagged feeding vessels.

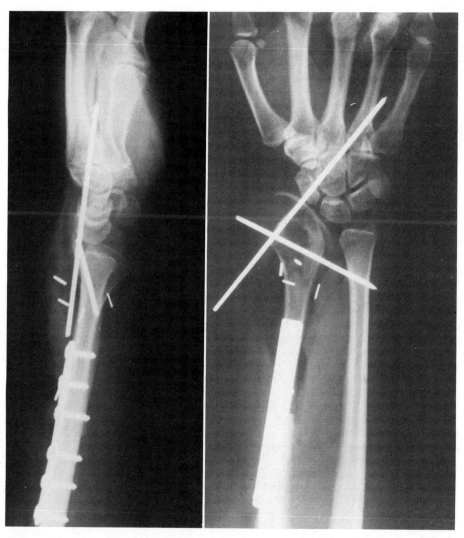

Fig. 19-10. Postoperative radiographs showing fixation of graft with plate and joint with Kirschner wire.

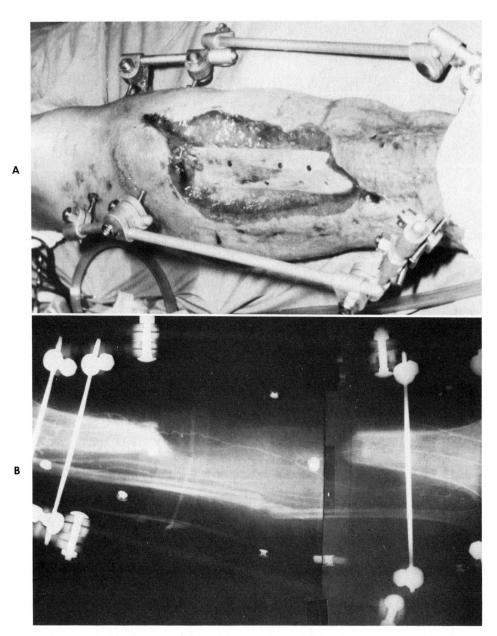

Fig. 19-11. A, Preoperative photo showing exposed tibia and large skin defect. **B,** Preoperative arteriogram performed in Tower apparatus of recipient site showing tibia defect and nonunion of fibula.

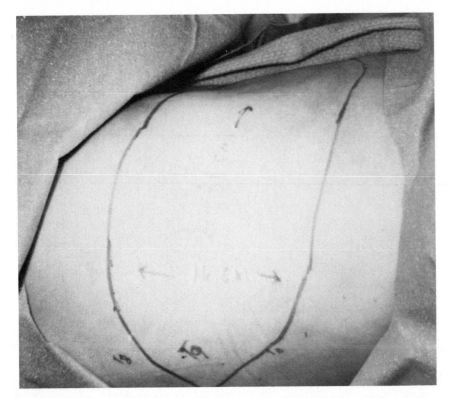

Fig. 19-12. First-stage procedure of raising rib flap is shown outlined in ink before incision is made.

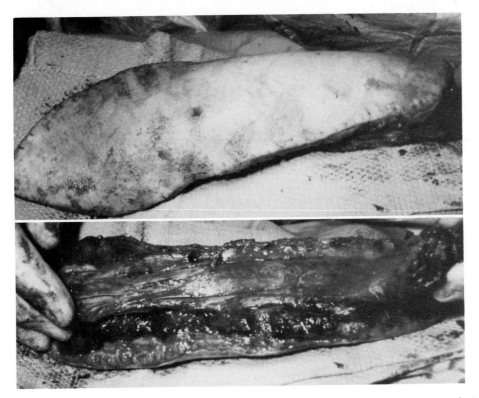

Fig. 19-13. Second-stage procedure performed 2 weeks later shows free rib (8 and 9) vascularized bone graft with surrounding muscle and skin.

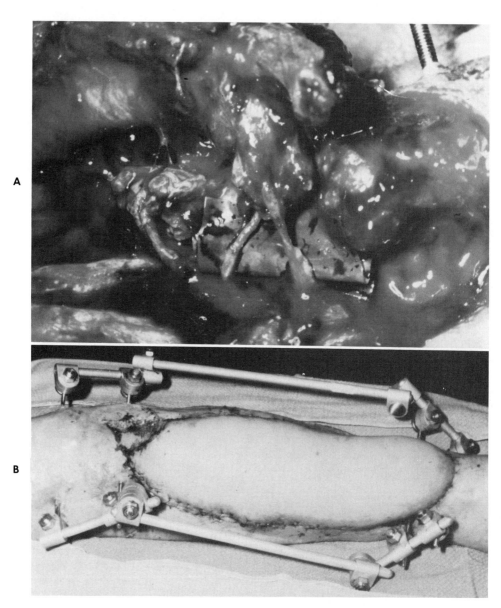

Fig. 19-14. A, Arteriovenous anastomosis at recipient site before wound closure. **B,** Clinical photograph taken 11 days postoperatively shows viability of skin flap and the absence of previous skin defect. Tower apparatus is in place.

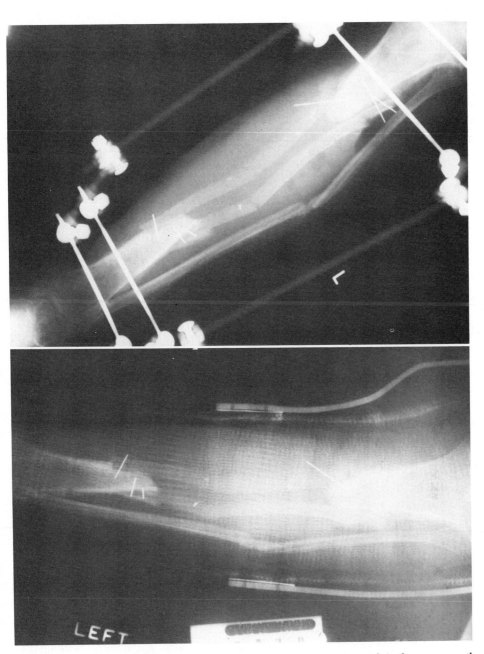

Fig. 19-15. A, Anteroposterior radiograph (10 days postoperatively) shows two rib segments secured in place by the use of multiple pins. The Tower apparatus was subsequently incorporated in the long leg cast, which was later applied. **B,** Recent radiograph shows G.P. fitted with a cast brace 3½ months postoperatively to begin ambulation.

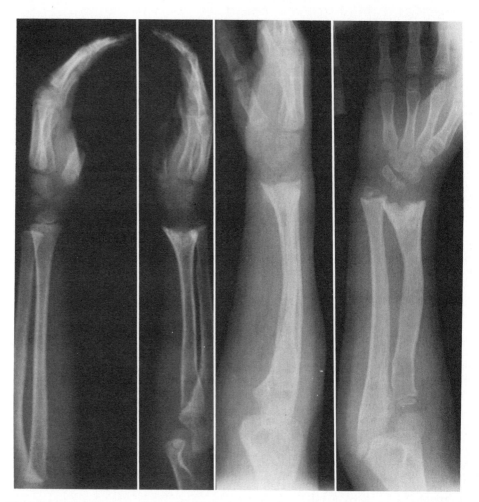

Fig. 19-16. Preoperative views showing absence of radial epiphysis in 1973 (S.S.) and 1975 with destruction and resorption of the radius. (From Weiland, A. J., Kleinert, H. E., Kutz, J. E., and Daniel, R. K.: Vascularized bone grafts in the upper extremity. In Serafin, D., and Buncke, H., editors: Microsurgical composite tissue transplantation, St. Louis, 1979, The C. V. Mosby Co.)

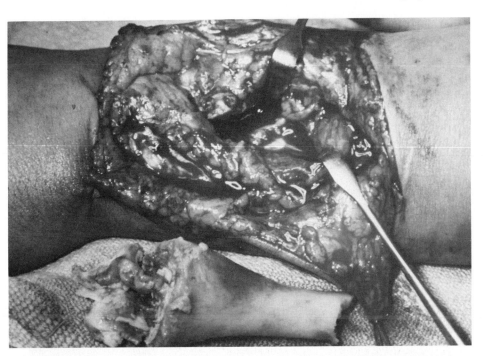

Fig. 19-17. S.S. at surgery showing specimen of radius excised. Note absence of epiphysis and large amount of granulation tissue. (From Weiland, A. J., Kleinert, H. E., Kutz, J. E., and Daniel, R. K.: Vascularized bone grafts in the upper extremity. In Serafin, D., and Buncke, H., editors: Microsurgical composite tissue transplantation, St. Louis, 1979, The C. V. Mosby Co.)

was followed and at age 7 was admitted for tendon transfer to correct a progressive radial deviation of the wrist. Radiographs showed absorption of the distal radial epiphysis. Clinically on measurement of the forearms on radiographs, there was a 6.2 cm limb-length discrepancy. Therefore at the age of 8 years she underwent a transfer of the proximal fibular epiphysis to the distal radius. The inferior lateral geniculate and radial artery (metacarpal branch) were anastomosed. Postoperatively the fibular epiphysis remained open for 15 months. On the last examination in June 1978, she was considered for a radial lengthening procedure to decrease the limb discrepancy, which remains. (See Figs. 19-16 to 19-21.)

Congenital disorders. A radial or ulnar clubhand might in the future be reconstructed by use of the microvascular fibula graft (Fig. 19-22).

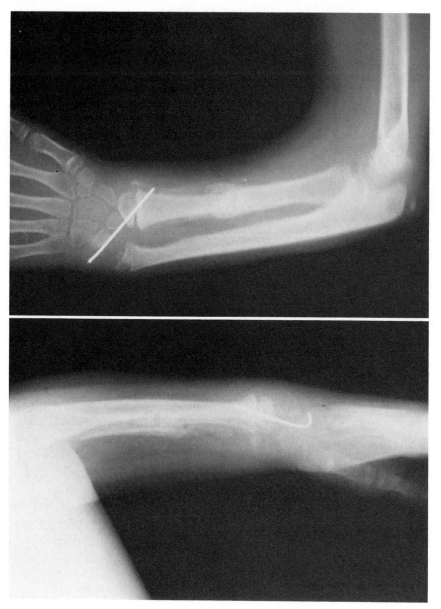

Fig. 19-18. Postoperative views showing position of fibula graft and callus formation at 5 weeks. (S.S.)

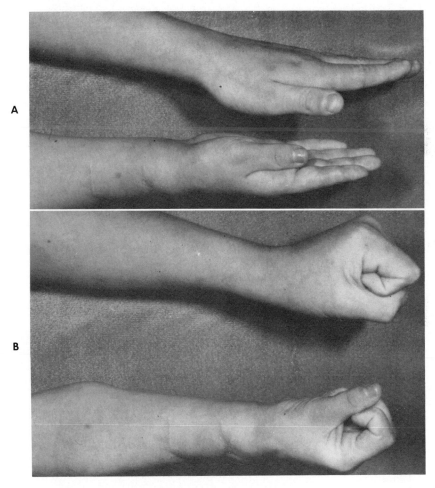

Fig. 19-19. Postoperative views. **A,** Limb-length discrepancy present preoperatively, and **B,** hand function.

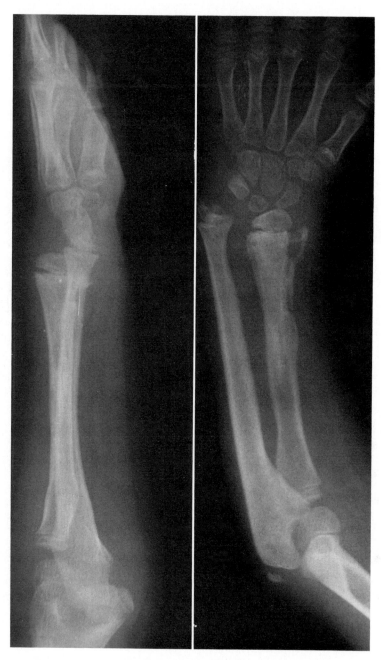

Fig. 19-20. Five months postoperatively, healed graft and open epiphysis.

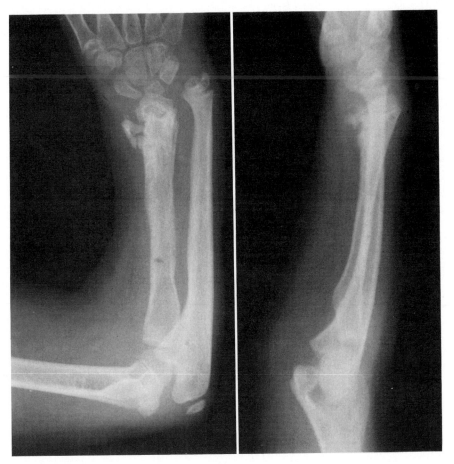

Fig. 19-21. Thirteen months postoperatively, radial epiphysis.

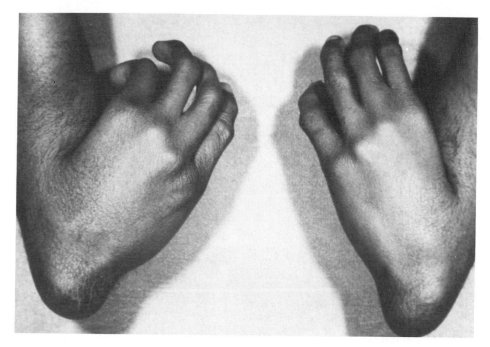

Fig. 19-22. Radial or ulnar clubhand might in the future be reconstructed by use of microvascular fibula graft.

REFERENCES

1. Acland, R.: Signs of patency in small vessel anastomosis, Surgery **72**:744, 1972.
2. McCullough, D. W., and Fredrickson, J. M.: Neovascularized rib grafts to reconstruct mandibular defects, Can. J. Otolaryngol. **2**:96, 1973.
3. Ostrup, L. T., and Fredrickson, J. M.: Distant transfer of a free living bone graft by microvascular anastomoses, Plast. Reconstr. Surg. **54**:274, 1974.
4. Strauch, B., Bloomberg, A. E., and Lewin, M. C.: An experimental approach to mandibular replacement: island vascular composite rib grafts, Br. J. Plast. Surg. **24**:334, 1971.
5. Taylor, I. G., Miller, G. D. H., and Ham, F. J.: The free vascularized bone graft, Plast. Reconstr. Surg. **55**(5):533, May 1975.
6. Taylor, I. G.: Microvascular free bone transfer. A clinical technique, Orthop. Clin. North Am. **8**(2):425, April 1977.

20. Microvascular free groin flap

James B. Steichen

Acquiring coverage for difficult problems of composite tissue loss, including skin and subcutaneous layers in the extremities, is occasionally a very challenging problem (Fig. 20-1). If distant flap coverage is required and conventional techniques of attached flaps are not suitable or are unavailable, the need arises for a flap that may be transferred to any part of the body to provide for immediate cover of exposed vital tissues. The development of microvascular surgical techniques and the development of axial pattern donor sites have paved the way for the free flap, which is an immediate one-stage composite-tissue transfer of skin and subcutaneous tissue with distant microvascular anastomoses and restoration of circulation to the transferred tissue.

The design of skin flaps, prior to microvascular transfer, and their corresponding length-to-breadth ratios have been based on their vascular anatomy and have been categorized as either random pattern flaps without any significant predictable vascular pattern or axial pattern flaps based on a predictable arteriovenous trunk supplying the direct axis of the flap.

The vascular supply to certain areas of the skin may be by musculocutaneous vessels, which penetrate the skin through the muscle and supply directly only a small segment of skin overlying the muscle, or by direct cutaneous vessels, which supply a large expanse of skin. Isolated areas of the body have been identified as being supplied by direct cutaneous vessels, and these areas of composite tissues are available for flaps with greater freedom from vascular compromise and also for free-flap donor tissue.

Conventionally attached random-pattern flaps, such as abdominal, chest, and cross-leg flaps, have many limitations based on their random vascular supply. The length of the flap may need to be closely related to a ratio of its width, which means that if a flap is long, it may have to be much wider than needed. The flap must be attached for several weeks to the donor site, an operation that may cause adjacent joint stiffness, such as a frozen shoulder. In the lower extremity, cross-leg flaps have been used if available, and multiple procedures may be necessary over a long period of time so that this type of flap may be successfully transferred. The lower extremities may be immobilized

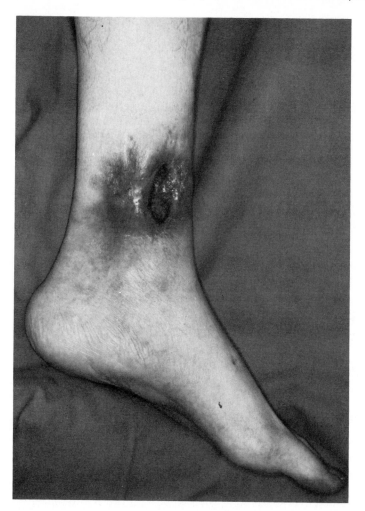

Fig. 20-1. A 47-year-old man with a 4-year history of an open draining osteomyelitis of the left medial distal tibia unresponsive to débridement and skin grafting.

together for a prolonged period of time, which is not ideal. Occasionally, there may not be an opposite lower extremity available for this type of transfer, as in the case of amputation, peripheral vascular disease, or venous stasis bilaterally. There are, therefore, many cases where the random-pattern flap is not advisable.

Attached axial-pattern flaps, such as groin, deltopectoral, and hypogastric flaps, have given the freedom to use these donor areas to cover a wider range of difficult skin-coverage problems. These axial-pattern flaps based on direct cutaneous vessels can be very long and narrow and the base easily tubed to transfer skin to distant recipient sites that would be difficult to cover correctly by a random-pattern flap. These flaps, however, still must be attached for several weeks, a period of time compounding the problem of stiffness of immobilized joints, and they may also not be able to reach the recipient area.

INDICATIONS FOR A FREE FLAP

There are physically many anatomic areas that are very difficult to reach if necessary by either a random-pattern flap or an attached axial-pattern flap. The lower extremity especially is difficult to provide coverage to by attached flaps. There are also many patients who because of either previous injury, medical condition or age may develop serious and irreversible problems of stiffness if they were required to be immobile for a 2- to 4-week period of time.

The indications, then, for free one-stage flaps to the extremities are many.

The greatest indication and usefulness of a free flap is for a composite tissue defect of the extremities with bone or other vital tissue exposed, whether created by trauma or iatrogenically during a reconstructive procedure. If a random-pattern flap or an attached axial-pattern flap is unavailable or, even more importantly, may have been tried and failed, then a free flap is the treatment of choice.

If the patient is elderly or may have injury to adjacent joints, the position of immobilization and length of immobilization for an attached flap may be impossible and a free flap may be able to provide coverage and not compound the existing problems.

ADVANTAGES OF FREE FLAPS VERSUS ATTACHED
AXIAL-PATTERN FLAPS

There are many reasons why a free flap may be preferable to an attached axial-pattern flap, as many reasons have already been outlined why an attached axial-pattern flap may be preferable to an attached random-pattern flap.

A free one-stage flap coverage may require only one operative procedure and only one anesthetic procedure for the patient in order to achieve total skin coverage.

As there will be a totally closed wound at the end of the procedure, other reconstructive procedures may be accomplished at the same time if necessary, such as bone, tendon, or nerve grafts.

Unless there are other complications either preoperatively or postoperatively, the total period of hospitalization and the hospital expense will be much less than with multiple-staged procedures of skin coverage.

As the recipient is not attached to the donor site, mobilization may be maintained in adjacent joints almost fully and thus one would hope to prevent any additional stiffness or contracture.

The patient is less confined, more independent, and better able to take care of himself both physically and psychologically.

What may be the most important advantage of the free one-stage transfer with microvascular anastomoses, however, may be that it delivers fresh tissue to the recipient area with improved vascular supply, which is usually needed, and the flap does not draw on the surrounding skin for its own vascularity.

DISADVANTAGES OF FREE-FLAP TRANSFERS

Obviously, if there are advantages there are a few disadvantages.

The initial operative time and anesthetic time is usually longer than would be required for a conventional attached flap.

It is also not possible to successfully perform the procedure unless there is a satisfactory recipient artery present with normal flow to provide blood to the flap and adequate competent veins to drain the flap after revascularization.

Finally, there is a greater risk of complete loss of a free flap versus an attached flap if there is irreversible vascular compromise after the free transfer.

FREE-FLAP DONOR SITES

There have been many axial-pattern donor sites anatomically defined and clinically used for free innervated and noninnervated skin flaps to the extremities, such as groin or iliofemoral, deltopectoral, dorsum of the foot, first web space of the foot, scalp or forehead, and axillary. Many more donor sites are being investigated and used today, and more will become available with more anatomic research.

ADVANTAGE OF THE GROIN AS A FREE-FLAP DONOR SITE

The groin or iliofemoral flap is a desirable choice as a donor tissue for several reasons over other possible axial-flap donor sites. There are always axial vessels of predictable location and adequate size for transfer. The size of the flap that may be raised is essentially unlimited, and the axial vessels will support small as well as large flaps greater than at least 25 cm in length. The donor site can almost always be closed primarily with flexion of the hip and knee, eliminating the need for skin grafting the donor area. Most importantly, the donor defect and scar is cosmetically and functionally acceptable to the patient. The area is not on an exposed area of the body and is covered by clothing during almost all activities in which the patient would participate. This donor area also eliminates the possibility of a tender area created at other donor sites that might affect function, such as shoe wear on the dorsum of the foot.

SURGICAL ANATOMY OF GROIN FLAP

The anatomy of the groin flap has been well illustrated by several authors, including McGregor and Jackson.

The superficial circumflex iliac artery (SCIA) and vein (SCIV) are the direct cutaneous vessels that supply the groin flap.

The superficial circumflex iliac vein is the most superficial structure in the medial dissection of the flap and can be identified at the location of the saphenous bulb as it enters the fatty tissue in the femoral triangle region several centimeters distal to the inguinal ligament. The SCIV then joins the SCIA as it progresses laterally.

Additional predictable venous drainage from the flap is always present with the venae comitantes of the SCIA, which are always found deep to the SCIA at the femoral artery, arise from the femoral vein, and pass deep to the femoral artery as they drain the area of the flap.

Deeper dissection will reveal the femoral artery, and the SCIA will usually arise from the anterolateral side of the femoral artery about 1 cm distal to the inguinal ligament. The SCIA may arise separately or from a short common trunk associated with the superficial epigastric artery (SEA). The SCIA will then usually be found in a course parallel to the inguinal ligament, and as it progresses laterally, it may become slightly superior as it nears the anterior superior iliac spine.

The vessels may be superficial to the sartorius fascia or may be deep to it to the lateral level of the sartorius and then pierce the fascia lata and become more superficial as they progress laterally.

PREOPERATIVE EVALUATION

Careful evaluation of the vascular status of the donor groin area as well as the recipient site in the extremity is essential for planning of a successful free transfer. If the recipient site is on the upper extremity, the contralateral groin is selected as the initial donor site. This choice is made to prepare for the possibility of failure of the initial transfer, and thereby the ipsilateral flap would still be available for secondary coverage either as another free transfer or as an attached groin flap. One must evaluate the donor skin to be certain that there are no previous surgical or traumatic scars present that may have disturbed the axial flow of the superficial circumflex iliac vessels.

The vascular supply, arterial and venous, to both the donor and recipient areas is thoroughly defined and mapped out prior to the operation by use of clinical palpation, ultrasonic Doppler monitoring, and contrast arteriography.

The donor groin vessels can be evaluated by palpation of the femoral artery and auscultation if necessary to determine the clinical status of the vessel. The possible presence of flow abnormalities in the vessel may be elicited in this manner.

The ultrasonic Doppler monitor may be the best instrument for accurately determining the precise location of the superficial circumflex iliac artery (Fig. 20-2). One can identify the vessel's anatomic course by correct Doppler auscultation techniques and by finding the vessel just distal to the inguinal ligament as it leaves the femoral artery and tracing it laterally. The course and location of the vessel should then be accurately marked on the skin with indelible ink to be used later in determination of the location of the flap.

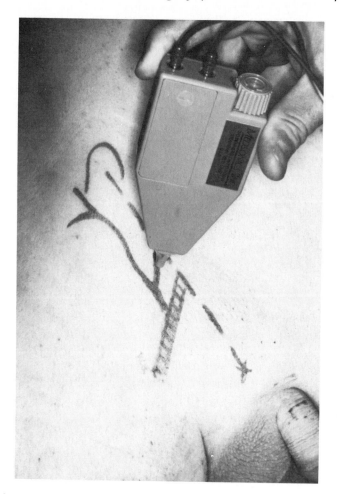

Fig. 20-2. Ultrasonic Doppler monitor used to preoperatively outline the anatomic path of the superficial circumflex iliac artery in the right side of groin.

The use of arteriography may contribute additional information about the arterial supply to the groin flap, but it is most beneficial in outlining the vascular status of the recipient area. If the technique of a femoral puncture is used for the arteriogram, the radiologist must be instructed not to use the femoral artery of the donor groin for the examination. When in the past, the same groin was used for the femoral puncture that was to be used the next day for the free flap, the dissection of the donor vessels in the femoral area was exceedingly difficult and time consuming because of the hematoma present and the difficulty in dissection of the SCIA and SCIV without damaging the small vessels.

One can identify the SCIA on the arteriogram by placing the pelvis in an oblique position (Fig. 20-3). The information obtained in the groin is helpful

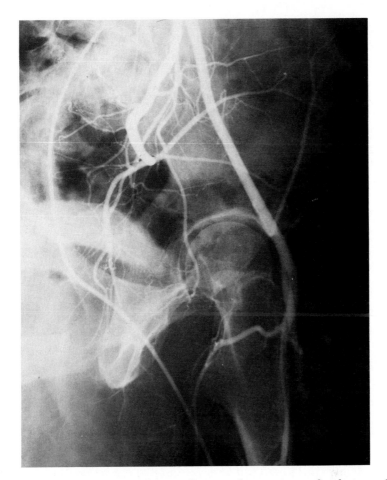

Fig. 20-3. Contrast arteriogram of femoral artery showing superficial circumflex iliac artery progressing laterally from the femoral artery with the patient in a slightly oblique position.

in the identification of any anatomic abnormalities to the vessel but is not so helpful in localization of the vessel as the information obtained with the ultrasonic Doppler monitor.

Peripheral arterial spasm at the time of arteriography may be relieved by the intra-arterial injection of tolazoline (Priscoline), which aids in the definition of the peripheral vessels.

The recipient area for the flap must be evaluated with even more care because the vascular success of the transfer is dependent on both a normal arterial vessel present to deliver flow to the transferred flap and competent veins nearby to drain the flap. We have preferred to perform end-to-end vascular anastomoses whenever possible to increase the patency rates. Therefore an exact knowledge of the total arterial supply to the recipient area distal to the flap is of paramount importance.

If the recipient site is in the upper extremity, clinical palpation of the vessels and use of Allen's test yields much useful information. The ultrasonic Doppler monitor, as outlined previously, may add more information. Prior to the performing of arteriography on the upper extremity, an axillary block is given to relieve vasospasm, which results in better peripheral definition.

A recipient site in the lower extremity may need, in addition to the attention to arterial definition, careful evaluation of the venous system to verify that competent venous drainage is available.

If there are any signs of venous insufficiency present, venography should be performed to verify that if the superficial system might be incompetent, the deep system will adequately drain the flap.

Finally, the patient must be evaluated systemically as to his medical status to be able to withstand the prolonged operative procedure. His bleeding and clotting mechanism should be in order and adequate blood replacement available for the surgery.

OPERATIVE TECHNIQUE

Whenever possible, a two-team approach to this operation is beneficial. This allows the dissection of the donor and recipient sites to proceed simultaneously so that the anesthetic time is shortened for the patient as well as the operative time for the surgeon. As one team dissects the groin, another team approaches the recipient site. Under tourniquet control, when possible, the recipient artery and veins are dissected over an ample distance and thorough débridement of all involved skin and deep tissues is performed to a peripheral border of normal skin, and the defect size is then measured. The recipient artery is then temporarily clamped with a removable vascular clamp and the tourniquet deflated. If there is adequate and prompt revascularization of the extremity distal to the operative site, a decision is made as to whether the vessel can be ligated and used for an end-to-end anastomosis to the flap vessel or whether it should be spared and an end-to-side anastomosis be accomplished. If the vessel can be spared, it should be sectioned and the flow from the proximal vessel evaluated. If the vessel appears normal and there is normal flow from the proximal vessel, the operation can proceed as a free microvascular transfer. If there is doubt as to whether the vessel is possibly damaged or abnormal at the operative site, it can be resected more proximally until normal flow occurs and the distance back to the operative site be bridged later with an interpositional vessel graft. Hemostasis should be obtained with the tourniquet deflated to prevent later flap hematoma and possible vessel compression.

The surgical team assigned to the groin dissection first establishes the superficial landmarks that were determined preoperatively. The pubic tubercle (PT), anterosuperior iliac spine (ASIS), and femoral artery (FA) are identified and marked on the skin (Fig. 20-4). The previously outlined SCIA

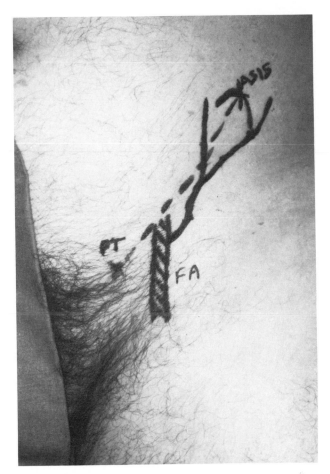

Fig. 20-4. Left groin with important landmarks outlined on the skin for flap orientation.

is redrawn on the skin as it proceeds laterally from the femoral artery and the inguinal ligament is also noted.

A linear incision is made to overlie the femoral artery from superior to the inguinal ligament proceeding distally. The dissection can be performed adequately with operative loupes of 4.5 magnification. The SCIV will be the most superficial distal vessel identified draining from the flap to the saphenous bulb. This vessel must be carefully protected during the remainder of the dissection. The femoral sheath is opened, and the femoral artery dissected proximally. Just deep and slightly distal to the inguinal ligament the vessel to the flap can be identified. This may be the superficial circumflex iliac artery arising directly from the anterolateral side of the femoral artery, (Fig. 20-5, *A*) or it may be a short common trunk (Fig. 20-5, *B*) that will soon bifurcate into the superficial epigastric artery (SEA) and the SCIA. The arteries should be dissected far enough laterally for later anastomosis. The venae comitantes of

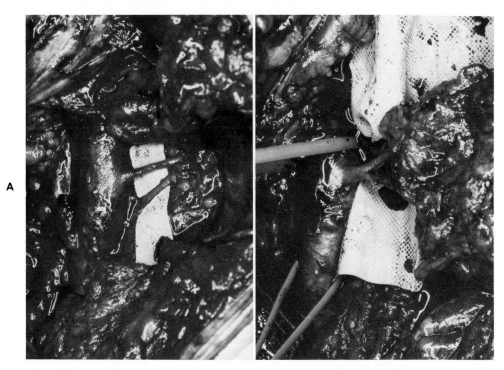

Fig. 20-5. A, Single superficial circumflex iliac artery (SCIA) arising from the anterolateral side of left femoral artery with accessory SCIA just distal to it. **B,** Common origin of SCIA and superficial epigastric artery (SEA) from short common trunk from the anterolateral side of the left femoral artery.

the SCIA can now usually be identified deep to the vessel and should be transferred with the flap for anastomosis, since we prefer to anastomose as many veins as possible.

If at this point the recipient team has determined that satisfactory vessels are available to revascularize the flap, then the operation proceeds. A template of the exact size is measured of the recipient defect with the location of the vessel anastomoses being identified.

This template is then transferred to the groin. The recipient vessels are lined up with the SCIA and SCIV, and then the flap is centered over the path of the SCIA, which is usually about 1 cm distal to and parallel to the inguinal ligament. The flap is outlined and then raised from lateral to medial.

Hemostasis should be obtained and preferably bipolar coagulation only used on the flap to prevent injury to the axial vessels. The flap may be thinned laterally through the fatty layer until the dissection medially has reached the ASIS and the lateral border of the sartorius. At this point, the dissection should go deep and carefully include the superficial sartorius fascia with the flap, since the SCIA and SCIV may lie directly superficial to the fascia or a branch of the SCIA may be on its deep surface. The risk of possible damage to these vessels is greater if the fascia is not raised with the flap from this point medially.

The lateral femoral cutaneous nerve should be identified and spared and then with the flap vessels in direct vision medially, the flap can be isolated now from its tissues and attached only by its vascular supply. The flap now exists only on the SCIA and the intact veins, and it should be examined to verify that it is still adequately vascularized. If there is fresh arterial bleeding from the distal margin of the flap and the capillary blanching of the skin is adequate, it can be considered ready for transfer.

Control should be obtained of the femoral artery, and then the SCIA or common trunk can be ligated with a suture or a vessel clip and sectioned. If the recipient vessel lumen diameter is much greater than the flap artery, a cuff of the femoral artery can be taken with the SCIA and the arteriotomy closed transversely.

The veins are then ligated, and the flap removed and taken directly to the recipient site. The vessels to the flap are not sectioned until the recipient site is ready for the transfer to decrease the ischemic time of the flap.

When adequate hemostasis is secured in the groin wound and there is no bleeding from the femoral artery, suction drains are placed in the depths of the wound prior to closure. The donor sites have always been closed primarily by acute flexion of the hip and knee and undermining of the skin as necessary.

As the donor site is being closed by one team, the other team is attaching the flap to the prepared recipient site.

Drains are placed, the flap is positioned, and the peripheral skin margins are sutured in place. The peripheral attachment of the flap is important to the prevention of later possible accidental separation or avulsion of the anastomoses.

The operating microscope is now brought to the field, and the vessel repairs are performed by careful adherence to established microvascular techniques of anastomosing only normal vessels under no tension with interrupted suture usually of 10-0 or 9-0 monofilament nylon or polypropylene. Interpositional venous or arterial grafts are used whenever necessary to achieve the above conditions. The arterial repair is performed first and then as many venous repairs as possible. One vein will drain the flap, but several venous anastomoses establish better drainage and provide insurance against venous thrombosis and postoperative problems. Intravenous low molecular weight dextran (dextran 40) is started after the arterial repair. The flap color, temperature, and peripheral bleeding should be satisfactory before the surgeon leaves the operating room.

OPERATIVE PROBLEMS

Immediately after the arterial anastomosis has been performed, the flap should show a bright pink flush with immediate capillary blanching and peripheral margin bleeding. If this does not occur, the anastomosis must be reevaluated and revised if necessary. Two percent lidocaine or papaverine can be applied topically and locally to the exposed anastomosed vessels to relieve local vasospasm. The papaverine will give a whitish cast to the adventitial layers, which may be distracting, and therefore lidocaine may be preferred.

The recipient artery must have normal brisk uninterrupted bleeding and be allowed to demonstrate this prior to the anastomosis to the flap being made. Experience has shown that whenever this was not able to be accomplished, the procedure would go on to failure not because of surgical failure or a poor anastomosis but rather because of inadequate delivery of arterial blood flow to the flap. This observation should be made before the flap is raised and the procedure changed to other methods of coverage rather than a free microvascular tissue transfer.

Skin closure over the site of the anastomoses and the thick part of the groin flap at its most medial border is sometimes a problem at the end of the procedure.

The flap may become severely engorged by the end of the procedure and the surrounding recipient skin may not be able to reach easily over the engorged subcutaneous tissue to the groin skin and should not be forced closed under tension. If this is done, it may cause pressure on the anastomoses, possibly leading to thrombosis. The exposed area may be covered nicely with a split-thickness skin graft if necessary. The noticeable engorgement and swelling of the flap, which is attributable largely to the lymphedema present, will subside nicely during the first postoperative month.

POSTOPERATIVE REGIMEN

The immediate postoperative care of the patient is centered on observation of the transferred flap for any problems of arterial or venous thrombosis, and therefore the flap is left visible in the dressing. The involved extremity is elevated slightly, and the flap is observed clinically for any signs of arterial or venous compromise such as change in color, temperature, or tissue consistency. Normal groin skin is pale with poor capillary blanching, and this must be appreciated as the immediate postoperative blush disappears.

Medication consists of oral aspirin for a 3-week period and a 5-day course of intravenous low molecular weight dextran. The dextran may not be necessary if the anastomoses are performed well and there are no vascular flow problems. With large flaps, the donor area is usually closed with some tension and the hip and knee must be kept flexed in bed for several days after surgery. The joints are then slowly brought into extension, and the patient is allowed to bear weight as he desires. This usually allows the donor site to heal uneventfully, and hip contracture is not a problem. If there are no postoperative problems, the patient is discharged on the sixth postoperative day and there have been no vascular problems with the flap after this period of time.

POSTOPERATIVE PROBLEMS

If problems of arterial or venous compromise are noticed, the patient is returned to the operating room for revision. Postoperative problems are rare if there were no problems in the operating room.

Stellate blocks may be helpful, but in these elective cases, a return visit to the operating theater may be indicated as initial treatment and may be the most beneficial therapy and, if done, should be done as early as possible.

Clinical evaluation of the vascular status of the flap is complicated by the "bruising" of the flap that occurs in the margins occasionally and also by the ecchymosis that may discolor the flap but not affect the normal postoperative course.

Partial-thickness skin loss may occur in the distal margins but usually heals without incident or may be aided by a split-thickness skin graft, if necessary.

There have been patients on dextran postoperatively who bled into their donor groin wound, but this bleeding stopped with discontinuance of the dextran and could probably have been prevented by no postoperative use of dextran.

CASE REPORTS

The following case reports illustrate a variety of indications for the successful use of free one-stage microvascular groin flap transfers.

Case 1 (Fig. 20-6)

E.W., a 56-year-old man on July 12, 1977, sustained an open, severely contaminated dislocation of the right wrist that was thoroughly debrided and reduced with loose closure. Two days later he had a fever, tachycardia, and a foul-smelling wound. In surgery the wound clinically resembled gas gangrene with massive tissue necrosis, which was radically debrided. *Clostridium perfringens* was cultured, and after large doses of appropriate antibiotics and almost daily débridements, the infection was controlled but left a large open volar wound with the intact ulnar artery and nerve and profundus tendons and bone exposed.

Because of his age and the location of the defect, a free groin flap was selected as the proper method of coverage to prevent a stiff shoulder and elbow and was performed on July 21, 1977. The radial artery, which had been severed in the original injury, was identified in the proximal forearm along with its venae comitantes and the cephalic vein.

At the same time another team was identifying the left groin vessels through a medial linear incision. The SCIV was isolated and then the SCIA and the SEA were seen to arise from a short (3 mm) common trunk. Two venae comitantes were also isolated. The flap was outlined according to the defect size, which measured 12 × 23 cm, and raised from lateral to medial, including the sartorius fascia, and then detached

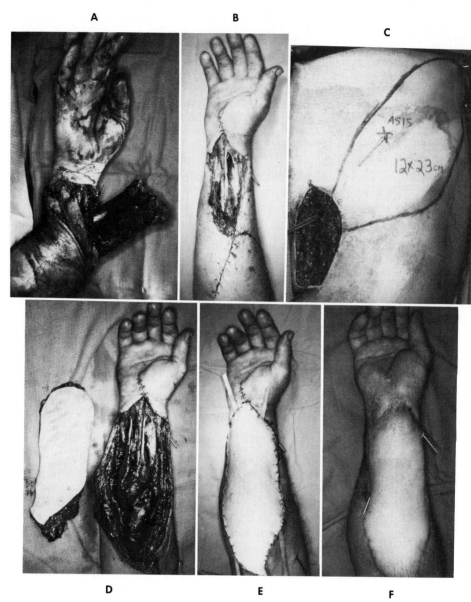

Fig. 20-6. A, Man, 56 years old, with contaminated open dislocation of right wrist with viable hand. **B,** Gas gangrene developed, and the patient and the hand survived after multiple débridements as shown here 9 days after the injury. All deep structures are exposed and require composite tissue coverage to survive. **C,** After the recipient area was dissected, a defect of 12 × 23 cm was created. The femoral vessels and the SCIA and SCIV have been dissected and the flap centered on the SCIA. **D,** The flap has been detached from the groin and lies next to the defect site ready to be attached and have the microvascular anastomoses performed. **E,** Immediately after revascularization. **F,** Three months postoperatively with complete coverage of the wound.

from its vascular pedicle along with a cuff of the femoral artery, which was then closed, primarily followed by direct closure of the donor site.

The flap was secured distally followed by direct end-to-end anastomosis of the common trunk of the SCIA and SEA to the radial artery with immediate revascularization of the flap. Three subsequent venous repairs were then done by anastomosis of the SCIV to a vena comitans of the radial artery and then the two venae comitantes of the flap to the cephalic vein and then the other radial artery vena comitans. Drains were placed.

After operation the patient was placed on aspirin and low molecular weight dextran. The flap healed uneventfully, but the groin donor area bled and the dextran was stopped with resolution of the bleeding. The flap remained well and provided good skin coverage.

Case 2 (Fig. 20-7)

W.N., a 55-year-old man, had an open fracture of his right distal tibia and fibula in 1944 with multiple surgical procedures until 1966. He developed chronic venous stasis and ulceration of the lateral malleolar area that was controlled until August 1976, when the wound broke down and resisted healing. Degeneration of the ankle joint, causing pain and preventing gainful employment, contributed to the problem. An ankle prosthesis or fusion was being considered, but adequate skin coverage was required prior to this possibility.

On examination in November 1976, there was a 2 cm open venous stasis ulcer over the lateral malleolus with 6 cm of surrounding unstable skin. Posterior tibial and anterior tibial pulses were good. The opposite leg had similar changes of chronic venous stasis, which eliminated the possibility of conventional cross-leg flap coverage.

Preoperative arteriograms showed intact anterior and posterior tibial vessels continuing to the foot. Venograms showed incompetent superficial veins but competent deep veins, and therefore it was elected to attempt a free groin flap to the ankle. The patient was placed on complete bed rest with elevation. Six months later the ulcer had closed and on June 10, 1977, a free groin flap was transferred to the right ankle area with many operative problems. One team explored the leg and excised 10 × 12 cm of unstable skin with slight peripheral undermining to better accept the flap. Dense scar tissue was encountered, and only one deep vein, which was firmly adherent in scar tissue, was identified. The anterior tibial artery was identified and clamped with the tourniquet deflated and the posterior tibial artery adequately perfused the leg. The anterior tibial artery was ligated.

Simultaneously along with the leg dissection, another team dissected the left groin through a linear incision medial to the femoral artery. A common trunk was identified emptying the superficial circumflex iliac vein and the superficial epigastric vein into the saphenous bulb. A common trunk from the anterolateral side of the femoral artery also divided into the superficial epigastric artery and the superficial circumflex iliac artery. A flap was then designed, centered on the inguinal ligament, and made 12 × 14 cm, a size that was slightly larger than the recipient defect in case more unstable skin needed to be resected. The flap was then raised from lateral to medial and included the fascia from the lateral border of the sartorius medially. When the recipient area was ready, the flap was raised on its vascular pedicle with a cuff of the femoral artery being included with the common arterial trunk for better apposition of the later anastomosis. The femoral artery arteriotomy was closed primarily, the veins were clipped, and the flap was removed. The donor site was able to be closed primarily with flexion of the hip and knee. The flap was sewn in distally at the ankle to prevent possible accidental dislodgment and disruption of the anastomoses. The anterior tibial artery then revealed

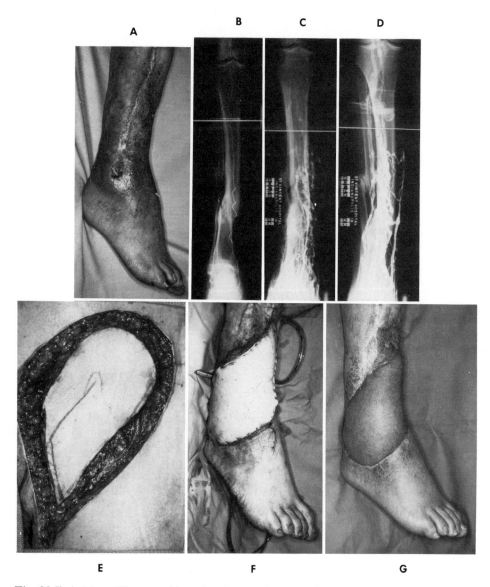

Fig. 20-7. A, Man, 55 years old, with a 22-year history of right leg and ankle problems after an open distal tibia and fibula fracture. Patient has had bilateral chronic venous stasis problems with ulcerations, swelling, and superficial venous incompetency. Adequate skin coverage was required before open procedures could be performed on the ankle. **B,** Preoperative arteriograms showed abnormal but intact anterior and posterior tibial vessels to the foot. **C,** Preoperative venogram showed superficial incompetency of the venous system. **D,** Preoperative venogram with the calf compressed shows adequate drainage through the deep system. **E,** After the ankle defect had been created, a 12 × 14 cm flap was raised from the left side of groin. **F,** Groin flap after revascularization in the ankle. **G,** Four months postoperatively the flap has provided adequate coverage without any further open wounds.

no pulsation or flow, and it was necessary to identify the normal anterior tibial artery proximally in the calf and then use an arterial interpositional graft of 10 cm length to bridge the gap distally to the flap vessels. The common arterial trunk of the flap was then sewn end to end into the interpositional graft with prompt revascularization of the flap with peripheral bleeding. The single venous anastomosis was then sewn, and drains were placed.

Postoperatively the patient was placed on aspirin and low molecular weight dextran. By 6 days postoperatively the unstable skin around the periphery of the free flap underwent necrosis complicated by a *Pseudomonas* infection. Four subsequent procedures were necessary, including débridement, defatting and advancement of the free flap, and split-thickness skin grafting to close the peripheral wound. The patient was discharged 5 weeks postoperatively with complete viability of the flap.

At 2 months postoperatively the flap was developing venous stasis, becoming deeper in color and scaly, but by 4 months it was recovering and there has been no further change in the flap.

Case 3 (Fig. 20-8)

L.C., a 47-year-old man, had an open fracture of his left distal tibia and fibula in July 1973, with the subsequent development of an open (2 × 5 cm) continually draining and painful *Pseudomonas* and *Staphylococcus aureus* osteomyelitis with a healed fracture. He had had multiple débridements, saucerizations, and skin-grafting procedures without success. Because of his continual pain, he was unable to bear weight on the involved extremity or work. A free groin flap was proposed to bring in fresh vascularized tissue after wide scar excision and saucerization.

Preoperative arteriograms and venograms revealed patent normal arteries and competent veins. Ultrasonic Doppler examination localized the vessels in the donor and the recipient sites.

On June 3, 1977, a team excised a 9 × 14 cm area of involved scarred skin from the left distal tibial area with sequestrectomy and wide saucerization. The posterior tibial artery was identified with its venae comitantes and another superficial vein. With the tourniquet deflated, temporary clamping of the posterior tibial artery did not interfere with the circulation to the foot, which was supplied by the anterior tibial artery. Drains were placed.

Simultaneously another team was dissecting the right groin through an incision medial to the femoral artery. The superficial circumflex iliac vein was identified draining into the saphenous vein, and the superficial circumflex iliac artery arose from the anterolateral side of the femoral artery. A 9 × 14 cm flap was designed, centered over the course of the superficial circumflex iliac artery, and raised from lateral to medial including the sartorius fascia from the lateral border of the muscle medially. Since the recipient site was ready, the vascular pedicle was detached, including a cuff of the femoral artery. The arteriotomy was closed primarily, as was the donor site.

The flap was sewn in distally, and then the superficial circumflex iliac artery was anastomosed end to end to the posterior tibial artery with immediate revascularization of the flap. The venae comitantes of the superficial circumflex iliac artery were anastomosed to the venae comitantes of the posterior tibial artery, and the superficial circumflex iliac vein was anastomosed to a branch of the saphenous vein.

Postoperatively, the patient was placed on aspirin and low molecular weight dextran for 5 days. He was given a 21-day course of intravenous gentamicin for the *Staphylococcus aureus* and *Serratia* infection that was cultured, and he was discharged 1 month postoperatively.

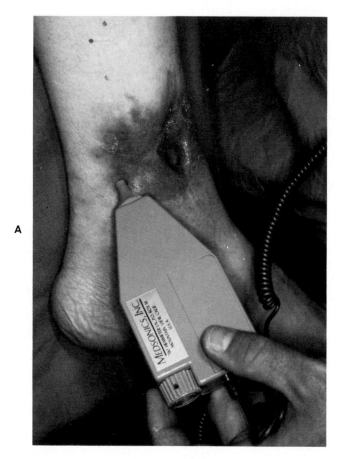

A

Fig. 20-8. A, Man, 47 years old, with a 4-year history of an open draining osteomyelitis after an open fracture of the left distal tibia and fibula that had not healed with multiple surgical procedures. **B,** Donor area of right side of groin after excision of a 9 × 14 cm free groin flap. The donor area was closed primarily by flexion of the hip and knee resulting in a linear scar. **C,** Free groin flap ready to be sewn to the recipient defect. **D,** Immediately after revascularization of the free flap. **E,** Four months postoperatively the flap is here shown healed and has remained so.

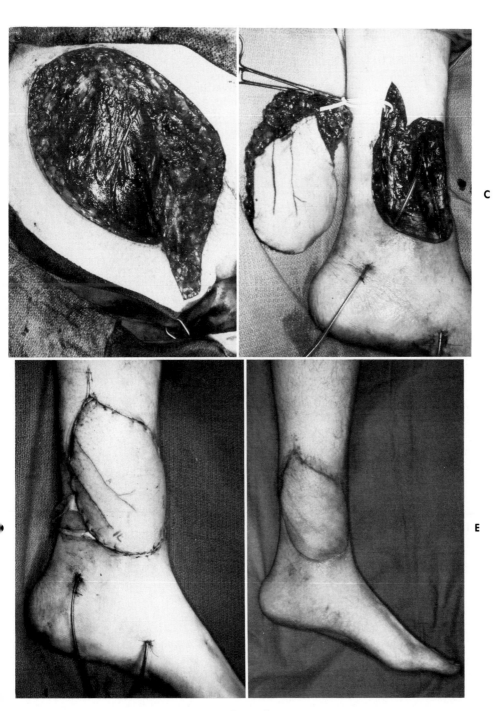

C

E

Fig. 20-8, cont'd. For legend see opposite page.

One month later he had spontaneous drainage from the flap that responded to antibiotics and has had no further problems since then.

Case 4 (Fig. 20-9)

E.S., a 57-year-old man, had an industrial crushing injury to his right hand and wrist on August 25, 1973, with subsequent infection, gangrene, and loss of the thumb at the carpometacarpal level. On December 2, 1974, pollicization of the index digit was attempted, but there was partial necrosis leaving a short inappropriate stump with some drainage. Several débridement procedures were performed, and then on May 5, 1975, it was elected to elongate the stump with a fibular bone graft of 5 cm. This created a difficult skin defect to cover by conventional means. The choice of a free groin flap was made to resurface the composite-tissue defect and to prevent stiffness in the shoulder and elbow.

The recipient site was dissected, the radial artery and two superficial veins were identified, the bone graft obtained from the left fibula was inserted and stabilized, and then a skin defect of 7.5 × 12.5 cm was outlined.

Simultaneously with the dissection of the hand another team was dissecting the

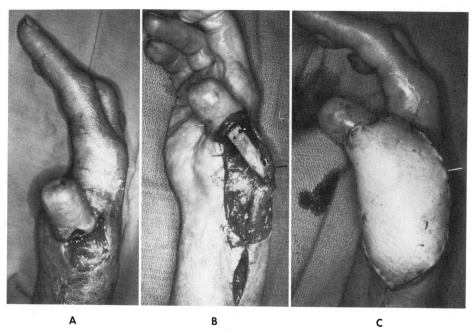

A **B** **C**

Fig. 20-9. A, Five months after attempted pollicization of the right index digit in a 57-year-old man who 21 months previously had had a traumatic amputation of the thumb. The proximal portion of the index digit necrosed and left a distal sensitive stump in wide abduction. **B,** At surgery, the viable and sensitive tip was extended with a fibular bone graft creating a large iatrogenic defect of 7.5 × 12.5 cm in size. **C,** To prevent stiffness in the shoulder and elbow, a free right-side groin flap was transferred at the same procedure and provided total skin coverage. Partial defatting was done several months later at a secondary procedure.

right groin. An incision medial to the femoral artery revealed the superficial circumflex iliac vein draining into the saphenous bulb. The superficial circumflex iliac artery was identified on the anterolateral side of the femoral artery with its venae comitantes in proximity. The flap was outlined, centered on the inguinal ligament, and raised from lateral to medial. When the recipient site was ready, the flap was detached from its vascular pedicle with the donor site closed primarily by flexion of the hip and knee. The groin flap was sewn in peripherally, and then a vena comitans of the superficial circumflex iliac artery was anastomosed to a superficial vein. The superficial circumflex iliac artery was anastomosed end to side to the radial artery. After topical lidocaine was applied to the arterial anastomosis, the flap revascularized promptly with good peripheral bleeding. The superficial circumflex iliac vein was then anastomosed to a superficial recipient vein with good flow.

Postoperatively, the patient was placed on aspirin, dipyridamole (Persantine), and low molecular weight dextran. He developed some chest pain, and for preventive measures, the cardiology service gave him heparin, which caused some ecchymosis of the flap, but it did not interfere with its complete survival. He was discharged 2 weeks postoperatively. Some partial defatting was done as a secondary procedure.

Case 5 (Fig. 20-10)

C.G., a 53-year-old man, had third-degree burns to his right upper extremity from the wrist to the axilla with radial and ulnar nerve loss on September 22, 1976. His initial treatment of skin grafting and an abdominal flap had provided wound closure, except for the medial epicondylar area of his elbow, which had been open and draining for 8 months by the time he was first seen by us. The elbow had a flexion contracture, and radiographs showed an osteomyelitis of the medial epicondyle. Because of the unavailability of adjacent flap donor sites, a free groin flap was selected to resurface and revascularize the infected exposed area.

Preoperative arteriograms of the elbow and groin revealed normal vasculature, and on July 28, 1977, a free groin flap was transferred.

Dissection of the arm revealed the superior ulnar collateral artery to supply the recipient area. Two venae comitantes and the basilic vein were also isolated. The exposed bone and unstable skin were resected with a defect measuring 9 × 18 cm being created. Simultaneously, the left groin was dissected with an incision medial to the femoral artery, and the superficial circumflex iliac vein was identified as it emptied into the saphenous bulb. The superficial circumflex iliac artery was isolated as it arose directly from the anterolateral side of the femoral artery, and there was an accessory artery 1 cm distally also going to the flap. The venae comitantes of the SCIA with two medial branches were also identified. The 9 × 18 cm defect size was then outlined, centered slightly distal to the inguinal ligament, and then raised from lateral to medial. The flap was thinned from the lateral border of the flap to the lateral border of the sartorius, and then the fascia was included in the flap continuing medially. The vessels could be visualized just superficial to the sartorius fascia as it was raised.

The flap was suspended on its vascular pedicle until the recipient site was ready and the vessels were clipped. Because of the larger recipient artery, a cuff of the femoral artery was excised with the SCIA and the arteriotomy closed. The donor site was closed primarily by flexion of the hip and the knee.

The flap was sewn into the arm distally, and then the SCIA (1.5 mm) was anastomosed end to end to the superior ulnar collateral artery with immediate revascularization and venous engorgement of the flap. The two venae comitantes of the SCIA were then anastomosed to the two venae comitantes of the recipient artery and the

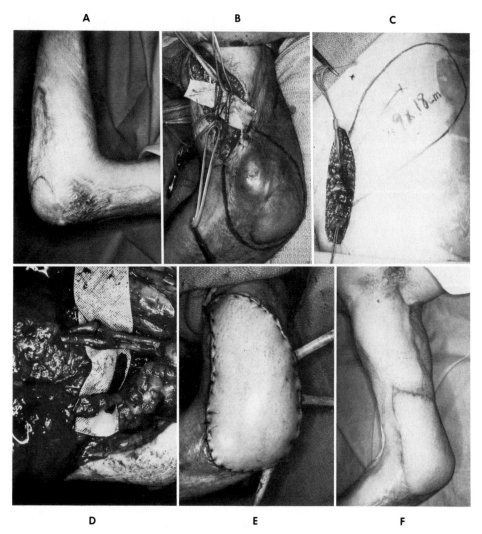

Fig. 20-10. A, Man, 53 years old, 10 months prior to being referred to us, had had full-thickness burns to the right elbow, arm, and forearm with coverage achieved by split-thickness skin grafts and a small abdominal flap. He now had an open draining area over the medial epicondyle with bone exposed. **B,** At surgery, the superior ulnar collateral artery was dissected and the defect area outlined. **C,** A 9 × 18 cm free groin flap was raised and the defect was closed primarily. **D,** One artery and three veins after microvascular anastomoses. **E,** Flap immediately after revascularization. **F,** Nine months postoperatively the flap has decreased in size and provides excellent cosmetic and functional coverage.

superficial circumflex iliac vein (2 mm) was anastomosed to the basilic vein. Drains were placed.

The patient was on antibiotics, aspirin, and low molecular weight dextran for 5 days postoperatively and was discharged on the sixth postoperative day. He has had no problems postoperatively with skin coverage or drainage and has returned to work.

SUMMARY

With a very high percentage rate of success of elective microvascular free-tissue transfers now possible by experienced microsurgeons, the use of free-tissue transfers has become an available choice for coverage of difficult problems of composite-tissue loss in the extremities. There are many instances in the upper extremity when a free-tissue transfer is preferable to an attached transfer. Especially in the lower extremity, however, the indications may be much greater than for conventional methods of advancing tubed flaps or cross-leg flaps.

The groin flap is an ideal flap for this free transfer and has advantages over other donor sites in that it leaves the most cosmetically pleasing scar compared to other possible axial-pattern donor sites, its size available for transfer is almost unlimited, and a single axial vessel nourishes it.

The main disadvantage to the groin flap is its requisite thickness at its medial border and the overall thickness of the flap as compared to other parts of the body where the subcutaneous tissue is much thinner.

Experience has shown, however, that as long as the flap is not made larger than the defect size at the time of the surgery, the flap will decrease in size and be cosmetically pleasing, and defatting and size reduction will not be necessary. Defatting may be done several months later if desired, but it has been rare for patients to want this done because the graft very nicely blends into the recipient area.

Perhaps one of the greatest advantages of this method of coverage of old areas of scar, inadequate skin coverage, and osteomyelitis is that it brings fresh tissue with its own blood supply to these areas of tissue ischemia and possible infection. This allows the better delivery of blood and antibiotics to these areas as needed.

The free one-stage microvascular groin flap has provided us with an excellent method of composite-tissue coverage of difficult problems.

ACKNOWLEDGMENT

I wish to thank my associate, Dr. James W. Strickland, for having provided some of these patients, for his invaluable help and assistance during these difficult cases, and for making the team concept work.

READINGS

Acland, R. D.: Outlining a free flap exactly, Plast. Reconstr. Surg. **59**:113, 1977.

Aoyagi, F., Fujino, T., and Ohshiro, T.: Detection of small vessels for microsurgery by a Doppler flowmeter, Plast. Reconstr. Surg. **55**:372, 1975.

Bakamjian, V. Y.: A two-stage method for pharyngoesophageal reconstruction with a primary pectoral skin flap, Plast. Reconstr. Surg. **36**:173, 1965.

Baudet, J., and LeMaire, J.-M.: Le lambeau abdominal en chirugie de la main. Que faut-il en penser? Ann. Chir. Plast. **20**:215, 1975.

Baudet, J., LeMaire, J.-M., and Guimberteau, J.-C.: Ten free groin flaps, Plast. Reconstr. Surg. **57**:577, 1976.

Boeckx, W. D., de Coninck, A., and Vanderlinden, E.: Ten free flap transfers: use of intra-arterial dye injection to outline a flap exactly, Plast. Reconstr. Surg. **57**:716, 1976.

Boo-Chai, K.: John Wood and his contributions to plastic surgery: the first groin flap, Br. J. Plast. Surg. **30**:9, 1977.

Brownstein, M. L., Gordon, L., and Buncke, H. J., Jr.: The use of microvascular free groin flaps for the closure of difficult lower extremity wounds, Surg. Clin. North Am. **57**:977, 1977.

Buncke, H. J.: Hand reconstruction by microvascular island flap transplantation, J. Bone Joint Surg. **57**:729, 1975.

Daniel, R. K., and Taylor, G. I.: Anatomy and hemodynamics of free flap donor sites. In Daniller, A. I., and Strauch, B., editors: Symposium on microsurgery, St. Louis, 1976. The C. V. Mosby Co., Vol. 14:32.

Daniel R. K., Cunningham, D. M., and Taylor, G. I.: The deltopectoral flap: an anatomical and hemodynamic approach, Plast. Reconstr. Surg. **55**:275, 1975.

Daniel, R. K., and Taylor G. I.: Distant transfer of an island flap by microvascular anastomoses, Plast. Reconstr. Surg. **52**:111, 1973.

Daniel, R. K., and Terzis, J. K.: Free tissue transfer by microvascular anastomoses. In Daniel, R. K., and Terzis, J. K., editors: Reconstructive microsurgery, Boston, 1977, Little, Brown & Co., p. 191.

Daniel, R. K., and Williams, H. B.: The free transfer of skin flaps by microvascular anastomoses, Plast. Reconstr. Surg. **52**:16, 1973.

Daniel, R. K., and Terzis, J. K.: Reconstructive microsurgery, Boston, 1977, Little, Brown & Co.

Daniel, R.: Toward an anatomical and hemodynamic classification of skin flaps, Plast. Reconstr. Surg. **56**:330, 1975.

Daniller, A. I., and Strauch, B., editors: Symposium on microsurgery, St. Louis, 1976, The C. V. Mosby Co.

de Coninck, A., and Vanderlinden, E.: Thoradorsal skin flap: new possible donor sites in distant transfer of island flaps by microvascular anastomoses, Ann. Chir. Plast. **20**:163, 1975.

Finseth, F. J.: Anatomy and design of flaps. In Krizek, T. J., and Hoopes, J. E., editors: Symposium on basic sciences in plastic surgery, St. Louis, 1976, The C. V. Mosby Co., p. 263.

Finseth, F., Kavarana, N., and Antia, N.: Complications of free flaps transfers to the mouth region, Plast. Reconstr. Surg. **56**:652, 1975.

Finseth, F., May, J. W., and Smith, R. J.: Composite groin flap with iliac-bone flap for primary thumb reconstruction. Case report, J. Bone Joint Surg. **58**:130, 1976.

Fujino, T., Harashina, T., Tanino, R., Ohshiro, T., and Aoyagi, F.: Clinical success of distant transfer of free skin flaps in hand and neck regions by microvascular anastomosis, Keio J. Med. **23**:47, 1974.

Fujino, T.: Contribution of the axial and perforator vasculature to circulation in flaps, Plast. Reconstr. Surg. **39**:125, 1967.

Fujino, T., Harashina, T., and Nakajima, T.: Free skin flap from the retroauricular region to the nose, Plast. Reconstr. Surg. **57**:338, 1976.

Fujino, T.: Microvascular transfer of free deltopectoral dermal-fat flap, Plast. Reconstr. Surg. **55**:428, 1975.

Fujino, T., and Saito, S.: Repair of pharyngoesophageal fistula by microvascular transfer of free skin flap, Plast. Reconstr. Surg. **56**:549, 1975.

Gilbert, A., and Morrison, W.: First web space neurovascular free flap transfer, Lettre d'Information #3 of the Groupe pour l'Avancement de la Microchirurgie, Paris. 1976.

Goldwyn, R. M., Lamb, D. L., and White, W. L.: An experimental study of large island flaps in dogs, Plast. Reconstr. Surg. **31:**528, 1963.

Hackett, M. E. J.: The use of thermography in the assessment of depth of burn and blood supply of flaps with preliminary reports of its use of Dupuytren's contracture and treatment of varicose ulcers, Br. J. Plast. Surg. **27:**311, 1974.

Harashina, T., Nakijima, T., and Yoshimura, Y.: A free groin flap reconstruction in progressive facial hemiatrophy, Br. Plast. Surg. **30:**14, 1977.

Harashina, T., Fujino, T., and Aoyagi, F.: Reconstruction of oral cavity with free flap, Plast. Reconstr. Surg. **58:**412, 1976.

Harashina, T., Mikata, A., Epstein, L. I., and Fujino, T.: Rejection phenomena after homotransplantation of skin flaps in dogs by microvascular technique, Plast. Reconstr. Surg. **52:**390, 1973.

Harii, K.: Composite tissue transfer by microvascular anastomoses, Asian Med. J. **17:**264, 1975; **17:**417, 1975.

Harii, K.: Current clinical experiences in vascularized free skin flap transfers. In Daniller, A. I., and Strauch, B., editors: Symposium on microsurgery, St. Louis, 1976, The C. V. Mosby Co., p. 45.

Harii, K., and Ohmori, K.: Direct transfer of large free groin skin flaps to the lower extremity using microanastomoses, Chir. Plastica (Berlin) **3:**1, 1975.

Harii, K., Ohmori, K., and Ohmori, S.: Free deltopectoral skin flaps, Br. J. Plast. Surg. **27:**231, 1974.

Harii, K., and Ohmori, K.: Free groin flaps in children, Plast. Reconstr. Surg. **55:**588, 1975.

Harii, K.: Free groin flaps, Plast. Reconstr. Surg. **58:**120, 1976.

Harii, K., Ohmori, K., Torii, S., Murakami, F., Kasai, Y., Sekiguchi, J., and Ohmori, S.: Free groin skin flaps, Br. J. Plast. Surg. **28:**225, 1975.

Harii, K., Ohmori, K., and Sekiguchi, J.: The free musculocutaneous flap, Plast. Reconstr. Surg. **57:**294, 1976.

Harii, K., and Ohmori, K.: Free skin flap transfer, Clin. Plast. Surg. **3:**111, 1976.

Harii, K., Ohmori, K., and Ohmori, S.: Hair transplantation with free scalp flap, Plast. Reconstr. Surg. **53:**410, 1974.

Harii, K., Ohmori, K., and Ohmori, S.: Successful clinical transfer of ten free flaps by microvascular anastomoses, Plast. Reconstr. Surg. **53:**259, 1974.

Harii, K., and Ohmori, S.: Use of the gastroepiploic vessels as recipient or donor vessels in the free transfer of composite flaps by microvascular anastomoses, Plast. Reconstr. Surg. **52:**541, 1973.

Ikuta, Y.: Free flap transfer by end-to-side arterial anastomosis. In Daniel, R. K., and Terzis, J. K., editors: Reconstructive microsurgery, Boston, 1977, Little, Brown & Co., p. 248.

Ikuta, Y., Watari, S., Kawamure, et al.: Free flap transfers by end-to-side arterial anastomosis, Br. J. Plast. Surg. **28:**1, 1975.

Joshi, B. B.: Neural repair for sensory restoration in a groin flap, Hand **9:**221, 1977.

Kahn, S.: Terminology of flaps, Plast. Reconstr. Surg. **47:**485, 1971.

Kaplan, E. N., Buncke, H. J., and Murray, D. E.: Distant transfer of cutaneous island flaps in humans by microvascular anastomoses, Plast. Reconstr. Surg. **52:**301, 1973.

Karkowski, J., and Buncke, H. J.: A simplified technique for free transfer of groin flaps by use of a Doppler probe, Plast. Reconstr. Surg. **55:**682, 1975.

Krizek, T. J., Tani, T., Desprez, J. D., and Kiehn, C. L.: Experimental transplantation of composite grafts by microsurgical vascular anastomoses, Plast. Reconstr. Surg. **36:**538, 1965.

Krizek, T. J., and Hoopes, J. E., editors: Symposium on basic science in plastic surgery, St. Louis, 1976, The C. V. Mosby Co.

Kutz, J. E., Hyland, W. T., Stott, W. G., and Kleinert, H. E.: Free groin flap to the hand with end-to-side vessel anastomosis. Case report, South. Med. J. **69:**1240, 1976.

Lanier, V. C., Jr., Serafin, D., Kleinert, H. E., et al.: Microvascular procedures in reconstructive surgery, South. Med. J. **69:**1595, 1976.

Liggins, D. F., and Mehrotra, O. N.: Petechial haemorrhages in a free flap anastomosed to abnormal vessels, Br. J. Plast. Surg. **30:**138, 1977.

Lister, G. D., McGregor, I. A., and Jackson, I. T.: The groin flap in hand injuries, Injury **4:**229, 1973.

McCraw, J. B.: On the transfer of a free dorsalis pedis sensory flap to the hand, Plast. Reconstr. Surg. **59:**738, 1977.

McCraw, J. B., Myers, B., and Shanklin, K. D.: The value of fluorescein in predicting the viability of arterialized flaps, Plast. Reconstr. Surg. **60:**710, 1977.

McGregor, I. A., and Morgan, G.: Axial and random pattern flaps, Br. J. Plast. Surg. **26:**202, 1973.

McGregor, I. A.: Basic principles in skin flap transfer, Surg. Clin. North Am. **57:**961, 1977.

McGregor, I. A., and Jackson, I. T.: The groin flap, Br. J. Plast. Surg. **25:**3, 1972.

Maass, D.: Significance of microsurgery in the surgery of extremities. II. Free transplantation of composite tissue with microvascular connections, Helv. Chir. Acta **43:**679, 1976.

May, J. W., Jr., Chait, L. A., Cohen, B. E., and O'Brien, B. M.: Free neurovascular flap from the first web of the foot in hand reconstruction, J. Hand Surg. **2:**328, 1977.

May, J. W., Chait, L. A., O'Brien, B. M., and Hurley, J. V.: The no-reflow phenomenon in experimental free flaps, Plast. Reconstr. Surg. **61:**256, 1978.

Nickell, W. B.: Special considerations in resurfacing hand injuries with the groin flap, South. Med. J. **67:**567, 1974.

O'Brien, B. M., Sharzer, L. A., and MacLeod, A. M.: Clinical experiences in microvascular free flap transfer. In Daniller, A. I., and Strauch, B., editors: Symposium on microsurgery, St. Louis, 1976, The C. V. Mosby Co. p. 41.

O'Brien, B. M., and Shanmugan, N.: Experimental transfer of composite free flaps with microvascular anastomoses, Aust. N.Z. J. Surg. **43:**285, 1973.

O'Brien, B. M., Morrison, W. A., Ishida, H., MacLeod, A. M., and Gilbert, A.: Free flap transfers with microvascular anastomoses, Br. J. Plast. Surg. **27:**220, 1974.

O'Brien, B. M.: Microvascular free flap and omental transfer. In O'Brien, B. M.: Microvascular reconstructive surgery, Edinburgh, 1977, Churchill Livingstone, p. 205.

O'Brien, B. M., MacLeod, A. M., and Morrison, W. A.: Microvascular free flap transfer, Orthop. Clin. North Am. **8:**349, 1977.

O'Brien, B. M.: Microvascular reconstructive surgery, Edinburgh, 1977, Churchill Livingstone.

O'Brien, B. M., MacLeod, A. M., Hayhurst, J. W., and Morrison, W. A.: Successful transfer of a large island flap from the groin to the foot by microvascular anastomoses, Plast. Reconstr. Surg. **52:**271, 1973.

Ohmori, K., and Harii, K.: Free dorsalis pedis sensory flap to the hand, with microneurovascular anastomoses, Plast. Reconstr. Surg. **58:**546, 1976.

Ohmori, K.: Free flaps in children. In Daniel, R. K., and Terzis, J. K., editors: Reconstructive microsurgery, Boston, 1977, Little, Brown & Co., p. 248.

Ohmori, K., and Harii, K.: Free groin flaps: their vascular basis, Br. J. Plast. Surg. **28:**238, 1975.

Ohmori, K., Harii, K., Sekiguchi, J., and Torii, S.: The youngest free groin flap yet? Br. J. Plast. Surg. **30:**273, 1977.

Ohtsuka, H., Fujita, K., and Shioya, N.: Replantations and free flap transfers by microvascular surgery, Plast. Reconstr. Surg. **58**:708, 1976.

Ohtsuka, H., Kamiishi, H., Saito, H., Ito, M., and Shioya, N.: Successful free flap transfers with diseased recipient vessels, Br. J. Plast. Surg. **29**:5, 1976.

Orticochea, M.: The musculocutaneous flap method: an immediate and heroic substitute for the method of delay, Br. J. Plast. Surg. **25**:106, 1972.

Panje, W. R., Krause, C. J., and Bardach, J.: Microsurgical techniques in free flap reconstruction, Laryngoscope **87**:692, 1977.

Panje, W. R.: Reconstruction of intradural defects with the free groin flap, Arch. Otolaryngol. **103**:78, 1977.

Panje, W. R., Bardach, J., and Krause, C. J.: Reconstruction of the oral cavity with a free flap, Plast. Reconstr. Surg. **58**:415, 1976.

Repair of facial defect with large island flap from the groin by microvascular anastomoses. A case report, Chin. Med. J. [Engl.] **1**:297, July 1975.

Rigg, B. M.: Transfer of a free groin flap to the heel by microvascular anastomoses, Plast. Reconstr. Surg. **55**:36, 1975.

Schenck, R. R.: Free muscle and composite skin transplantation by microvascular anastomoses, Orthop. Clin. North Am. **8**:367, 1977.

Serafin, D., Villarreal-Rios, A., and Georgiade, N.: Fourteen free groin flap transfers, Plast. Reconstr. Surg. **57**:707, 1976.

Serafin, D., Shearin, J. C., and Georgiade, N. G.: The vascularization of free flaps, Plast. Reconstr. Surg. **60**:233, 1977.

Sharzer, L. A., O'Brien, B. M., Horton, C. E., et al.: Clinical applications of free flap transfer in the burn patient, J. Trauma **15**:766, 1975.

Sinclair, S. W., and Blake, G. B.: The groin flap in hand injuries, N.Z. Med. J. **84**:393, Nov. 1976.

Smith, P. J., Foley, B., McGregor, I. A., and Jackson, I. T.: The anatomical basis of the groin flap, Plast. Reconstr. Surg. **49**:41, 1972.

Tan, E., O'Brien, B. M., and Brennen, M.: Free flap transfer in rabbits using irradiated recipient vessels, Br. J. Plast. Surg. **31**:121, 1978.

Taylor, G. I., and Daniel, R. K.: The anatomy of several free flap donor sites, Plast. Reconstr. Surg. **56**:243, 1975.

Taylor, G. I., and Daniel, R. K.: The free flap: composite tissue transfer by microvascular anastomoses, Aust. N.Z. J. Surg. **43**:1, 1973.

Thorvaldsson, S. E., and Grabb, W. C.: The intravenous fluorescein test as a measure of skin flap viability, Plast. Reconstr. Surg. **53**:576, 1974.

Vecchione, T. R.: Hair growth as a late sequela in skin grafts from the groin, Br. J. Plast. Surg. **30**:52, 1977.

Wells, J. H., and Edgerton, M. T.: Correction of a severe hemifacial atrophy with a free dermis-fat flap from the lower abdomen, Plast. Reconstr. Surg. **59**:223, 1977.

GENERAL DISCUSSION

Dr. Wilgis: The skin of a toe has a two-point discrimination of around 8 to 10 mm normally. When you put a toe onto a hand or thumb, does the toe have the potential to improve that two-point discrimination or is there anything we can do to the toe to improve that once we do the nerve suture?

Dr. Kutz: Theoretically, the sensation on the end plate is only going to be as good as its trained. I think we all know and we've all seen patients who have been born without hands who have developed a sensitivity in their toes almost as good as that in the hand. They have been able to grasp objects, pick up objects, identify coins, and so on just with their toes. So I really believe there is a potential to increase sensibility in the transferred tissues. The younger children we've done who have been completed over a year or a year and a half have been down to as little as 4 to 6 mm in some parts of the toe, but I really feel the potential of the end plates are there and that they can be reeducated to give them much better sensation.

Dr. Wilgis: I think this is true too. We put them on a preoperative education program to try to improve the sensation in the toes before we shift them. Dr. Kutz, is there any experience in free bone grafts in congenital partial bone loss problems such as tibial pseudoarthrosis?

Dr. Kutz: Yes, but they have been done too recently for me to give you any results; in fact, one of them is only 2 weeks old; so we can't really tell you. We have been using them in congenital defects of the tibia and some other areas and hope to see if we can get the growth potential.

Dr. Steichen: We have a case that was done early in 1975 of a young girl with congenital pseudoarthrosis of the tibia, and so we did a free vascularized rib graft. She has had four previous conventional grafting procedures that all had failed, and amputation was being considered. After the vascularized rib graft was done, the tibia united and she has been walking without the use of any external braces. This was done when I was with Harry Buncke in California. The patient has been followed by Bill Murray, and she's doing well.

Dr. Wilgis: Jim, do you use fluorescein?

Dr. Steichen: No, I have not done that yet, but I think that it is probably an excellent idea and we may start doing it.

Dr. Wilgis: Joe, what happens to the ankle motion when you take the fibular head?

Dr. Kutz: We've had no problem with ankle motion. If you stabilize the fibula, it has no effect on the lower portion of the fibula. We have never taken the full fibula.

Dr. Kutz: If you take too much of the fibula as Ian Taylor did (half of the fibula or more), it is necessary to screw the fibula to the tibia. Then you have, in effect, a single bone rather than a double bone.

Dr. Wilgis: Jim, do you anastomose nerves in the free groin flap, and if so, which ones?

Dr. Steichen: No, we haven't done it. It's obviously the big disadvantage to that kind of skin coverage. The nerve supply is variable, and I don't think it is covered by a single solitary nerve supply. If we need an area that requires innervation, we have other areas that we can use, such as the dorsal foot flap, which has been proved to be excellent except for the problem with the donor site. I think this is something you have to consider. The inner side of the toe that Joe Kutz showed is also an excellent area to supply sensation. If we have an area that needs innervation, we have to go to another area other than the groin.

Dr. Kutz: I think you can look for a nerve. We had only one case out of our series in which we found a nerve that fit this area, and I used it to graft the back of the hand. I hooked it up to the radial nerve and sensation has returned to it, but it was a fortunate event, not something you see regularly.

Dr. Wilgis: Joe, what happens to the perineal nerve in bone grafts?

Dr. Kutz: Nothing; you avoid it. If you carefully dissect away from it, you can easily remove the bone without interfering with the nerve at all. I think this has to do with your knowing anatomy and dissection technique. We've never had any problems.

Dr. Wilgis: Jim, is infection a contraindication to free groin flap? How much will the graft dissolve even though vascularized in an infected bed?

Dr. Steichen: The question refers to how much infection, such as how much during pregnancy?

Dr. Wilgis: Yes, I suppose so.

Dr. Steichen: Doctor Harii in Tokyo first introduced me to the idea in 1974. He told me that he was doing transfers to the area of chronic osteomyelitis in order to bring increased vasculature to these areas, and he was able to control the osteomyelitis. This points out another benefit of free-tissue transfers; that is, we bring skin along with a whole new blood supply to these chronically scarred and possibly osteomyelitic area. Three of the flaps that I showed you today were done in areas where there was chronic osteomyelitis. The most severe one was obviously the first one. I believe that over a period of time this possibly can give us an avenue to introduce enough antibiotics along with the surgical débridement at the time of surgery to help control osteomyelitis over a period of time. I am still laboring under that illusion, and we are doing some of the flaps specifically for chronic osteomyelitis. Only time will tell whether this is folly. The answer to the second part of the question is that the grafts have not dissolved underneath the flap.

Dr. Wilgis: Joe, do you reanastomose veins when you transfer bone grafts?

Dr. Kutz: No, we have reanastomosed veins when we take the center portion or the total bone. When we did the ones with terminal vessels, we have not. When you hook up the blood supply, you see the bleeding through the bone and you also see some bleeding in the canal, and so far we have not hooked up the vein. There has been enough going through the marrow cavity that it has bled enough to stay alive. I don't think you have that much blood loss. Of the ones that we take the full fibula or the larger segments, we have hooked up the veins because you can take a portion of muscle and there are usually veins that you can see.

Dr. Wilgis: The next two questions are related to that. In your last slide you talked about revascularizing bone, and one says tubular bones are blood vessels. Is there any work exploring the vascular capabilities of tubular interposition bone grafts without vascular pedicles? Do you have enough follow-up on your patients to show if they have benefited from this procedure?

Dr. Kutz: In answer to the first part, you have bone of "pick-up" blood supply that we all have had experience in using. your best results in bone grafting are using cancellous bone or soft bone, rather than the outside of the bone. The cortical bone works as a strut and does pick up its supply from the surrounding tissue. To use it as a tubular supply, we've done it this way in the hope that it would work. In replants where I just put back the bone, which functions as a tubular unit, and hope to get them together, I've never been able to demonstrate any return or blood supply going through this bone to a replant or to another portion of bone. I believe the blood supply around it gives enough vascularity so that capillaries grow into the bone rather than the bone by itself acting as a tube.

The answer to the second question is no.

Dr. Wilgis: Jim, obese people are the enemy of many surgeons. How does the degree of obesity influence you in the decision to do groin flaps?

Dr. Steichen: I start earlier in the morning. It is nice if you can get them to lose weight. The best flaps are on thin Orientals; if you can do free flaps on Orientals you win every time. Obesity is not a contraindication because I believe the groin is the best donor site. If the indications are present for free flap, we will continue to do it. I tell the patient that it's not going to be a cosmetically pleasing flap, because their groin is not cosmetically pleasing, and that it will probably be necessary to do one or two defatting procedures. I emphasize this to them; I explain to them that when they look at their leg or their arm or wherever it's going to be and they see an enormous flap sticking out there, they should look down at the other side of the groin and see the same enormous flap sticking out there and realize that if they wanted it equal we would have to defat that too. People accept this.

Dr. Wilgis: Joe, do you have any problem with hallux valgus after removing the second toe, and, if so, how do you prevent that?

Dr. Kutz: In the slides, the patient's toes pointed to one another like the hoof of an animal, but with time, we've had, more or less, kind of a meeting of the two. The third toe meets the great toe, therefore stopping at that particular area. The whole foot has been narrowed and there really is not that noticeable a discrepancy because you've narrowed the whole midfoot as well as removing the toe. We have not had the same problem that I've seen in patients who have had amputated toes at the head of the metatarsal. Then the big toe suddenly flops right over and covers up the end of the metatarsal. We have not seen that because there is a uniform narrowing of the forefoot.

Dr. Steichen: Shaw, if I might, I have a case I'd like to show that might illustrate a point brought up today. The question was brought up that when one does toe transfers in young children it might be better not to take the big toe because we're not sure what's going to happen to the push-off, gait, and running. We have a 2-year follow-up now on a 4-year-old boy who sustained an injury to both hands and one knee with total loss of this thumb and index finger on the right side. It happened that his grandparents had been driving across the country and stopped at a diner somewhere in Iowa. A man walked in who had a toe-to-thumb transfer, which was not very common in 1974, and related his experience to the parents and boy. The parents presented asking for a toe-to-thumb transfer. We dissected out the great toe and the dorsal vasculature along with a fairly large dorsal flap because of previous skin loss, and then transferred this to the thumb. The adduction contracture of the first metacarpal was released. This picture was a couple of months after surgery. He has regained grasp. He is now 6 years old. With regard to the question about what is going to happen to his foot, he is independent. He can stand on the toes and support his whole body entirely on the foot that we operated on. He can run without any type of limp at all as fast as he could before the surgery. We have movies taken of his gait. In this particular child, with growth, the function in his legs has not changed.

There is another way to reconstruct the thumb. We saw a man with bad electrical injuries to his right hand. He lost his thumb and his index finger and burned out the dorsum of his forearm. On the left side, he had burned out the entire volar part of his forearm, all the nerves, and tendons. He had an insensitive painful left hand with no movement, and the left thumb had no sensation; there was no motion in the index finger. He came to us because he wanted his left upper extremity amputated and a prosthesis. He was totally incapacitated. He couldn't button his shirt and couldn't do anything with either hand with absence of his thumb and index finger on the right and the insensitive inflexible hand on the left. We agreed to amputate his left upper extremity, but at the same time, we transferred his left thumb to this right thumb. I believe if there is a perfect thumb re-placement, this patient may have fallen into that category. He developed good extension and flexion. He has been very pleased with this and has regained normal sensation. I might also add that the sensory return to the boy with the toe to thumb is doing well.

21. Use of electromagnetic flowmeters in experimental microvascular surgery

Barry S. Schonwetter
Anthony V. Seaber
James R. Urbaniak
Donald S. Bright

This chapter reviews the principles, theory, operation, and limitations of electromagnetic flowmeters with attention to our experiences with arteries of 0.5 to 2 mm in diameter. It also presents the results of studies performed in the microsurgical laboratory, which assessed aspects of microsurgical technique on blood flow and evaluated the use of vasodilators on vessels with experimentally induced vasospasm. Also, studies on the effect of vessel clamps on arterial blood flow are included. The results of this work provided not only sufficient evidence for continued application of flowmeter studies to microsurgical research, but also new information concerning the physiologic changes observed during certain aspects of most microsurgical procedures.

History and theory of electromagnetic measurement of blood flow

Electromagnetic blood-flow monitoring is not new.[2,23] Of the techniques available for measuring blood flow in intact vessels, that based on electromagnetic induction is probably the oldest and most widely used.

With the principle of electromagnetic induction, a potential is created whenever an electrical conductor moves across the lines of force of a magnetic field.[22,25] This potential, which can be measured with electrodes, is perpendicular to the magnetic field and direction of motion of the conductor. Using this idea, Michael Faraday at the Waterloo Bridge in London (1832), attempted to measure the induced voltage created by the flow of the river Thames through the earth's magnetic field.[11] Unfortunately he was unsuccessful in this attempt. Faraday did, however, live to hear of Woolasten's success in 1851 of measuring the voltages induced by the tidal currents in the English Channel. However, a number of years elapsed before practical applications were found for Faraday's idea.[22,27]

It was not until 1930 that Williams performed the first electromagnetic measurements of velocity using a conducting solution. He passed copper sulfate solutions along a nonconducting circular pipe under a magnetic field. He measured the voltage induced by the magnetic field and found it proportional to the flow rate.[27] Using this idea, Fabre suggested that electromagnetic flowmeters could be used as instruments for measurement of blood flow.[10] The flowmeters should have a rapid response and could be used to measure instantaneous flow. Another advantage included the fact that the induced voltage recorded by the meter was directly proportional to the flow rate. The history of the invention of the flowmeter remains somewhat unclear although it appears that Fabre's work received little attention.[33] In 1936, the electromagnetic flowmeter was independently introduced into physiological use by A. Kolin[19,20] of the United States and by E. Wetterer[33] of Germany in 1937.

Subsequent contributions to the development of blood flowmetry have been made by Kolin, whose work resulted in the use of alternating-current instead of direct-current amplifiers. This eliminated the polarization of electrodes seen in early models of the flowmeter. Other contributions in applied flowmetry have been made by Wetterer, Einhorn, Wyatt, and many others.[33,35]

Electromagnetic flowmeter measurements of blood flow have been exten-

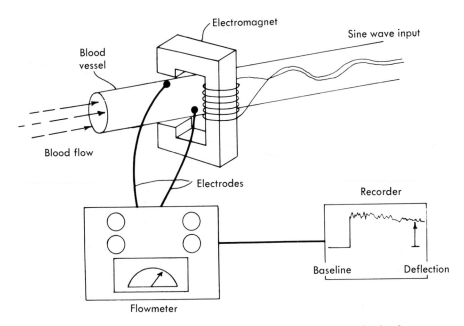

Fig. 21-1. Flow transducer, which encircles the artery, contains both electromagnet and measuring electrodes. The electromagnet creates a magnetic field. Blood, being a conductor, flows through the magnetic field, creating an induced voltage perpendicular to both the direction of the magnetic field and direction of motion. The induced voltage is picked up by electrodes located on the surface of the vessel.

sively used experimentally and clinically in reconstructive vascular surgery.[7,12,13,25,26]

The electromagnetic flowmeter is based on Faraday's law of electromagnetic induction:

$$E = ML\overline{V} \times 10^{-8}$$

where E is the potential difference in volts; M, the strength of the magnetic field in gauss; L, the lumen diameter in centimeters; and $\overline{V}$, the mean velocity of the conductor in cm/sec. If M and L remain constant, the potential difference varies linearly with the average velocity of flow across the tube or vessel.[22]

In accordance with this principle of arterial blood flow measurement, an electromagnet within a probe encircling the artery, creates a magnetic field in the vessel. Blood, being a conductor, flows through the magnetic field and generates an electromotive force (the potential difference in the above equation) in a direction perpendicular to both the magnetic field and direction of motion. This potential is picked up by electrodes located within the flow transducer, outside the vessel wall (Fig. 21-1). With this technique, the mean flow velocity can be measured without severance of the artery.[7] The principle behind electromagnetic flow measurement is simple. More complete theoretical treatments can be found in several reviews.[2,33,35]

Design of flowmeter systems

Flow probes (transducers) consist of both an electromagnet and an electrode assembled together with some suitable material such as plastic, epoxy resin, acrylic resin, or silicon rubber.[7] The probes contain a pair of electrodes located at opposite ends within the transducer. Many probes also contain a built-in ground wire, which could be sutured to the experimental subject to provide adequate grounding contact (Fig. 21-2).

As previously stated, a major difficulty in early measurement of blood flow was polarization of the electrodes. As a solution to this problem, magnets found within probe heads are energized with alternating current instead of direct current, which results in greater stability of the flow signal.[2]

Using alternating current does not eliminate all difficulties but creates a new problem—the transformer effect. The electrode leads, electrolyte, and electrodes form a conducting loop cutting through the lines of the magnetic field and create undesirable potentials.[2] Being several orders of magnitude greater than the flow-induced voltage, these potentials can interfere significantly with the transmission of the flow signal from probe to meter.[23]

The problems associated with alternating-current systems have resulted in the construction of meters with a variety of waveforms; the most common ones include sine-wave[21] and square-wave flowmeters.[8,25] With sine-wave systems,

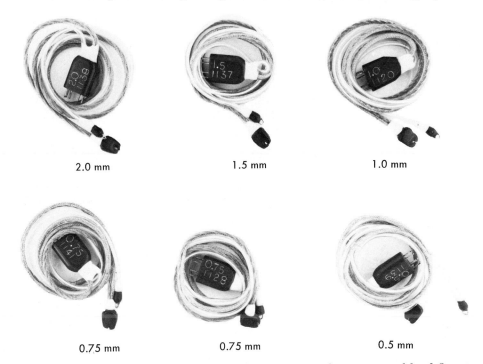

2.0 mm   1.5 mm   1.0 mm

0.75 mm   0.75 mm   0.5 mm

Fig. 21-2. Flow probes, often called transducers, are used to measure blood flow in arteries ranging from 2 to 0.5 mm. Pictured are the Howell flow probes, which have a grounding electrode sutured onto the surgical area for electrode grounding. The 0.75 mm probe (*center bottom*) is designed to eliminate arterial kinking when the surgeon measures blood flow by extending the area where the artery is placed into the probe. However, the increased bulk of this model necessitates larger dissection for probe insertion and may be inconvenient for vessels less than 1 mm in diameter.

the transformer voltage appears 90 degrees out of phase with the sinusoidal field waveform, whereas in square-wave systems, the transformer voltages take the form of a spike with an exponential decay occurring whenever the polarity of the magnetic field is reversed. To eliminate unwanted transformer voltages, flowmeters today are incorporated with appropriate balancing, gating, and filtering circuits to permit selective amplification of the flow signals and eliminate unwanted transformer potentials.[23]

The advantages of using sine-wave or square-wave flowmeters depends on both the preference and experience of the user and the situation in which the flowmeter is employed. Studies contrasting sine-wave and square-wave flowmeters can be found,[17,33] but attempts to demonstrate advantages of one system over another remain inconclusive. It appears that sine-wave probes are less bulky and produce less heat than do square-wave probes and thus may be more suitable to studies involving small or traumatized vessels. On the other hand, square-wave probes have been found to be less sensitive to changes in environment and provide greater stability than do sine-wave probes.

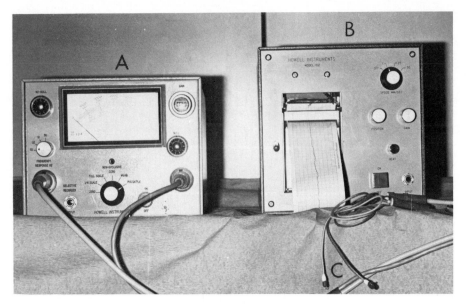

Fig. 21-3. A, Howell electromagnetic flowmeter. **B,** Chart recorder for permanent records. **C,** Flow probe and ground electrode.

Several commercial models of flowmeters are presently available. We have used models made by Statham,* Micron,† and Howell‡ manufacturers. Most of our experimental work involved the use of a Howell Model HMS 1000 fully transistorized sine-wave flowmeter with a pulsatile frequency response of 30 Hertz and a mean flow frequency of 0.1 Hertz (Fig. 21-3).

OPERATION AND LIMITATIONS

Blood flow measurement with the electromagnetic flowmeter is relatively easy to perform. It involves the following: calibration of the flow transducer, preparation of the experimental subject or model, establishment of a baseline of zero flow (no flow) that can be compared to subsequent flow recordings, and securing a stable baseline to ensure accurate measurements. Each of these procedures will be discussed in detail stressing the techniques used in our laboratory.

Calibration of probes

For the calibration of probes, in vivo,[1,3] in vitro,[9,30] and partial in vitro[14] calibration systems can be used. Our system consists of a partial in vitro flow system where saline flows through excised vessels (Fig. 21-4). It uses an

*Statham Laboratories, Hato Rey, Puerto Rico.
†Micron Instruments, Inc., 1519 Pontius Ave., Los Angeles, California 90025.
‡Howell Instruments, 1887 East Granger Street, Camarillo, California 93010.

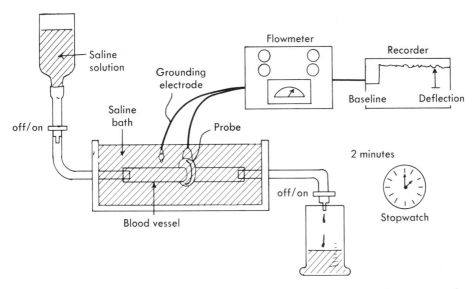

Fig. 21-4. Partial in vitro flow calibration system. The blood vessel used is an artery that is slightly larger than the probe size to be calibrated.

intravenous saline bottle, which serves as a constant pressure, gravity-feed reservoir. The fluid is collected in a graduated cylinder over a 2-minute interval, and at least four different flow rates are measured. The probe should be immersed in a saline bath to ensure adequate contact between probe and vessel while also preventing artifact potentials. The excised vessel must be a straight segment with no leaks or branches, since this will lead to inaccurate calibration. The probes are calibrated to check for linearity and to obtain quantitative flow rates (ml/min) during experimental studies. This calibration procedure is repeated on three successive days with different vessels to ensure probe stability. Once completed, the calibration of probes need only be performed periodically to ensure that the probes are operating adequately and the calibration factor remains constant.

Surgical preparation for blood flow measurements

Prior to measuring blood flow, the artery or vein is surgically exposed for up to 3 cm and lifted and fitted into a flow transducer of the appropriate size. All blood and fat must be removed from the site where the electrodes contact the vessel wall. Our laboratory used a 0.6 cm length of moistened umbilical tape to lift the vessel into the probe's lumen; thus trauma to the vessel was avoided. The fit should be snug for acute preparations and the vessel should be constricted slightly (approximately 10%) when the probe is applied,[2] so that adequate contact is ensured between the probe electrodes and the vessel wall. Constriction of the artery up to 20% does not affect pulsatile flow, whereas constriction greater than 50% can change mean flow recordings.[23] The area

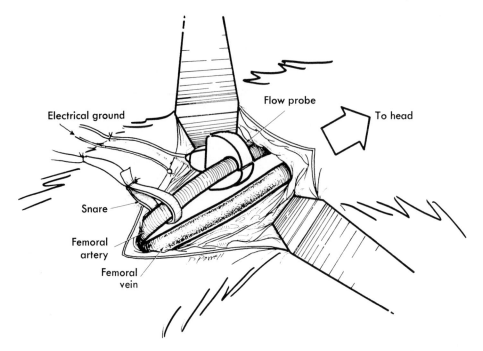

Fig. 21-5. The flow probe is placed onto the artery only after dissection of all the fatty tissues to ensure a snug fit. The ground electrode is sutured into the surrounding tissue.

surrounding the probe should be flooded with saline solution which improves stability and reduces interference. Large metal objects should be kept away from the probe since this may interfere with the magnetic field.[2] It is sometimes necessary to secure the probe by suturing it to the surrounding tissue. This prevents movement of the probe and the disruption of the waveform often seen when one uses sine-wave flowmeters with small vessels. Probes used in our laboratory contained a separate grounding electrode, which was also sutured to the experimental subject so that adequate grounding was ensured between the subject and the flowmeter (Fig. 21-5). Meticulous dissection without undue trauma to the vessel will complement a good study. Besides poor dissection, a major difficulty in performing flow studies is obtaining a reproducible baseline of zero flow when experiments are performed.

With both calibrations and in vivo blood flow measurements, it is necessary to obtain the level of baseline or zero flow before measured flow recordings are procured. Baseline flow determinations have been obtained by either of the following two methods: (1) occluding the vessel downstream to the probe to obtain a mechanical zero and (2) turning off the magnetic field to obtain an electronic zero.

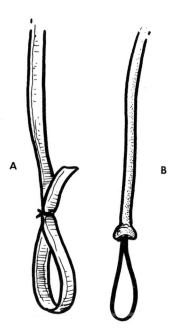

Fig. 21-6. A, Balloon-occluding snare. When placed around the artery, the loop is tied with a silk suture. A syringe is used to inflate loop when the vessel is to be occluded. B, Polyethylene tubing snare with 7-0 silk suture. When applied, the polyethylene tubing is fitted onto the artery that has been placed in the snare.

MECHANICAL ZERO

Although many methods can be used to achieve a mechanical zero,[15,16,29] in our laboratory we have used snares consisting of polyethelene tubing with the ends heat-flared to prevent damage to the vessel. After the snare is secured downstream to the probe, 6-0 or 7-0 silk suture is passed, encircling the vessel, and repassed through the tubing. This provides a simple loop for occlusion. We have also used balloon occluders consisting of Silastic or poly- ethylene tubing that had been heat-sealed and tied loosely around the vessel. This type of occlusive snare is readily inflated with a syringe attached to the tubing (Fig. 21-6). In experimental preparations, it is necessary to fasten the snare with sutures downstream to the probe to prevent movement when the vessel is being occluded. Also, when the snare is being attached to the vessel, care should be taken to ensure that there are no tributaries between the probe and snare. The snare placement and easy release are essential to a good flow study because they may be employed several times within the course of an experiment to ensure accurate baseline recordings.

ELECTRONIC ZERO

Many flowmeters are equipped with electronic zeroing devices. Electronic zeros consist of deenergizing the magnet to obtain zero flows. Several investigators, however, have reported that the electronic zero may not coincide at all times with the mechanical zero.[2,18] In our experiments, we obtain mechanical zeros with occlusive snares and find this method both simple and reliable for acute studies.

In addition to baseline stability, the probe's instability may be a source of error. The insulation of the probe should be maintained since any break in insulation may give erroneous readings. Additionally, probes should be cleaned after use to ensure that all foreign material is removed from the electrodes prior to reuse of the probe.

A frequent problem encountered with flowmeter usage is noise and electrical artifacts.[5,34] This may result from a poorly grounded room, extraneous sources such as lights or other machinery, or a careless experimental preparation. Care should be taken to locate all sources of electrical interference to ensure that all auxiliary equipment has sufficient grounding. The flowmeter should either have a built-in grounding system or should be manually grounded. The main limitation in flowmeter application is the operator; experience is necessary to obtain consistently satisfactory flow studies. Once mastered, however, the technique for measurement of flow in small vessels by means of an electromagnetic flowmeter remains relatively easy to perform.

EXPERIMENTAL USE OF ELECTROMAGNETIC FLOWMETERS— EVALUATION OF MICROSURGICAL TECHNIQUE
Effects of clamps and anastomoses on blood flow

This study was undertaken to evaluate the effects on blood flow of clamps used during replantation and to evaluate blood flow patterns after arterial anastomosis. All experiments were performed with the Howell 1 mm flow transducer. Microvascular clamps exerting 67 gm/mm² pressure were used for all procedures. Cats were anesthetized with sodium pentobarbital administered intraperitoneally and the femoral artery was exposed as previously described. Both flow probe and polyethylene snares were applied as described in the section concerning operation of the flowmeter. Additionally, all surgical techniques were performed by the same individual to maintain uniformity throughout the experiment.

Ten femoral arteries from cats were surgically exposed for 60 minutes to serve as controls. Measurements of blood flow were made at the start and conclusion of the experimental period. Nine additional cat femoral arteries were surgically exposed; however, in these preparations, microvascular clamps were applied for 60 minutes. Blood flow determinations were made prior to clamping and 5 minutes after the clamps were removed, avoiding the temporary rise in blood flow seen after mechanical occlusion. Throughout these experiments, all arteries were continuously moistened to prevent trauma from drying.

The 10 femoral arteries that were exposed for 60 minutes had a decrease in flow of approximately 17% when compared to initial flow measurement. On the other hand, the nine arteries that were clamped, in addition to being surgically exposed, had a decrease in mean flow of approximately 37%. Under controlled laboratory conditions, use of vascular clamps exerting 67 gm/mm² pressure resulted in approximately a 20% decrease in blood flow, in addition to the decrease that resulted from 60 minutes of surgical exposure. In part because of these studies and other clinical reports,[31,32] the use of clamps is avoided by our institution whenever possible, with inflating tourniquets being used during clinical anastomoses instead.

To study blood flow after arterial anastomosis, five cat femoral arteries were surgically exposed and clamped as previously described. These arteries were severed and anastomosed during the 60 minutes of clamping. When blood

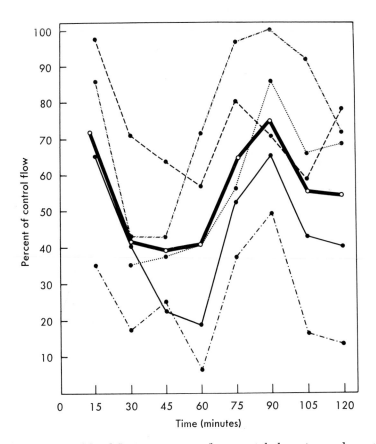

Fig. 21-7. Variations in blood flow in percent after arterial clamping and anastomoses. The mean is indicated with a heavy black line.

flow was monitored for 120 minutes after the release of clamps, there was a variable flow pattern with significant fluctuations of mean flow during the 2-hour interval (Fig. 21-7). The mean flow for the five determinations varied in a predictable pattern throughout the interval of the study. Since only five anastomoses were performed, it is difficult to make definite conclusions from this data. Besides assessment of specific aspects of microsurgical technique, the electromagnetic flowmeter can be used to evaluate the actions of various pharmacologic agents prior to their clinical application.

Use of lidocaine, reserpine, and papaverine in chemically mediated vasospasm

Vascular spasm has been identified as a major deterrent to successful limb replantation.[28] With use of the electromagnetic flowmeter, this experiment evaluated three potential spasmolytic agents: lidocaine, reserpine, and papaverine, with normal saline serving as a control against experimental epinephrine-induced arterial vasospasm.

Twenty femoral arteries from cats were exposed surgically, and both probe and snare were applied as described earlier in this chapter. Initial measurements of blood flow were recorded for all arteries after exposure. Two milliliters of epinephrine 1:2000 solution was sprayed locally on the artery distal to the snare. After 12 minutes, the area was irrigated with saline and blood flow measurements were recorded. After administration of epinephrine, flow recordings that were 60% or less of control blood flow levels, served as the criterion for arterial spasm. After spasm was confirmed, the cats were divided into four groups of five cats each, and either saline or one of the potential spasmolytic agents was applied to a specific group (Table 5). Measurements of blood flow were made for 30 minutes after application of the spasmolytic agent.

Table 5. Effect of spasmolytics on chemically induced spasm

Group	Number of subjects	Spasm induction	Spasmolytic applied locally where epinephrine was initially applied	Number of reapplications*
1	5	Epinephrine 2 ml 1:2000 solution	Saline 9% NaCl per 2 ml	5
2	5	Epinephrine 2 ml 1:2000 solution	Reserpine 5 mg per 2 ml	4
3	5	Epinephrine 2 ml 1:2000 solution	Papaverine 60 mg per 2 ml	0
4	5	Epinephrine 2 ml 1:2000 solution	Lidocaine 20 mg per 2 ml	2

*If no increase in blood flow was seen after 5 minutes, saline solution or the spasmolytic agent was reapplied.

In the five saline-treated control subjects, persistent vasospasm was seen throughout the experimental period with the exception of one animal, which showed a transient rise in blood flow 25 minutes after saline solution was applied. In the group treated with reserpine, the spasm reversed with a mean of 5 determinations measuring 95% of the initial blood flow levels within 30 minutes. The spasmolytic action of reserpine was gradual, with only minimal response seen within 5 minutes after topical reserpine application. Unlike the reserpine-treated group, the papaverine group showed a rapid reversal of spasm, with a mean of all subjects showing blood flow that was 60% higher than that of control values. With papaverine, the spasm not only reversed rapidly but also may have resulted in vasodilation. Unlike the group with papaverine, lidocaine was ineffective in reversing vasospasm with flows ap-

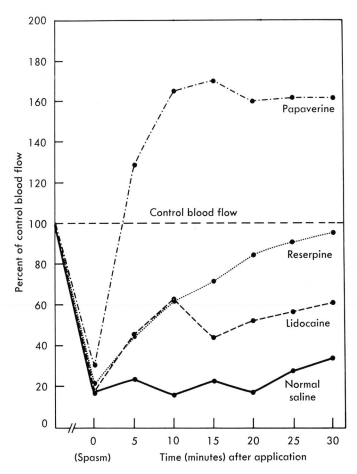

Fig. 21-8. Arterial blood flow recordings taken after drug application to measure the effects of various spasmolytic agents after chemically induced spasm of the femoral artery.

proximately 50% to 60% of prespasm levels obtained within a 30-minute period. A summary of the means of all experimental results can be found in Fig. 21-8. We have observed during pilot studies when using 1% lidocaine after papaverine that a white precipitate occurs around the vessel; thus the simultaneous use of papaverine and 1% lidocaine is contraindicated.

Since the electromagnetic flowmeter is a reliable method of blood flow, it can be used as a standard to compare with indirect measurements of blood flow. Thus Ramon et al.[24] compared the electromagnetic flowmeter recordings to data obtained by means of venous occlusion plethysmography when both instruments were used simultaneously. With complete venous obstruction, he reported the values were equal. However, his venous plethysmograph values were less than electromagnetically measured values prior to occlusion.

Use of electromagnetic flowmeter experimentally and clinically will lead to a better understanding of the pathophysiologic state of small vessels, together with new knowledge on how the peripheral vessels react after replantation or tissue transfer. This, in turn, will lead to refinements in microsurgical techniques. Many vascular surgeons presently use the electromagnetic flowmeter to monitor blood flow through reconstructed vessels and Dacron grafts.[4,6,26] Clinically, in this institution monitoring of blood flow through reconstructed vessels in replanted extremities is underway. With vast opportunities for both clinical and experimental microsurgery research, the electromagnetic flowmeter is a reliable technique for assessing blood flow in vessels of 2 mm down to 0.5 mm in diameter.

ACKNOWLEDGMENT

Work in this chapter was partly supported by NIH Grant no. 1 RO1 GM25666.

REFERENCES

1. Beck, R., Morris, J. A., and Assali, N. S.: Calibration characteristics of the pulsed-field electromagnetic flowmeter, Am. J. Med. Electronics, April-June, pp. 87-91, 1965.
2. Bergel, D. H., and Gessner, U.: The electromagnetic flowmeter, Methods Med. Res. **11**:70-82, 1966.
3. Bond, R. F.: In-vivo method of calibrating electromagnetic flowmeter probes, J. Appl. Physiol. **22**:358-361, 1966.
4. Cannon, J. A.: The clinical application of the electromagnetic blood flowmeter in direct arterial surgery. In Cappelen, C., editor. International symposium on electromagnetic flowmetry, new findings in blood flowmetry, Oslo, 1968, Universitetsforlaget, pp. 198-201.
5. Cappelen, C., Jr.: Relevant criteria for the evaluation of blood flowmeters, International symposium on electromagnetic flowmetry, new findings in blood flowmetry, Oslo, 1968, Universitetsforlaget, pp. 123-126.
6. Cappelen, C., Jr., Efskind, L., and Hall, K. V.: Electromagnetic flowmeter measurements of the blood flow in the ascending aorta during cardiac surgery, Acta Chir. Scand. Suppl. **356**:129-133, 1966.

7. Cappelen, C., Jr., and Hall, V.: Electromagnetic blood flowmetry in clinical surgery, Acta Chir. Scand. Suppl. **368**:2-27, 1967.
8. Denison, A. B., Jr., and Spencer, M. P.: Square wave electromagnetic flowmeter design, Rev. Sci. Instrum. **27**:707, 1956.
9. Engell, H. C., and Lauridsen, P.: The use of the square wave electromagnetic flowmeter in reconstructive vascular surgery, J. Cardiovasc. Surg. **7**:283-288, 1966.
10. Fabre, P.: Utilisation des forces électromotrices d'induction pour l'enrégistrement des variations de vitesse des liquides conduisant un nouvel hémomonographe sans palette dans le sang, C. R. Acad. Sci. **194**:1097, 1932.
11. Faraday, M.: Experimental researches in electricity, Phil. Trans. **15**:175, 1832.
12. Franklin, D. L.: Techniques for measurement of blood flow through intact vessels, Med. Electron. Biol. Eng. **3**:27-37, 1965.
13. Golding, A. L., and Cannon, J. A.: Application of electromagnetic blood flowmeter during arterial reconstruction results in conjunction with papaverine in 47 cases, Ann. Surg. **164**:662-677, 1966.
14. Gordon, A. S., Elazar, S., and Austin, S.: Practical aspects of blood flow measurement, Oxnard, 1971, Statham Instruments Press.
15. Hall, K. V.: Postoperative blood flow measurements in man by use of implanted electromagnetic probes, Scand. J. Thorac. Cardiovasc. Surg. **3**:135-144, 1969.
16. Jacobson, E. D., and Swan, K. G.: Hydraulic occluder for chronic blood flow determinations, J. Appl. Physiol. **21**(4):1400-1402, 1966.
17. Kayser, K.: Performance characteristics of two commercial blood flowmeters, Am. J. Med. Electronics **4**:113-116, July-Sept. 1965.
18. Khouri, E. M., and Gregg, D. E.: Miniature electromagnetic flowmeter applicable to coronary arteries, J. Appl. Physiol. **18**:224-227, 1963.
19. Kolin, A.: An electromagnetic flowmeter, principles of the method and its application to blood flow measurements, Proc. Soc. Exp. Biol. Med. **35**:53-56, 1936.
20. Kolin, A.: An electromagnetic flowmeter, Am. J. Physiol. **119**:355-356, 1937.
21. Kolin, A.: Circulation systems methods, blood flow determinations by electromagnetic method, Med. Phys. **3**:141-155, 1960.
22. McDonald, D. A.: Flowmeters for pulsatile flow. In McDonald, D. A.: blood flow in arteries, Baltimore, 1974, The Williams & Wilkins Co., pp. 209-217.
23. Naitove, A.: Electromagnetic flowmeters. In Swan, K. G., editor: Venous surgery in the lower extremities, St. Louis, 1973, Green Publishing Co., pp. 79-89.
24. Ramon, E. R., Vanhyse, V. J., and Jageneau, A. H.: Comparison of plethysmographic and electromagnetic flow measurements, Phys. Med. Biol. **18**(5):704-711, 1973.
25. Roberts, V. C.: Electromagnetic techniques in blood flow measurement, Part II, London, 1972, Sector Publishing Ltd., pp. 79-136.
26. Ross, G., Kolin, A., and Austin, S.: Electromagnetic observations on coronary arterial blood flow, Proc. Natl. Acad. Sci. Phys., **52**:692-699, 1962.
27. Shercliff, J. A.: Electromagnetic flow measurement since Faraday. In Baker, J., editor: Electromagnetic flow measurement, London, 1962, Cambridge University Press, pp. 1-9.
28. Swartz, W. M., Brisk, R. R., and Buncke, H. J.: Prevention of thrombosis in arterial and venous microanastomosis by using topical agents, Plast. Reconstr. Surg. **58**:478-481, 1976.
29. Swan, K. G., and Reynolds, D. G.: A miniaturized occluder for electromagnetic blood flow measurements, J. Thorac. Cardiovasc. Surg. **63**:3, 403-406, 1972.
30. Tetirick, J. E., and Mergol, L.: Calibration and use of square wave electromagnetic flowmeter, Surgery **54**:621-626, 1963.

31. Thurston, J. B., Buncke, H. J., Chater, N. L., and Weinstein, P. R.: A scanning electron microscopic study of microarterial damage and repair, Plast. Reconstr. Surg. **57**:197-203, 1976.

32. Urbaniak, J. R., Soucacos, P. N., Adelaar, R. S., Bright, D. S., and Whitehurst, L. A.: Experimental evaluation of microsurgical techniques in small artery anastomoses, Symposium on replantation and reconstructive microsurgery, Orthop. Clin. North Am. **8**:2, 249-263, 1977.

33. Wetterer, E.: Flowmeters: their theory, construction, and operation. In Field, J. (Hamilton, W. F., and Dow, P.), editors: Handbook of physiology, Circulation II, Baltimore, 1963, The Williams & Wilkins Co., pp. 1311-1318.

34. Wyatt, D. G.: Noise in electromagnetic flowmeters, Med. Biol. Eng. **4**:333-347, 1966.

35. Wyatt, D. G.: Theory, design and use of electromagnetic flowmeters. In Hwang, N. H. C., and Normann, N. A., editors: Cardiovascular flow dynamics and measurements, Baltimore, 1977, University Park Press, pp. 89-149.

22. Experimental microlymphatic surgery

Anthony V. Seaber
James R. Urbaniak
Hiroo Hiramatsu

Although many centers throughout the world are routinely anastomosing arteries and veins of 0.5 mm diameter, lymphatic anastomosis is seldom attempted. Today, lymphatic anastomoses are rarely performed during traumatic limb repair and only in selective cases during muscle or tissue transfer. Attempted microlymphatic surgery either by direct end-to-side anastomosis[5,6,11,18] or by lymphatic shunts has not yielded the best possible results. Recently O'Brien[19] reported encouraging findings after lymphaticovenous anastomoses, but long-term results have to be observed before these microlymphatic surgical techniques will be fully accepted.

This chapter will consider the animal models necessary to achieve lymphatic anastomosis and will outline technical and procedural developments necessary to conduct further research in this field.

IMMEDIATE POSTOPERATIVE PERIOD: LYMPH FLOW

Many have reported the regenerative powers of the lymphatic system.[4,7,9,20] The regeneration patterns of the lymphatic system were first reported by Billroth[3] in 1863. He wrote that lymphatics do not grow across scar tissue but localized blocks of scar tissue are bypassed and lymphatics grow along preexisting collateral channels. Occasionally a lymphaticovenous shunt will be established. Danese[8] in 1962 observed that after loose approximation of muscle and skin, the lymphatic flow was restored within weeks. He postulated regeneration of lymph vessels in 14 to 21 days. Other studies substantiated by Gray,[13] Nanson,[17] and Olszewski[20] show the remarkable regeneration of lymphatic vessels.

Recent studies in our microsurgery research laboratory using the rabbit ear have shown that only after complete severance of all the lymph vessels does significant lymphedema occur. Also, by the tenth postoperative day, the ear thickness had receded to preoperative values (Fig. 22-1).

The first 10 days of a tissue transfer or replant is believed to be the "critical

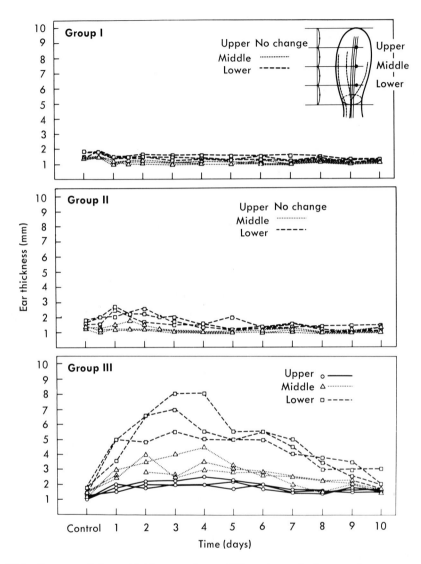

Fig. 22-1. By use of the rabbit's ear, three different surgical procedures were per-formed. In group I, a circumferential skin incision was made at the base of the ear. In group II, the skin and musculature was severed to arrest the dorsal and capillary lymph network. In group III, the rabbit's skin, musculature, and all lymph vessels were severed to leave intact the artery, vein, and nerve.

In all groups, the skin was loosely approximated by a 4-0 suture. The rabbit's ear was divided into three equal parts from the tip of the ear to the circumferential incision (*top right inset*). These areas were designated upper, middle, and lower. Twelve-hour measurements were taken of the thickness of the ear by a modified ECG caliper. The only significant change in ear thickness was measured in group III, which had returned to preoperative values by the tenth day.

stage" for survival. Based on the previous experiment, if lymph anastomosis can be achieved, it may be of greatest benefit during the acute postoperative period. During this stage, the maximum cellular clearance and washout of waste, metabolic products, and toxins needs to occur. The establishment of lymph vessels together with restoration of arterial and adequate venous flow may well be a deciding factor in survival of the replanted part during this critical period. Also if cadaveric limb transplantation is to be achieved, anastomosis of the lymphatic vessels may have to be performed.[1,2,14]

General lymphatic system

The lymphatic system is only well developed in homotherms; thus the models available for research are limited. Lymph is a fluid very similar to blood plasma with similar proteins and salts. It is a clear, colorless fluid and usually contains no cells until lymphocytes are added in its passage through the lymphatic nodes. Lymph collected from the digestive tract may be milky in appearance after a meal because of contained fat particles. The cells of the lymph are almost entirely lymphocytes varying from 2000 to 20,000 per cubic millimeter in the thoracic duct of man.[10] Histologically the lymphatic capillaries are "closed-ended" endothelial tubes, highly permeable to macromolecules and particles. Apart from this, the lymphatic capillaries are similar to the vascular capillaries, and they are distributed among the tissue cells in the same way as the vascular capillaries. The peripheral channels do not communicate with blood vessels but form an extensive capillary network that collects lymph in the various organs and tissues. This is known as the superficial lymph system.[21] The deep lymphatic system is made up of a vast network of vessels that carries the lymph from the lymphatic channels into the blood system through the great veins within the thorax of man. These lymphatic vessels also contain lymph nodes, which are believed to work like filters in the path of the collecting vessels.[22]

The lymph nodes have a rich blood supply[16] containing phagocytes, which attack and destroy foreign material contained in the lymph fluid. They are also known to produce lymphocytes, plasma cells, and some antibodies.

Within the deep lymphatic vessels are to be found valves that are like the valves contained in the veins. They are formed of thin layers of fibrous tissue covered on both sides by endothelium. They are either monocuspid or bicuspid, and only permit lymph flow in one direction, toward the central veins.

The main difference between the valves of the lymphatic system and the veins is that the valves within the lymphatic system are placed at much closer intervals than those within the veins. More lymphatic valves can be found near the lymphatic nodes, and they are more frequent in the larger lymphatic vessels and upper extremities than in the lower extremities. The wall of the lymphatic vessel immediately above the point of attachment of the valve has been reported as appearing as a pouch, which, when the vessel is extended, has a beaded appearance.[25] This beaded appearance is seldom seen when microsurgery is performed, even under high power, perhaps because of the interruption of the lymphatic flow or because of the dissection of the perivascular tissue surrounding the lymphatics and veins.

The lymph is propelled by contractions of vessel walls in the larger vessels and only by the motion of surrounding structures in the smaller vessels.

MAJOR COMPOSITION OF LYMPH FLUID

In man, between 75 to 200 gm of protein return through the lymph channel to the bloodstream every 24 hours; this protein is contained in 2.5 to 4 liters of lymph.[10] Both the fluid and the protein of lymph are derived from the vascular bed as a result of filtration and diffusion across the capillaries. This slow but continuous circulation of tissue fluid protein from the blood and back to the blood through the lymphatics is an important factor in the maintenance of normal cell environment. The concentration of protein found in lymph varies according to the region or organ and the metabolic rate at a given time. For example, lymph from the leg at rest contains about 15% to 20% of the protein in plasma. But with heavy exercise, the protein concentration will decrease because of increased ultrafiltration and osmotic fluid transfer. About half of the total lymph flow is derived from the gastrointestinal tract and liver.

Lymph from the gastrointestinal tract contains 40% to 50% of the plasma protein concentration. The highest protein concentration is found in the liver, which is about 85% of that of plasma. Lymph contains fibrinogen and prothrombin and will form a gel-like clot if left standing at room temperature. However, lymph flow, when compared to plasma, has a remarkably low coagulability, which is in part attributable to the absence of platelets, especially in the superficial lymph network.[10]

Particular enzymes are known to be carried from their cells of origin by the lymph to the blood. The intestinal lymphatic channel carries some 60% of the lipid, mainly long-chain fatty acids, absorbed from the intestine after digestion. Alpha and beta lipoproteins and chylomicrons have been found in lymph fluid. These include amylase, alkaline phosphatase, and histaminase.[10]

CONDITION OF LYMPH FLOW

The pressures in the lymphatic system vary from 3 to 5 mm H_2O in peripheral trunks to near zero in the thoracic duct. The right thoracic duct delivers a smaller volume of lymph because it drains a smaller surface area of the body.[23] Considerable phasic changes in pressure occur with movements. These phasic changes in pressure in the lymph vessels are believed to compress the ducts and displace their contents.

Landis[15] in 1946 showed that venous obstruction greatly increased the lymph flow in man. The capillary pressure rises as a result of venous obstruction; therefore capillary filtration rates increase accordingly. Venous pressure of 60 to 70 mm Hg may increase lymph flow as much as tenfold. Recent work by Gnepp and Sloop[12] in 1978, using the dog's paw, showed that lymph flow rates could be halved if one decreases the frequency of paw pumping from 100 to 10 counts per minute.

Vasodilation, during muscle exercise, is known to increase both the capillary filtering surface and the filtration pressure. Hyperosmolarity of the activated muscles contributes to the fluid transfer, and lymph flow increases. Increased capillary permeability (which may be caused by locally released histamin), bacterial toxins, and foreign proteins are known to increase in lymph flow. Glandular secretion is usually accompanied by a sharp increase in lymph flow. During glandular secretion, kallidin is released in the salivary glands; thus the capillary pressure and capillary surface area are increased by its vasodilation action.

STRUCTURES OF LYMPHATIC VESSELS

In lymph vessels, smaller than 0.1 mm, there are no muscular or elastic fibers and the wall consists only of a connective tissue coat sparsely lined by endothelium. This makes it impossible to use conventional suturing techniques when one attempts to anastomose the vessel. In larger vessels above 0.1 mm, the vessels have three main structures.

1. The internal structure (intima) is thin, transparent, and elastic. It is composed of a layer of elongated endothelial cells that are dovetailed into one another. This cell network is supported by an elastic membrane.
2. The center structure (media) is composed of smooth muscle having fine elastic fibers orientated in a transverse direction.
3. The external structure (adventitia) has connective tissue and smooth muscular fibers that forms a protective covering. This covering serves to connect the vessel with the surrounding structures and should be preserved as much as possible when one dissects the lymph vessel free prior to anastomosis.

The lymphatic vessels under a high-powered operating microscope prior to dissection are pale yellow. After the vessels are dissected free, with the consequent arrest of most of the lymphatic flow, the vessels become completely white and need a dark blue background to distinguish them from their surroundings.

The larger lymphatic vessels such as a thoracic duct are more complex in structure than are the smaller lymphatic vessels. They are composed of a distinct subendothelial layer of branched cells similar to those found in the arteries, making them less difficult to repair than the smaller lymph vessels.

Identification of lymphatic vessels

For visualization of the lymphatic vessels under the microscope, an intradermal injection of blue-violet dye is used. In the rabbit's ear for example, 0.1 ml of the blue dye is injected into the tip of the ear with a 25-gauge needle.

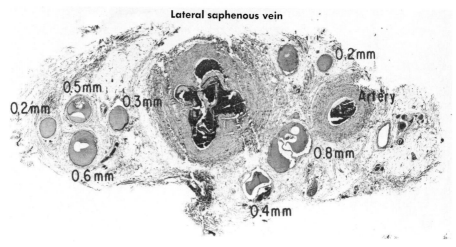

Fig. 22-2. In the hind leg of the canine, lymph vessels range in size from 0.8 to 0.2 mm. They are located in the perivascular tissue surrounding the lateral saphenous veins. For identification of the lymph vessels for pathophysiologic section they are filled with 0.5 ml of radiopaque material by cannulation of a distal lymphatic vessel.

For identification of lymphatic vessels in the canine's hind leg, 1 ml of dye is injected into the plantar pad. The dye is quickly absorbed into the lymphatic drainage system and permits visualization of the lymphatic vessels as a thin blue line seen under the high power of the operating microscope. As seen in Fig. 22-2, the main lymph vessels of the hind leg of a 23 kg canine are found in the perivascular tissue surrounding the lateral saphenous veins. The lymphatic vessels, unlike the single artery or vein contained in the fibrous body, are made up of various sizes; thus repair of all of them is impossible during the surgical procedure. Another method using x rays to identify the vessels distal to the proposed anastomosis site is by cannulation of a lymph vessel and injection of 1.5 ml of radiopaque material (Angio-Conray*) directly into the lymphatic network, as seen in Fig. 22-3. To facilitate lymph flow, the paw can be pumped 90 to 100 times per minute, a rate that will increase the lymph flow considerably.

ANIMAL MODELS FOR LYMPHATIC STUDIES
General lymphatic system in rabbit

The rabbit, partly because of his eating habits has developed a substantial general lymphatic system ranging in size of 0.5 mm in the abdomen vessels to 0.1 mm in the femoral area. Because of the initial low cost, the low per diem rates, together with the accessibility and the general knowledge of this re-

---

*Mallinckrodt Chemical Works, St. Louis, Missouri 63160.

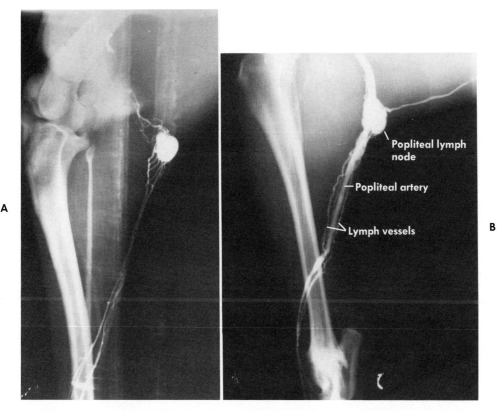

Fig. 22-3. A, Distinct network of the lymphatic system in the hind leg of a 22.5 kg canine is seen. The lymphatic vessels were identified by an intradermal injection of blue dye and the lymphatic vessels cannulated by use of the microscope with a polyethylene catheter whose outside diameter was 1.1 mm. The popliteal lymph node is well developed in the canine hind leg. **B,** Anatomic placement of the popliteal artery is shown. The relationship of the artery to the lymphatic vessels is identified by an arterial lymphogram.

search animal, the rabbit becomes an attractive animal for lymphatic studies. Fig. 22-4 shows the general lymphatic system of a 3.6 kg rabbit.

Lymphatic vessels in rabbit's ear

The rabbit's ear is supplied by a central artery and vein with additional subcutaneous veins and is innervated by a central nerve, seen in Fig. 22-5. For identification of the lymphatic channels before surgery is attempted, the ear is injected at its tip intradermally with blue dye. Time is allowed for visualization of the lymphatic channels, which is brought about by shining a flashlight on the surface of the ear, where the blue color is clearly seen. Apart from lymphatic anastomosis and grafting, nucleotide clearance studies and the effect of temperature on lymphatic flow can be measured in this model mainly

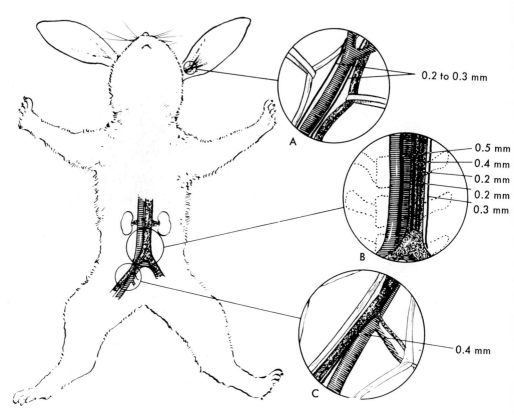

Fig. 22-4. A, The two main lymph vessels in the ear measure 0.2 to 0.3 mm in a 3.6 kg rabbit. In larger sized rabbits, the lymph vessels of the ear can measure 0.4 mm. **B,** Abdominal lymph vessels, the largest of them being 0.5 mm. **C,** The size of the lymph vessels in the femoral region is 0.4 mm. Because of their anatomic location, the lymph vessels in this area of the femoral range receive too much tension for a routine end-to-end anastomosis.

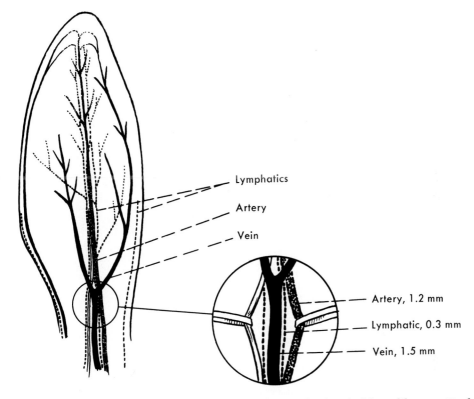

Lymphatics

Artery

Vein

Artery, 1.2 mm

Lymphatic, 0.3 mm

Vein, 1.5 mm

Fig. 22-5. Two lymphatic vessels are routinely seen at this level of the rabbit ear. *Circle on right,* Vessels are embedded in perivascular tissue formed around the vein and range in size from 0.4 to 0.2 mm in rabbits weighing 3.6 to 4.5 kg.

because of the low amount of musculature in the ear and the good visualization of the vascular bed.

Lymphatic vessels in cat

The domestic cat, which is often bred in large quantities for research purposes, is an easily acquired and relatively inexpensive research animal. The ease of handling and low per diem rates permit long-term experiments. Its mode of walking and the use of the hind quarters with well-developed musculature in its hind legs make this species attractive for replantation and muscle transfer. Problems encountered with anesthesia in the cat can be overcome by anesthetization and tracheotomy and by placement of the animal on a respirator using halothane as an anesthetic.

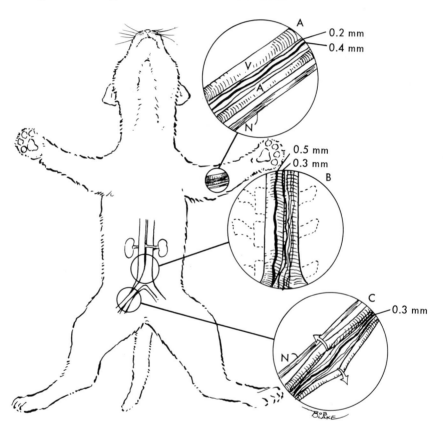

Fig. 22-6. Lymphatic system in the cat (4 kg) is similar to that of the rabbit and canine. **A,** The upper forearm has two main vessels; the larger one is found in the perivascular tissue between the artery and vein. In the abdomen, **B,** the lymphatic vessel measured 0.5 mm. It is easily visible after an injection of blue dye and is located midline on the inferior vena cava. Also between the inferior vena cava and the aorta are located many smaller lymphatic vessels. In the hind leg, **C,** the lymphatic vessels are 0.2 and 0.4 mm in size, and also there are many smaller vessels in the perivascular tissue.

Lymphatic vessels in the cat are much the same as those found in the rabbit and canine but are smaller in size as seen in Fig. 22-6. If lymphatic experimental work is planned for this species, a high level of expertise in microsurgical techniques should precede any experimental attempts, since the largest vessel in the abdomen is only 0.5 mm in size.

Lymphatic vessels in rhesus monkey

The rhesus monkey's ability to coordinate his arms and especially his hands makes him a desirable research species. Unfortunately the cost is extremely high, both for initial purchase and for board and special handling requirements. Additionally elaborate precautions against infection are required both to protect the animal and investigator. The largest vessels of the rhesus monkey used for the dissection was 0.3 mm in the thoracic cavity (Fig. 22-7). The animal was in excellent health and had been in captivity approximately half his life.

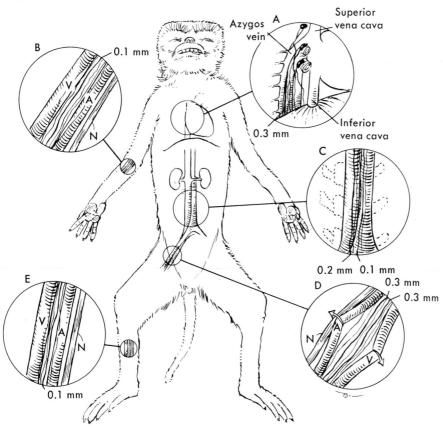

Fig. 22-7. In a rhesus monkey *(Macaca mulata)* 12 years old with a weight of 14.4 kg, the largest lymphatic vessel was 0.3 mm in the thoracic cavity, **A.** All other vessels were from 0.3 to 0.1 mm in diameter seen in **B** to **E.**

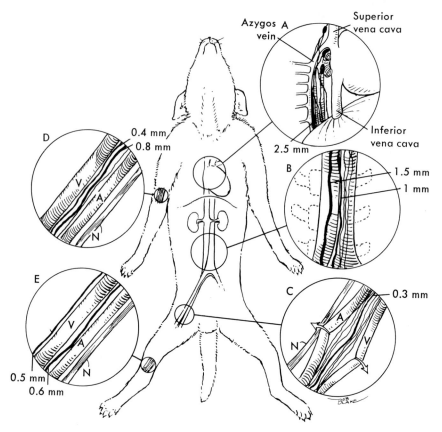

Fig. 22-8. A, The thoracic duct of a 23.4 kg canine measures 2.5 mm. **B** to **D,** The lymphatic vessels vary in size from 0.3 mm to 0.4 and 0.8 mm. **E,** At the level where most experimental amputations and replantations are carried out, the lymphatic vessels are 0.5 to 0.6 mm in diameter with many vessels larger than 0.1 mm, as shown in Fig. 22-2.

Lymphatic vessels in the canine

A great amount of knowledge has already been collected regarding the anatomy and limitations of the canine as an experimental model. Seen in Fig. 22-8, the largest lymphatic vessels in a 23 kg dog range in size from 2.5 mm in the thoracic cavity to 0.3 mm in the femoral area. The 0.8 mm lymphatic vessels found in the upper forearm and the well-developed lymphatic network of the hind leg, as seen in Fig. 22-9, allow this model to be used for lymphatic vessel grafting, lymphatic-venous grafting, and most microlymphatic experimental protocols. Also amputations of the hind leg and reanastomosis of the artery, veins, nerves, and lymphatic vessels are possible. Although it is not possible to anastomose all the lymphatic vessels in the hind leg, the two main vessels of 0.5 and 0.6 mm in size may be sufficient for lymphatic drainage of that area. The large skeletal muscle mass and the ability to postoperatively

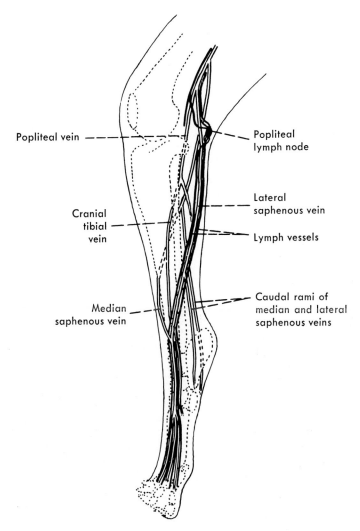

Popliteal vein

Popliteal
lymph node

Lateral
saphenous vein

Cranial
tibial
vein

Lymph vessels

Median
saphenous vein

Caudal rami of
median and lateral
saphenous veins

Fig. 22-9. In the hind leg of the canine, the anatomic relationship of the popliteal lymph node to the lateral saphenous vein and lymphatic vessels is shown.

monitor this animal for metabolic and pathologic studies, together with lymphograms and nucleotide clearance studies, allow the canine to be used for most experimental microlymphatic surgery procedures.

LYMPHATIC END-TO-END ANASTOMOSIS—THREE-SUTURE TECHNIQUE
General considerations

Most lymphatic vessels in the animal models described are approximately 0.8 to 0.3 mm. Although lymphatic vessels smaller than 0.5 mm can be anastomosed, the difficulties encountered during surgery become proportionally greater partly because of the lack of structural composition of the vessel walls. Although, frequently, approximating vascular clamps are used during vein and arterial anastomosis, because of the fragility of lymphatic vessels, these clamps are never used during lymphatic anastomosis. Also, the need for clamping lymphatic vessels becomes unnecessary because of the low flow and minimal pressure in the lymphatic vessels.

Although the lymphatic channels are extremely extensible and can be stretched to twice their size, the traumatic damage done to the lumen, especially the elastic membrane that supports the lumen, may be the reason for poor lymphatic flow after anastomosis. Also, the natural tendency is for lymphatic vessels to lie relatively dormant within soft perivascular tissue. The stretching of the vessel to greater than one third its original size may be detrimental to future lymphatic flow along that vessel. The criteria that the vessel circumference only be dilated by one third of its original size should be

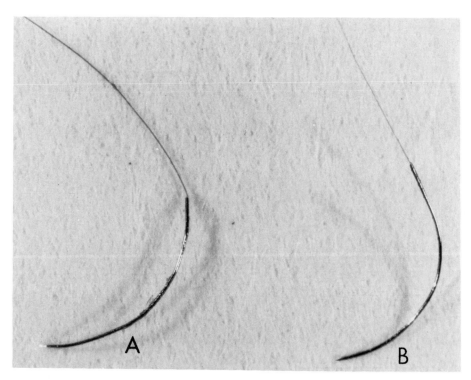

Fig. 22-10. A, An 11-0 Ethilon BV-8 micron needle (by Ethicon, Inc.). In comparison, **B** shows a 12-0 Vasculature suture (by S & T Chirurgische Nadeln GmbH) with a 50-micron needle. With the 12-0 suture, approximately half the suture material is used when compared to 11-0. Although the 12-0 suture with a 50-micron needle is suitable for lymphatic anastomosis, mainly because of the low pressure in the lymphatic system, this needle and suture may be contraindicated when a vein and an artery are anastomosed because of the large hole made from the 50-micron needle.

adhered to during lymphatic anastomosis. Likewise, the rule of longitudinal stretching of lymphatic vessels no more than 1 cm in either direction should be adhered to. It is the nonexposed area of the lymphatic vessels being anchored to the surrounding tissue that receives most of the tension; thus a breakdown of the lumen and lymphatic vessel proximal and distal to the anastomosis site is caused. Because of the intrinsic supply to the lymphatic channels from the perivascular tissue, a minimal amount of dissection should be carried out during exposure. Surgical techniques involving dissection of the lymphatic vessels are relatively the same as those used in small-vein anastomosis, but the removal of the perivascular tissue surrounding the lymphatic channel should only be adequate to allow for placement of the suture and for good exposure of the back wall. Because of the extremely thin wall of the lymphatic vessels, the suture mass becomes an important variable. The use of a 12-0 suture, such as that seen in Fig. 22-10, becomes paramount during anastomosis. Also, the number of sutures placed in the lymphatic vessel also becomes an important item.

We have found that a one-third suture anastomosis technique has merit. The suture material is less, and the ease of placing the sutures in a one-third configuration can be less time consuming. Also use of continuous irrigation and a dilator for suture placement has enabled us to achieve lymphatic anastomosis with relative ease.

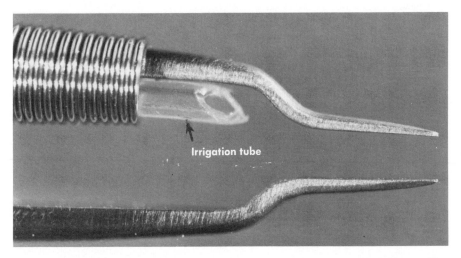

Irrigation tube

Fig. 22-11. Microirrigation forceps (by Edward Weck & Co., Inc.) having a 0.24 mm inside-diameter tube inserted into one shaft, with the tips being straight for approximately 4 mm to allow for greater control when the surgeon is tying or dissecting. When closed, the microirrigation forceps directs the fluid onto lymphatic vessels that are being anastomosed. The control that this forceps affords during tying and dissection is attributable to the large surface area of the tips compared to that of the conventional no. 5 jewelers' forceps now used. The microirrigation forceps can also be used for general microsurgery by removal of the irrigation tube, which can be easily replaced when irrigation is necessary.

Instrumentation for lymphatic anastomosis

Because of the "stickiness" of the lymphatic vessels and their continuous leaking of a high-protein fluid into the operating site, continuous irrigation is necessary. This is brought about by use of a forceps capable of irrigating the operating site and specially designed for microdissection and microsuture holding (Fig. 22-11). The irrigation tube is situated into the shaft of the forceps that is connected to a polyethylene tube connected to a bottle of saline (Fig. 22-12). A 25-gauge needle is inserted into the intravenous tube to allow for an adequate amount of irrigation fluid throughout the anastomosis. This fluid is removed from the operating site by suturing of a gauze swab in one corner of the incision and placement of a suction cannula into it. If more suction is

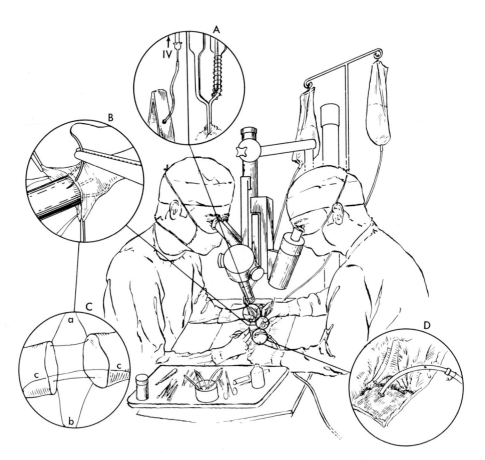

Fig. 22-12. In addition to the general microinstruments, lymphatic anastomosis requires the following: The animal should be placed on a heating pad and maintained at normal temperature. Fluid loss should be replaced by the establishment of an intravenous tube at the time of giving the anesthetic. **A,** Microirrigation forceps. **B,** Vessel dilator. **C,** Three 12-0 sutures are placed between the arms of the dilator. **D,** Suction cannula is placed in a swab in one corner of the field to remove irrigation fluid.

required than is being carried out, pressing on the swab will enhance filling of the gauze, thus quietly emptying the field of excess fluid (Fig. 22-12). The microlymphatic forceps are usually held by the surgeon with the assistant having the task of removing excess irrigation fluid. The placement of a suture in each one-third sector of the vessel is accomplished by use of a Storz* ocular foreign body instrument (Fig. 22-13) that is approximated to the lumen of the lymphatic channels and then used as a dilator for placing the sutures. Three sutures are placed at the proximal end of the lymphatic vessels, and the dilator

---

*Storz Instrument Co., 3365 Tree Court Industrial Blvd., St. Louis, Missouri 63122; no. E1969 Wilson Foreign Body Vitreous Forceps.

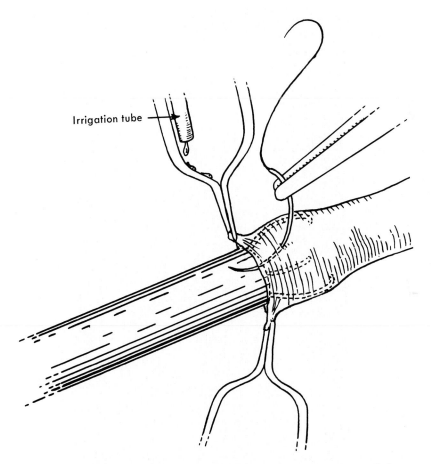

Irrigation tube

Fig. 22-13. The dilator is approximated to the lymphatic vessels, and the required finger pressure is applied to the instrument for the arms to dilate and stretch the vessel wall as needed. The sutures are then placed in a one-third circumferential pattern, and the same suture is used on the other vessel end. After all the sutures have been placed, two sutures are tied simultaneously.

can then be moved and placed at the distal portion where the same sutures are used (Fig. 22-12).

Three-suture surgical technique

With use of a 12-0 nylon suture with a 50-micron needle, three sutures are placed between the arms of the dilator (Fig. 22-13) at the proximal end of a lymphatic vessel. The dilator is then removed and placed at the distal end of the vessels where the same sutures are placed between the arms of the dilator (Fig. 22-12). After sutures have been placed with the dilator and have been designated A, B, and C, the surgeon and the assistant simultaneously approximate the lymphatic vessels by simultaneously tying A and B sutures. The

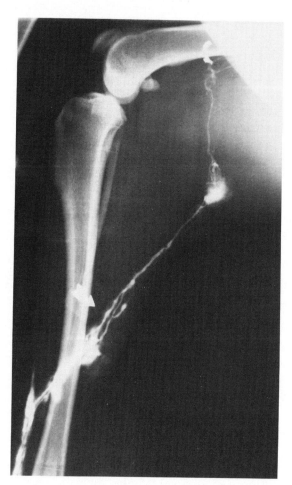

Fig. 22-14. *Arrow,* Location of the lymphatic anastomosis in a 22.5 kg canine. The lymph channels were cannulated distal to the anastomosis site, and the same technique of filling the channels with the radiopaque material was used as in Fig. 22-2. The study was carried out 48 hours postoperatively.

third suture is then tied. Compared to conventional venous- and arterial-anastomosis surgical techniques where the initial stitch has to sustain all the stretch in one small longitudinal direction of the vessel as the first stitch is tied, the simultaneous tying of two sutures in the lymphatic vessel allows the tension to be concentrated over a much greater surface area. Results in using this technique are shown in Fig. 22-14.

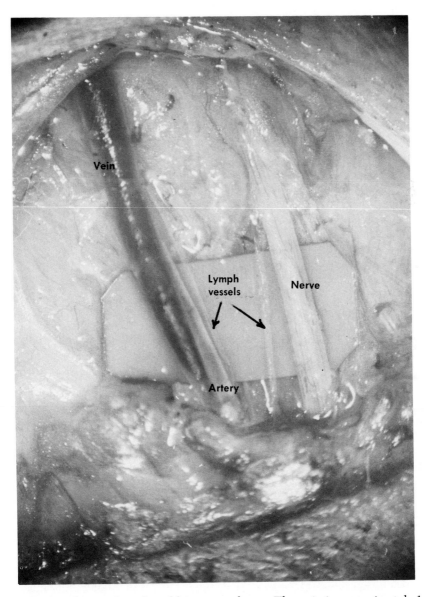

Fig. 22-15. Lymph vessels in the rabbit ear are shown. The vein is approximately 1 mm, and the two lymphatic vessels are approximately 0.3 and 0.2 mm in size.

CONCLUSION

During most replantation procedures or tissue transfer, the lymphatic vessels are usually ignored when anastomoses are performed to achieve blood flow. The anatomic location of the main lymphatic vessels in relationship to the vein and artery seen in Fig. 22-15 can be appreciated. They are easy to locate and can be anastomosed by suturing if they are 0.3 mm or larger. With the thrust in developing tissue adhesives and new and improved techniques for application, lymphatic anastomoses may well be routinely done during most microvascular procedures. Although long-term lymphedema after replantation has not been a problem, anastomosing or approximating the lymph vessels at time of surgery could enhance the success of the replant in the early postoperative period.

If cadaveric transplantation becomes possible, the anastomosis of the lymph vessels at the time of surgery may have to be achieved. If this can be achieved, then the cadaveric limb may survive the additional reaction phenomena and remain a viable and functional replanted part.

ACKNOWLEDGMENTS

The authors wish to thank William Joyner, Senior Technician, for his assistance in performing part of the lymphatic studies.

Work in this chapter was partially supported by NIH grant no. 1 RO1 GM25666.

REFERENCES

1. Barker, C. F., and Billingham, R. E.: The role of regional lymphatics in the skin homograft response, Transplantation (Suppl.) 5(4):962, 1967.
2. Barker, C. F., and Billingham, R. E.: The role of afferent lymphatics in the rejection of skin homografts, J. Exp. Med. **128**:197, 1968.
3. Billroth, T.: Die allgemeine chirurgische Pathologie und Therapie in 50 Vorlesungen, Berlin, 1863, G. Reimer.
4. Blalock, A., Robinson, C. S., Cunningham, R. S., and Gray, M. E.: Experimental studies on lymphatic blockade, Arch. Surg. **34**:1049, 1937.
5. Calderon, G., Robert, B., and Johnson, L. L.: Experimental approach to the surgical creation of lymphaticovenous communications, Surgery **61**:122, 1967.
6. Clodius, L., and Wirth, W.: A new experimental model for chronic lymphoedema of the extremities (with clinical considerations), Chir. Plast. (Berlin) **2**:115, 1974.
7. Danese, C. A.: Experimental lymphedema. In Mayerson, H. S., editor: Lymph and lymphatic system, Springfield, Ill., 1968, Charles C Thomas, Publisher.
8. Danese, C. A., Howard, J. M., and Brower, R.: Regeneration of lymphatic vessels, Ann. Surg. **156**:61, 1962.
9. Drinker, C. K., Field, M. E., and Homans, J.: The experimental production of edema and elephantiasis as a result of lymphatic obstruction, Am. J. Physiol. **108**:509, 1934.
10. Folkow, B., and Neil, E.: Circulation, New York, 1971, Oxford University Press.
11. Gilbert, A., O'Brien, B. M., Vorrath, J. W., Sykes, P. J., and Baxter, T. J.: Lymphaticovenous anastomosis by microvascular technique, Br. J. Plast. Surg. **29**:355, 1976.
12. Gnepp, D. R., and Sloop, C. H.: The effect of passive motion on the flow and formation of lymph, Lymphology **11**:32-36, 1978.

13. Gray, H. J.: Studies of the regeneration of lymphatic vessels, J. Anat. **74:**309, 1939-1940.
14. Lambert, P. B., Howard, A. F., Bellman, S., and Farnsworth, D.: The role of the lymph trunks in the response to allogeneic skin transplants, Transplantation **3:**62, 1965.
15. Landis, E. M.: Capillary permeability and the factors affecting the composition of capillary filtrate, Ann. N.Y. Acad. Sci. **46:**713-731, 1946.
16. Lundgren, O., and Wallentin, I.: Local chemical and nervous control of consecutive vascular sections in the mesenteric lymph nodes of the cat, Angiologica (Basel) **1:**284-296, 1964.
17. Nanson, E. M.: A study of the powers of reanastomosis of the lymphatic vessels and nodes in the dog, Can. J. Surg. **5:**329, 1962.
18. Nielubowicz, J., and Olszewski, W.: Surgical lymphaticovenous shunts in patients with secondary lymphoedema, Br. J. Surg. **55**(6):440, 1968.
19. O'Brien, B.: Microvascular reconstructive surgery, New York, 1977, Churchill Livingstone.
20. Olszewski, W., Machowski, J., Sokolowski, J., and Nielubowicz, J.: Experimental lymphedema in dogs, J. Cardiovasc. Surg. **9:**178, 1968.
21. Romanes, G. J., editor: Cunningham's textbook of anatomy, ed. 11, London, 1974, Oxford University Press.
22. Warwick, R., and Williams, P.: Gray's anatomy, ed. 35, Philadelphia, 1973, W. B. Saunders Co.
23. Woodbruner, R. T.: Essentials of human anatomy, ed. 6, New York, 1974, Oxford University Press.

ADDITIONAL READINGS

Burn, L. L., Rivero, O. R., Pentecost, B. L., and Calnan, J. S.: Lymphographic appearances following lymphatic destruction in the dog, Br. J. Surg. **53:**634, 1966.
Calderon, G., Robert, B., and Johnson, L. L.: Experimental approach to the surgical creation of lymphaticovenous communications, Surgery **61:**122, 1967.
Calnan, J. S., and Pentecost, B. L.: Lymphoedema. In Irvine, W. T., editor: Modern trends in surgery, London, 1966, Butterworth & Co. (Publishers), vol. 2.
Calnan, J. S., Reis, N. D., Rivero, O. R., Copenhagen, H. J., and Mercurius Taylor, L.: Natural history of lymph node to vein anastomosis, Br. J. Plast. Surg. **20:**134, 1967.
Casley-Smith, J. R.: The lymphatic system in inflammation. In Zweifach, B. W., Grant, L., and McClusky, R. C., editors: The inflammatory process, ed. 2, New York, 1965, Academic Press, Inc., vol. 2, pp. 161-204.
Casley-Smith, J. R.: The entrance of material into initial lymphatics and their relationship with fenestrated blood capillaries. In Witte, M., and Witte, C., editors: Proceedings of the IVth International Congress on Lymphology, Tucson, 1973, University of Arizona Press.
Casley-Smith, J. R.: The action of the benzopyrones on the blood tissue-lymph system, Folia Angiol. **14:**7, 1976.
Clodius, L., Uhlschmid, G., and Madritsch, W.: Chirurgische Möglichkeiten der Lymphödembehandlung, Folia Angiol. **11:**304, 1973.
Clodius, L., and Wirth, W.: A new experimental model for chronic lymphoedema of the extremities (with clinical considerations), Chir. Plast. (Berlin) **2:**155, 1974.
Cockett, A. T. K., and Goodwin, W. K.: Chyluria: attempted surgical treatment by lymphatic-venous anastomosis, J. Urol. **88:**566, 1962.
Collard, M.: Pharmacotherapie des Lymphgefäss-systems. In Gregl, A., editor:

Lymphographie und Pharmacolymphographie, Stuttgart, 1975, Gustav Fischer Verlag.

Danese, C., Bower, R., and Howard, J.: Experimental anastomoses of lymphatics, Arch. Surg. **84**:6, 1962.

Danese, C., Georcalas, M., and Morales, L.: A model of chronic post-surgical lympho-edema in dogs' limbs, Surgery **64**:814, 1968.

Drinker, C. K., and Field, M. E.: Lymphatics, lymph and tissue fluid, Baltimore, 1933, The Williams & Wilkins Co.

Firica, A., Ray, A., and Murat, J.: Les anastomoses lympho-veineuses, étude expérimentale, Lyon Chir. **65**:384, 1969.

Foldi, M.: Diseases of lymphatics and lymph circulation, Springfield, Ill., 1969, Charles C Thomas, Publisher.

Gilbert, A., O'Brien, B. M., Vorrath, J. W., Sykes, P. J., and Baxter, T. J.: Lymphatico-venous anastomosis by microvascular technique, Br. J. Plast. Surg. **29**:355, 1976.

Gimbrone, M. A., Aster, R. H., Cotran, R. S., Corkery, J., Jandl, J. H., and Folkman, J.: Preservation of vascular integrity in organs perfused in vitro with a platelet rich medium, Nature **222**:33, 1969.

Jacobson, J. H.: Discussion of Danese et al.: Experimental anastomoses of lymphatics, Arch. Surg. **84**:6, 1962.

Jacobsson, S.: Studies of the blood circulation in lymphedematous limbs, Scand. J. Plast. Reconstr. Surg. Suppl. **3**:1, 1967.

Laine, J. B., and Howard, J. M.: Experimental lymphaticovenous anastomosis, Surg. Forum **14**:111, 1963.

Lundgren, O., and Wallentin, I.: Local chemical and nervous control of consecutive vascular sections in the mesenteric lymph nodes of the cat, Angiologica, **1**:284-296, 1964.

MacDonald, I.: Resection of axillary vein in radical mastectomy: its relation to mechanism of lymphedema, Cancer **1**:618, 1948.

Mayall, R. C., and Witte, M. H.: Progress in lymphology, New York, 1977, Plenum Press.

Mayall, R. C., and Witte, M. H.: Progress in lymphology, New York, 1973, Plenum Press.

Mayerson, H. S.: The physiologic importance of lymph. In Field, J., editor: Handbook of physiology, Circulation II, Baltimore, 1963, The Williams & Wilkins Co., 1035-1074.

Mislin, H.: Die Wirkung von Cumarin aus *Melilotus officinalis* auf die Funktion des Lymphangioms, Arznei Forsch. **21**:833, 1971.

Mistillis, P., and Skyring, A. P.: Intestinal lymphangiectasia—therapeutic effect of lymph-venous anastomosis, Am. J. Med. **40**:634, 1966.

Neyazaki, T., Kupic, E. A., Marshall, W. H., and Abram, H. L.: Collateral lymphatico-venous communications after experimental obstruction of the thoracic duct, Radiology **85**:423, 1965.

Nielubowicz, J., and Olszewski, W.: Surgical lymphatico-venous shunts in patients with secondary lymphoedema, Br. J. Surg. **55**(6):440, 1968.

Oden, B.: Micro-lymphangiographic studies of experimental skin autografts, Acta Chir. Scand. **121**:219, 1961.

Ohara, I., and Taneichi, N.: Lymphaticovenous anastomosis in a case with primary lymphoedema tarda, Angiology **24**:668, 1973.

Olszewski, W., and Nielubowicz, J.: Surgical lymphatico-venous communication in the treatment of lymph stasis. Presented at the Forty-third Congress of Polish Surgeons, Lodz, 1966.

Pentecost, B. L., Burn, J. I., Davies, A., and Calnan, J. S.: A quantitative study of lymphovenous communications in the dog, Br. J. Surg. **53:**630, 1966.

Politowski, M., Bartkowski, S., and Dunowski, J.: Treatment of lymphedema of the lungs by lymphatic-venous fistula, Surgery **66:**639, 1969.

Reichert, F. L.: The regeneration of lymphatics, Arch. Surg. **13:**871, 1926.

Rivero, O. R., Calnan, J. S., Reis, N. D., and Mercurius Taylor, L.: Experimental peripheral lymphovenous communication, Br. J. Plast. Surg. **20:**124, 1967.

Rusznyak, I., Foldi, M., and Szabo, G.: Lymphatics and lymph circulation, London, 1967, Pergamon Press.

Sedláček, J.: Lymphovenous shunt as supplementary treatment of elephantiasis of lower limbs, Acta Chir. Plast. (Praha) **11:**157, 1969.

Threefoot, S. A., and Kossoner, H. T.: Lymphaticovenous communication in man, Arch. Intern. Med. **117:**213, 1966.

Yamada, Y.: The study on lymphatic venous anastomosis in lymphoedema, Nagoya J. Med. Sci. **32:**1, 1969.

Yoffey, J. M., and Courtice, F. C.: Lymphatics, lymph and lymphoid tissue, Cambridge, 1956, Harvard University Press.

23. Concepts of peripheral nerve repair with emphasis on management of small and large nerve gaps

J. Leonard Goldner

The management of peripheral nerve injuries depends on recognition of the unique anatomic, biochemical, and physiologic characteristics of nerve tissue. During the last hundred years, an understanding of the peripheral nerve problem has improved as information from the laboratory has become available, and a better use of clinical models has been adapted by those treating patients with traumatized nerves.[1,2,4,5,8,11,16-18,20,23-26]

The description St. Anthony's fire designates the hyperesthesia of peripheral neuropathy.[3] Causalgia described by Mitchell during the Civil War referred to the severe burning of the extremity associated with nerve trauma.[18] Our present experience documents a definite relationship between nerve damage and vascular insufficiency and does explain certain aspects of this particular pain syndrome and its response in a positive or negative way to sympathectomy.[12] The percussion test described by Tinel during World War I provided a method of recognition of regeneration of nonmyelinated nerve fibers. This reliable test has proved to be helpful in determining the quality of axon regrowth, even though the information derived from the test is gross and provides only a limited amount of information in assessment of a complex problem associated with peripheral nerve injuries.

The data collected by Seddon and his colleagues during World War II emphasized the importance of postinjury muscle testing, preoperative sensory assessment, and persistent and careful recording of information during a long follow-up.[22] Nerve grafting was undertaken by these investigators between 1945 and 1950, but the results were disappointing.[23] In retrospect, the limited use of magnification and nonavailability of microsuture and microinstruments accounted, in part, for the discouraging results that provided only minimum protective sensation and a limited degree of motor recovery, both in the child and in the adult.

Woodhall and his associates during World War II provided a team approach

348

to the management of peripheral nerve injuries.[16,26,27] These publications emphasized not only the clinical aspects of the preoperative and postoperative management, but also accumulated a large amount of information by use of light microscopy and special staining techniques.[16]

The material prepared by Woodhall served as a guide to encourage recognition of normal and abnormal neural tissue at the time that nerve repair was performed. Sunderland, in his all-inclusive book concerning peripheral nerves, defined the complexity of the problem and emphasized the funicular patterns of a peripheral nerve. Other authors contributed to the total understanding of the problem by emphasizing the fascicular alignment during nerve repair,[14] anomalous motor and sensory innervation as it affects assessment of nerve regeneration,[9] compression lesions of intact and repaired nerves, the use of electromyography in assessment of peripheral nerve injuries,[4] and the value of electrical stimulation in the awake and the anesthetized patient in the recognition of motor and sensory elements of the intact peripheral nerve or the severed peripheral nerve.[14]

Omer observed casualties from the Korean War and drew certain conclusions about the results of nerve repair.[21] Correlation of end results at different centers and in different parts of the world has not been clearly accomplished.[12] A definition of a result is essential before a particular method or methods can be selected as the best form of treatment for a particular lesion.[12] Spinner, in his book on peripheral nerves,[25] clarified many of the anatomic aspects, presented clinical examples, and reemphasized the changes caused by compressive lesions. The publication by the Veterans Administration, motivated by Beebe and Woodhall,[30] includes a large amount of information from World War II as a bench mark for future comparison. The results of treatment of casualties after the Korean war and after the Vietnam war, when compared with those after World War II, demonstrated the same pattern of results.

There are many unanswered questions related to the physiology of neural regeneration, the patterns of blood supply, the relationship of blood supply to nerve regeneration, the importance of a nonfibrotic environment for the nerve, and an understanding of the inherent elastic properties of peripheral nerves and the relationship of this elasticity to the management of nerve gaps.[6-12]

Smith[24] stimulated interest in the operating room microscope and reemphasized the importance of magnification in peripheral nerve repair. Millesi[17] modified the techniques of nerve grafting advocated by Seddon and others and took advantage of the operating room microscope, newly developed instrumentation, and sophisticated suture material to stimulate a renewed interest in nerve grafting. Narakas[19] has presented his wide experience with brachial plexus injuries managed by exploration, nerve grafting and nerve repair. Kline[15] has documented the value of evoked action potentials in primates and in humans and has a controlled study in primates comparing epineurial repair and fascicular repair. Cabaud and Rodkey[2] have a controlled study comparing epineurial and fascicular repair in cats and other studies in primates. They also show that *reasonable tension in mobilization making up a nerve gap is not detrimental to the outcome.*

I have drawn certain conclusions after reviewing the literature related to peripheral nerve injuries, listening to presentations by all the individuals listed and many more, and observing several hundred patients with peripheral nerve injuries who have been treated and followed at Duke University Medical Center during the past 25 years.[6-8,12] These conclusions are influenced by information provided by neurophysiologists and other investigators who have provided data concerning sensory receptors; neuromuscular end-plate activity; special characteristics of slow and fast muscle fibers; sprouting activity of damaged nerves; multiple connections between major peripheral nerves, particularly the segments of the brachial plexus; effect of the sympathetic nerves on temperature control, pain, blood flow, and sweating of the extremity; and changes in the sensory ganglion and the anterior horn cells after peripheral nerve injury. The movement of protein within the axon, the occurrence of abnormal painful sensations, and the biochemistry of myelinization, demyelinization, and alterations of the characteristic of collagen reflect results of trauma and affect the degree of regeneration.

Total physiologic recovery after nerve laceration does not occur. Functional recovery of both motor and sensory elements, however, is a reasonable goal, and our efforts in that direction must continue.[29,30]

SUMMARY OF GUIDELINES FOR MANAGEMENT OF PERIPHERAL NERVE INJURIES

1. In regard to *age,* nerve regeneration in children and adolescents, with all other things being equal, occurs with greater speed and greater axon volume than in the adult. As an individual grows older, the process of axon regeneration is overall less successful than in the child.

2. *The anatomic location of injury and the mechanism of injury control the severity of nerve damage.* Concomitant vascular injury affects the degree of nerve regeneration. Stretch injuries, high-velocity injuries, and multiple lacerations in the same nerve diminish the likelihood of a desirable result. Restitution of arterial input and venous outflow within 4 hours after injury and decompression of the involved muscle compartments is essential as the first step in maintenance of muscle function and prevention of ischemic necrosis of muscle.[26]

3. *Preoperative assessment of the hand and forearm after nerve injury by muscle testing, detailed sensory examination,* and *peripheral nerve block and assessment of arterial and venous input* are required in order to establish a baseline prior to definitive treatment and to aid in determining undesirable changes that occur after the initial injury.[6,9,12]

4. *The decision concerning primary repair of a lacerated nerve, early*

delayed repair at 3 to 5 days, late delayed repair from 5 to 21 days, or secondary repair from 21 to 42 days is dependent on the nature of the initial injury, the likelihood of infection, and the experience and state of fatigue of the surgeon.[7,10] A reasonable period of delay is not detrimental to the result. Funicular orientation may be easier, but not necessarily so, at the time of the acute injury. A reasonable delay of a few days to several weeks or even longer will not affect the result if the majority of the axons of the nerve are motor fibers. An attempt should be made to repair mixed nerves within 72 hours if all factors involved are in keeping with this decision. This will allow electrical stimulation of the distal segment in an awake, cooperative patient and may aid immeasurably in the orientation of sensory segments to sensory fibers and motor fibers to motor segments.

5. *Epineurial suture done immediately or delayed or secondarily* has certain technical and time advantages over fascicular suture or funicular repair. Experimental and clinical evidence indicates that a fascicular suture has no advantage over an epineurial suture if the nerve ends are congruous and if it is done by an experienced surgeon.[25,27]

At certain anatomic locations, fascicular suture is mandatory, such as laceration of the median nerve at the base of the palm of the hand at the point where the median nerve branches into the common digital nerves. The same concept is true if the ulnar nerve is lacerated distal to the pisiform bone.[2]

6. There is *inherent elasticity in a peripheral nerve*. Extremity-lengthening procedures demonstrate that a nerve can be stretched 1 to 2 mm a day without harm, provided that certain clinical tethering points do not impale the nerve. Clinical and laboratory experiments indicate that a minimum of 10% of the length of the nerve can be made up by *mobilization* of the nerve and realignment of the proximal and distal segments without application of excessive tension to the site of repair. Flexed joints will protect the repair. Clinical examples of repair of gaps of 15% of the total length have shown acceptable sensory and motor regeneration, and this has been my experience also. Nerve defects in the median, ulnar, or radial nerve varying from 4.5 to 7 cm (2 to 3 inches) have been possible with acceptable clinical results.[12]

7. After careful assessment of published information, examination of patients at many centers in the country who have had *nerve grafting* or *nerve gaps* made up by mobilization and a review of the patients treated at Duke University during the past 25 years, I believe that every effort should be made to obtain a *congruous* repair by *end-to-end* epineurial suture of a motor, sensory, or mixed nerve if this is reasonably possible. If this is not possible, because of a great loss of neural tissue or an excessive amount of peripheral fibrosis or incongruous ends with a large gap, then nerve grafting with or without bone shortening should be considered.[12,17]

Nerve grafting should also be considered if the defect is greater than 6 cm and if this defect cannot be diminished by mobilization of the proximal and distal nerve segments[17,22,23] or shortening of the osseous skeleton. Isolated defects in sensory nerves that cannot be repaired by mobilization and relaxation by bending of adjacent joints should be grafted. However, repair of a gap in a sensory nerve under moderate tension is usually successful.[2]

If tendon transfers are possible in order to reestablish satisfactory motor function such as in an isolated radial nerve injury, and if humeral shortening is not likely to provide an end-to-end epineurial suture, then nerve grafting may or may not be indicated in the management of an isolated radial nerve injury. Nerve injuries associated with open fractures can be managed by moderate bone shortening at the time that the open fracture is treated definitively.[13]

8. *Nerve grafts should not be sutured under tension.*[17]

9. *Maximum blood flow to the extremity before or after nerve repair is essential.* Cold tolerance is greater if blood flow approaches normal. Causalgia, or the burning pain associated with incomplete nerve lesions or a combination of nerve injury and vascular insufficiency, is diminished in intensity if blood flow is increased.[5]

10. *In regard to the electrical stimulation of denervated muscle during the period of regeneration,* there is no clinical or laboratory evidence available at this time that indicates that electrical stimulation of a repaired peripheral nerve or stimulation of a denervated muscle will affect the result favorably.

11. *Assistive splinting,* to maintain the range of motion of joints and to assist in protection of denervated skin during the period of regeneration, is necessary.

12. *Sensory reeducation* of the denervated extremity or part of the extremity should be considered and attempted, although there is no clear controlled evidence that alterations of the central synapsis or peripheral cross-over pathways occur because of this environmental effort. Nerve sprouting occurs distally after nerve injury but does not necessarily respond to improved sensory or motor function by behavioral reeducation. The effort is not harmful, however, and if the patient and the therapist are willing, the program should be undertaken.

13. *Tendon transfers after a peripheral nerve repair* has been accomplished should not be done hastily. As long as there is evidence of progressive improvement of sensory and motor regeneration, and reasonable function is possible, tendon transfer should be delayed. However, extremities affected by irreparable nerve lesions should be managed by early tendon transfer, provided that the tendons to be transferred are of maximum strength. Many times, multiple nerve injuries exist and sufficient time must elapse for the muscle-tendon units to be used for transfer to obtain maximum strength.[13]

Maximum sensory recovery requires a period of time varying from 3 to 5 years, although evidence of regeneration occurs within a few weeks after a satisfactory nerve suture. Signs of motor recovery can be detected first by electromyography and later by clinical evidence of muscle contractions. A laceration of the ulnar nerve at the elbow, for example, may require 3 to 4 years before maximum motor recovery occurs. Within 1 year, however, definite evidence of motor recovery is obvious.[12] Both motor and sensory recovery follow a steady state and begin directly after nerve repair or soon after nerve trauma that has not resulted in total loss of continuity of the nerve. The admonition to wait for sensory and motor regeneration implies that steady progression of regeneration is occurring very early after injury.

A laceration of the median nerve at the midarm level will usually show no motor recovery in the hand for a period of at least 6 months; 2½ to 3 years must elapse before maximum recovery occurs. Decisions concerning tendon transfer will depend on the rate of motor recovery and the functional impairment, and the relationship between the transfer and physiologic recovery. Occasionally, excessive strength will result, such as occurs when early tendon transfers are done for total radial nerve injury even after a satisfactory nerve repair. Two years later, when all muscles supplied by the radial nerve have recovered, there is insufficient flexion strength of the wrist, fingers, and thumb to allow balanced motor activity.[4,13]

14. *Assessment of end results has been clearly defined,* but the guidelines are not used uniformly throughout the world. This assessment requires the utilization of two-point discrimination, response to the tuning fork, the patient's recognition of varying degrees of heat and cold, the occurrence of sweating, the measurement of skin temperatures, and the use of object pick-up tests in order to define sensory recovery. Grasp and pinch testing and recording and descriptions of motor function are also essential in the determination of results after nerve repair, as well as after tendon transfer.

A "good result" in one center, which defines results in a vague, general way, may be considered as a "fair or poor result" in another center, depending on the methods used in defining the end results.

NERVE REPAIR—WHEN AND HOW?

Primary repair may be done if a pure sensory nerve is involved, such as a digital nerve; or a pure motor repair, such as the motor branch of the ulnar nerve; or a mixed nerve if the circumstances involving the nerve injury are ideal. The object causing the injury should be thin and sharp, there should be little or no stretch involved, there should be no rotational or forceful avulsion, and there should be no obvious loss of neural tissue. However, if adequate arterial and venous flow cannot be established, nerve repair should not be done.

Attempted primary repair without a liberal cutback of the ends of the proximal and distal nerve segments will fail. Analysis of primary repair of digital nerves associated with replantation[5] demonstrated a spectrum of results ranging from excellent to poor, with a direct relationship between both the vascular supply and the mechanism of injury.[28,29]

An alternate to primary repair is a nondefinitive end-to-end suture to maintain physiologic elasticity. However, even if the nerve ends are not "tagged," the nerve can be easily mobilized to its optimum length at an early or late delay interval, depending on the circumstances involved.

From my experience, there is no difference in the end result if the nerve is repaired ideally immediately or at 5 days after injury, or even 5 weeks after the initial trauma. The main advantage of primary or early repair, however, is more accurate configurational alignment; although once the nerve ends are cut back, even that alignment is only speculative.[4]

The advantages of primary nerve repair are as follows:
1. Only one operation.
2. Less risk in returning to the site of the original injury if vascular repair is done simultaneously.
3. Most accurate configurational alignment.
4. Early initiation of nerve regeneration.

Advantages to early delayed repair, that is, 3 to 5 days, are as follows:
1. Less chance of infection.
2. Nonviable axons are more readily recognized at the time, and proximal and distal ends are cut back.
3. Distal segment may respond to electrical stimulation for orientation purposes.
4. A rested surgeon working under ideal circumstances on a rested patient.[12,29]

Discussion of nerve fragment alignment

In regard to *configurational alignment,*[10] even sensory nerves should, if possible, be realigned; although the importance of exact alignment of sensory fibers, as compared with the undesirable procedure of suturing motor fibers to sensory fibers, is less significant. We have performed motor nerve "mapping" of median, ulnar, and radial nerves in the upper extremity and the sciatic nerve and its branches in the lower extremity.[20] Circular nerve maps have been prepared to show the location of the motor segments of the peripheral nerve, which, when stimulated, cause isolated action of peripheral muscles. Numerous mappings of the median nerve at the wrist, which were done when the transverse retinacular ligament was released, demonstrated the location of the motor fibers innervating the thenar muscles and just adjacent to that location a nerve segment that, when stimulated, caused isolated action of the first lumbrical.[8-10,13,25]

This information has been helpful in performing early repairs of lacerated mixed peripheral nerves such as the median and ulnar nerves, or in repairing nerves that are primarily made up of motor fibers with only a small percentage of sensory fibers such as the radial nerve. The exact pattern of nerve fibers varies every few millimeters throughout the course of the nerve, but the overall configurational alignment is reasonably constant when one patient is compared to another.[27] Elective nerve repairs in the past have been planned so that the anatomic area usually considered to be made up of motor fibers, that is, the radial aspect of the median nerve at the wrist, is joined to the same region proximally or distally, depending on mobilization of both fragments. Blood vessel alignment, funicular recognition, and mobilization of the proximal and distal ends for at least 2 to 3 cm will aid in providing alignment in the anesthetized patient.

Electrical stimulation in the awake patient will provide a sensory map that has been used in order to orient the proximal and distal sensory and motor fibers. If the repair is done during a 3-to-5 day period after the initial laceration, the patient may recognize distal stimulation of the nerve and be able to identify a sensory zone in the hand that corresponds with the fibers being stimulated in the distal nerve segment. The proximal segment is also stimulated, and the patient recognizes a phantom zone in the hand, and the locations in the proximal and distal nerve segments are then matched with a suture.[12,14]

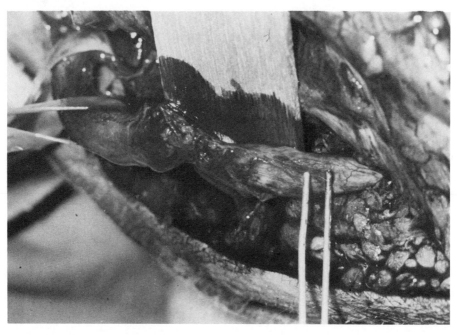

Fig. 23-1. Right ulnar nerve of a 28-year-old man who received an open injury 2 cm proximal to the medial epicondyle 2 weeks prior to this operation. The nerve is held together by a fibrous strand, but no axons traversed the area of trauma. The muscles usually supplied by the ulnar nerve below this level were nonfunctional and the sensory deficit was in keeping with a complete ulnar nerve transection.

Motor fibers may respond to stimulation in the distal segment; these are matched to a corresponding area of the proximal segment.[20]

Fig. 23-1 shows a traumatized ulnar nerve at the elbow of a 28-year-old male who forcibly struck his flexed elbow against the sharp edge of a 2-inch lead pipe. He noted immediate onset of numbness of the ring and little fingers, and profound weakness of grip and pinch. The initial skin laceration was treated in the emergency room and 2 weeks later I saw him for the first time for definitive management. The procedure was done under local anesthesia with supplementary analgesia. The plan was to isolate the ulnar nerve through a medial incision, to mobilize the injured segments of the nerve, and to determine if there was a grade IV lesion with interruption of conduction but with axon continuity with the nerve intact, or to determine if the nerve had been lacerated. The nerve was to be transferred anteriorly in order to gain length of approximately 2 cm, and the proximal and distal segments were to be mobilized so that the nerve suture could be done easily. Electrical stimulation was

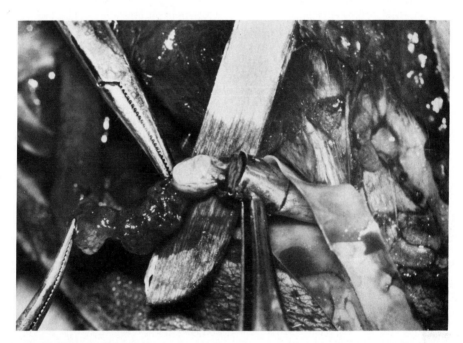

Fig. 23-2. "Nerve-holding" circular forceps is around the distal end of the nerve, and a right angle cut has been made through clearly defined fascicles. The proximal fascicles directly under the hemostat indicate that the nerve has been incised proximally to the fibrous neuroma. The remaining nerve defect was about 3 cm, which was measured with the elbow in extension, the arm away from the side, and the wrist in extension. This interval in the nerve was overcome by transposition of the nerve proximally and anteriorly by incision of the intermuscular septum and the surrounding fascia, and by mobilization of the distal segment by splitting of the fascia of the flexor carpi ulnaris and cutting of an articular branch of the ulnar nerve.

to be used in order to recognize the sensory fibers in the proximal fragment, and a distal dissection of the nerve was performed to recognize the offshooting motor fibers. Fig. 23-2 shows the proximal and distal segments being cut back to discrete fascicles. The epineurium was not removed, as I believe that epineurial suture, when possible, is preferable to funicular or fascicular suture. Also, the epineurium protects the funiculi from invasion by peripheral fibrous tissue.

The nerve was placed in the subcutaneous tissue rather than under the flexor muscle mass, as the latter has, in my experience, occasionally resulted in further compression of the ulnar nerve and increases the likelihood of injury to the motor branches of the flexor muscles. The flexor carpi ulnaris sheath was split 3 cm, so that angulation of the nerve distally was minimal. The intermuscular septum was incised so that the nerve was not compressed by this sharp edge, and the proximal restraining ligaments were not detected.

The technique of nerve repair included use of an ocular magnification of 3.5 times normal and sensory electrical stimulation of the proximal nerve, which was performed after excision of the proximal neuroma and distal fibroma using the nerve-holding forceps (Fig. 23-2). After electrical stimulation was completed and the sensory and motor fibers were oriented, a suture of 6-0 Ethibond was placed at a 12 o'clock position and a second at a 4 o'clock position (Fig. 23-3). Sutures of 7-0 nylon were placed in the epineurium so that wrinkling of the fascicles and excessive tightening would be avoided. The holding sutures were then switched, and the undersurface of the nerve was approximated with 7-0 nylon. During the placement of the sutures, a sharp probe was inserted between the nerve endings, so that any overlap would be obviated. The nerve was manipulated gently to avoid internal angulation of the fascicles.

A single layer of Surgicel, in addition to the subcutaneous fat, provides a biologic barrier from ingrowth of surrounding fibrous tissue, with less likelihood of adherence to the skin and muscle. After the nerve segments had been cut back, the 2½ cm defect, because of contraction of the proximal and distal segments, was made up easily by mobilization and transfer of the nerve anteriorly. Flexion of the elbow was used to eliminate any stress on the suture line. The amount of tension on the suture line could be easily tested by gentle and slow extension of the forearm. The elbow could be extended to plus 10 degrees before visible motion of the nerve occurred. The purpose of elbow flexion was to eliminate tension, to eliminate the force of gravity from the suture line, and to allow biologic healing to occur, in order to replace the holding strength of the sutures, which provide a temporary bond.

Even though there was no tension on this epineurial suture line, the patient was advised to avoid forceful stretch of the elbow for at least 6 weeks and to avoid a position of abduction of the shoulder, extension of the elbow, and forceful dorsiflexion of the wrist for at least 3 months.

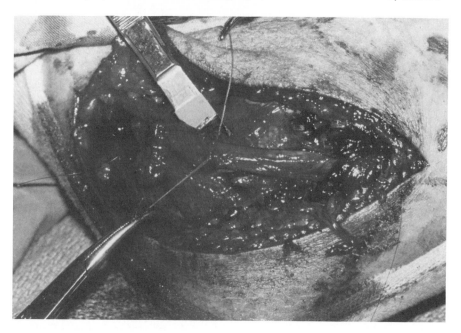

Fig. 23-3. Ulnar nerve has been transposed anteriorly and the proximal and distal segments have been mobilized. The 3 cm gap has been made up easily, and an end-to-end epineurial suture is being completed. The 5-0 Ethibond holding suture at 12 o'clock position was placed after configurational alignment was done by electrical stimulation. The second suture at 120 degrees in the clockwise direction was placed for epineurial fixation and congruous alignment. The proximal end was stimulated with the patient awake and with the nerve not affected by local anesthesia. *Sensory* alignment was possible in the proximal fragment by electrical stimulation, and in the distal fragment by dissecting out the outcropping of *motor* fibers. Stimulation of the distal nerve segment was not helpful because of the time period that had elapsed since the laceration. Recognition of the distal motor fibers by their anatomic location aided in reidentification of the sensory fascicles.

Figs. 23-4 and 23-5 show the position of the hand 14 months after nerve suture. The flexor digitorum profundus muscles to the ring, little, and one half of the long fingers had improved to a strength of 80% of normal (4/5 or G). The intrinsic muscles usually supplied by the ulnar nerve all showed evidence of clinical motion and action potentials by electromyography. The hypothenar muscles rated 40% of normal (fair minus) and were of sufficient strength to eliminate practically all of the claw deformity. The first dorsal interosseous muscle and the adductor muscle rated 35% of normal. Measurable pinch had increased from a preoperative pressure of 12 p.s.i. to 17 p.s.i., as compared to 28 p.s.i. on the normal side. Grip had progressed from 40 pounds preoperatively to 70 pounds, as compared to 100 pounds of the normal side. Sensory recovery on the dorsum and volar aspects of the forearm, hand, and ring and little fingers showed an even recovery with Tinel's sign having advanced at the rate of 1.5 mm per day, or 45 mm per month. The percussion test was out to the fingertips at about 9 months.

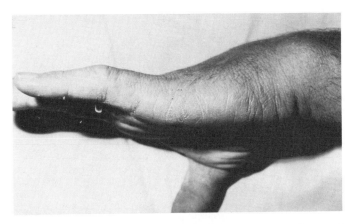

Fig. 23-4. Distance from the suture line to the fingertips was 45 cm. Regeneration occurred at a rate of 4 cm a month or approximately 2 mm a day. Percussion evidence of regeneration was evident within 2 weeks after nerve suture. The percussion test progressed distally at a steady speed, and motor regeneration followed with documentation by electromyography early and clinical detection of muscle action later. Extension of the fingers at 2 years after the high epineurial suture. The initial claw hand included wrist flexion of 30 degrees, metacarpophalangeal joint hyperextension of 45 degrees, and interphalangeal flexion of 50 degrees. As the strength of the intrinsic muscles increased, the claw appearance diminished and the pinch strengthened. The flexores digitorum profundi at 2 years were about 80% of normal. The ulnar innervated intrinsic muscles regained 60% of normal strength at 2 years and will continue to strengthen during the next 3 years. Early tendon transfer procedures were unnecessary. The patient has been working successfully as a plumber since 6 weeks after the operation.

Quantitative improvement occurs for the next 4 to 5 years, during which time all modalities of sensation improve and motor power continues to strengthen, so long as the pattern of improvement has been progressive and continuous. If early evidence of the percussion test (Tinel's sign) does not exist and if motor recovery of the forearm flexor muscles is not evident by clinical examination and electromyography within the first 6 months, then waiting for a longer period of time is not beneficial.

In an adult male doing manual work, this kind of recovery has been compatible with his occupation as a plumber and construction worker. Tendon transfers have not been necessary, fascicular suture was not done, nerve mobilization was used to provide appropriate approximation, and electrical stimulation did augment the concept of configurational alignment while the nerve ends were being united.

Preoperative determination of motor and sensory anomalous innervation is done by nerve block and by evoked potential with electrical stimulation. Accurate muscle testing is essential to provide a preoperative baseline of motor strength. Pinch testing, grip recordings, sensory examination, and vascular status aid in assessing the end result. Cold intolerance is defined for each patient.[5,8]

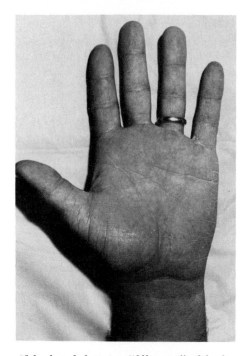

Fig. 23-5. Palm review of the hand showing "filling in" of the hypothenar muscles, skin lines, and skin markings, but incomplete adduction of the little finger against the ring finger. Sensory examination showed sweating, the presence of fingerprints, and the recognition of heat and cold. Two-point discrimination was greater than 10 mm but was improving slowly. Cold intolerance had diminished. Improvement would continue for at least 3 additional years. Tendon transfers would not be necessary.

Our experience at Duke University Medical Center during the last 30 years in the management of patients with peripheral nerve injuries has been that epineurial suture is performed when feasible. We have used magnifications of 2 to 6 times, careful cutback of nerve ends until good fascicles are evident, and liberal mobilization of proximal and distal nerve ends in order to unite most nerve interruptions. This method of repair continues to be our basic approach in the management of nerve injuries. Those nerve injuries associated with actual loss of nerve tissue caused by "blowout," stretch, or vascular infarct require nerve grafting or upper-extremity shortening to provide nerve continuity.

INHERENT ELASTICITY OF PERIPHERAL NERVES

There is an inherent elasticity in peripheral nerves, which is demonstrated by positioning of the extremity in abduction, external rotation of the shoulder, extension of the elbow, and dorsiflexion of the wrist and of the fingers. If the extremity is held in this position for several minutes, subjective tingling may occur in the fingertips. Gross motor weakness does not occur. Another example of biologic nerve stretch is noted in the loose-jointed individual who is able to extend the spine and place the elbows on the floor. The contortionist is able to roll up into a circle and stretch the femoral nerves and the median, ulnar, and radial nerves without motor or sensory damage. If the factor of compression is added, however, then sensory alteration recognized by paresthesias, hypesthesia, and dysesthesia indicate interruption of conduction. These changes are noted in the following: paresthesia in the thoracic-outlet syndrome with sagging of the shoulder and stretching of the neck in the opposite direction, weakness of the deltoid and external rotator muscles when the posterior shoulder girdle compresses the quadrilateral space, and paresthesia of the fingers with acute flexion of the elbow and wrist. These demonstrate the different mechanisms that affect conduction temporarily without alteration of the anatomy or proper function of the nerve.

The living model, observed hundreds of times, that demonstrates the potential of nerve stretch without causing motor or sensory alteration is in extremity-lengthening procedures. The upper extremity has been lengthened by placement of pins above and below an osteotomy done in the congenitally short ulna, and lengthening of the ulna at the rate of 1 mm a day for a total of as much as 25 mm has been possible. Complications have been nerve compression at a point where the ulnar nerve is tethered around the medial epicondyle of the humerus or at a point where the ulnar nerve enters the heavy fascia covering the origin of the flexor carpi ulnaris muscle. The median nerve may be affected by compression under the fascial origin of the flexor superficialis or by the lacertus fibrosus of the biceps muscle of the arm. The tethering or fixation points cause nerve damage, but if these are eliminated, the nerve can be stretched, provided that the elongation is done slowly.[13]

In the lower extremity the tibia has been lengthened at the rate of 1 to 2 mm a day, with the amount depending on the kind of lesion involved, on the age of the patient, and on the fixation of the peroneal and anterior tibial nerves by fascia around the proximal fibula and the interosseous membrane between the tibia and the fibula. The tibia has been lengthened numerous times, up to 5 cm, without evidence of nerve damage. This lengthening may represent up to 20% of the total length of the sciatic nerve components. Exploration of the peroneal nerve has been done in patients who develop pain and motor weakness during the lengthening and compression of the nerve by the fascia in the region of the head of the fibula, and the biceps tendon has accounted for the tethering rather than overstretching of the nerve.

As the tibia is lengthened, the foot is placed in the equinus position in order to allow more rapid separation of the tibia and fibula and elongation of the nerves, muscles, and blood vessels. After adequate lengthening of the bone has occurred, the foot is brought up gradually to right angles. This elevation of the foot over a period of several days demonstrates additional elongation of the elastic component of the nerves without development of motor weakness or sensory change.

The femur can be lengthened in a 10-year-old child 6 cm over a period of 30 days without evidence of motor or sensory loss. If the length of the sciatic nerve is considered to be 35 cm, an elongation of 20% of the nerve has been done without obvious sensory or motor loss.[12]

Experimental evidence suggests that a peripheral nerve can be lengthened slowly up to 20% of its total nerve length without damage, whereas rapid stretch done forcibly and quickly will interfere with nerve conduction, vascular supply, and membrane potential. Femoral lengthening has not been associated with nerve tethering as frequently as has tibial lengthening because of the anatomic arrangement and course of the sciatic nerve.

On the basis of our clinical experience in overcoming nerve defects (gaps) and in observing patients who have had ulnar, tibial, and femoral nerve lengthening, we conclude that nerve defects of 5 to 7 cm are safely made up by transfer of the nerve, by mobilization of the nerve from surrounding soft tissue, and by modest degrees of positioning of the extremity and joint flexion. Current literature implies that any defect over 2 cm should be grafted. *I disagree with this statement and have evidence to show both sensory and motor recovery in patients who have had 5 to 7 cm defects made up by multiple techniques that allow end-to-end suture under minimal tension but depend on slow elongation of the nerve after the suture line has matured.[12]*

MEASUREMENTS AND METHODS OF OVERCOMING NERVE DEFECTS (GAPS)

The goal after nerve repair is restoration of motor and sensory function so that it approaches the preinjury condition. The method of treatment selected must be weighed with the probable result. Our belief is that epineurial suture completed without excessive tension will provide the maximum degree of sensory and motor recovery. Nerve grafting done in lieu of mobilization and transfer of nerve and joint flexion may provide a similar result although statistics from the experimental study of Cabaud and Rodkey and McCarroll with short grafts showed no statistically significant difference.[2] Thus there are the disadvantages of taking a donor nerve graft, insertion of an avascular piece of tissue, the use of two suture lines, and the complete loss of orientation as the length of the defect increases.

To discuss methods of correcting a nerve defect, I must clarify the method of measuring the interval between proximal and distal end. The ulnar nerve defect illustrated in Fig. 23-1 was measured after the nerve ends were cut back to normal fascicles, with the nerve lying in its usual course prior to any proximal or distal mobilization and with the arm at the side, the elbow extended, the wrist in neutral position, and the fingers flexed. A fresh or an old nerve injury should be measured with a centimeter ruler in the same way.

Procedure for lacerated ends. A nerve that has been cleanly lacerated and examined within 48 hours after laceration will show separation of the nerve ends of at least 1 cm. These nerve segments can be mobilized minimally, cut back a millimeter or two on either side, and sutured easily and without tension by flexion of the wrist in order to relieve tension on the suture line while the sutures are being placed. Once the sutures are in place, the wrist may be returned to the zero-degree position without excess tension on the suture line. The suture material holds, and the nerve endings do not separate. In this instance, wrist flexion of 45 degrees is used to make up for the natural elastic retraction of the separated nerve ends and to eliminate any tension on the sutured ends, as well as to avoid sudden extension motion in the splint. Flexion of the elbow is also done to protect the proximal end of the nerve and to eliminate the action of gravity on the suture line. When the splint is removed at 2 weeks, the wrist can be gently extended about 20 degrees but the elbow remains flexed for an additional 2 weeks, or a total of 28 days. Elbow flexion is allowed at 21 days, as is wrist and finger flexion, but forcible extension is not allowed for 8 weeks. The patient gradually extends without force until the elbow and wrist are straight.

Procedure for fibrosis. If the nerve has been injured in an irregular fashion and internal and external fibrosis involve the proximal and distal segments, trimming of the nerve ends may require removal of 1 cm from the proximal and distal segments. This nerve gap may then measure 4 cm because of contraction of the nerve, peripheral fibrosis, and actual removal of 2 cm of nerve tissue. A 4 cm gap at the elbow does not require nerve grafting but can be made up by consideration of the following points.

1. *Elongation of intact nerve.* An intact nerve can be elongated up to 20% of its total length if done slowly and at the rate of 1 to 2 mm a day. If the ulnar nerve measures 62 cm from the axilla to the wrist, this nerve can tolerate 6 to 8 cm of lengthening if intact. Alternatives to stretching 1.5 mm a day are mobilization and transferal. (a) *Mobilization* of the ulnar nerve proximally to the anterior axillary crease will not interfere with the blood supply significantly. The remaining nerve, with its intrinsic blood supply, and with blood vessels coming in from segmental vascularization will certainly have proportionately more blood supply in view of the size of the nerve than will sural nerve grafts. Proximal mobilization will provide at least 1 cm of nerve elongation without excess tension. Distal mobilization of the ulnar nerve by releasing it at its entrance into the flexor carpi ulnaris and by cutting an intra-articular branch will provide an additional 1 cm elongation. (b) *Transferring both segments* anterior to the epicondyle subcutaneously and in a direct line from the upper arm to the upper forearm will give a relative elongation of 2 cm. The mobilization and the transfer will then make up the 4 cm defect measured with the elbow in extension and the wrist at neutral with the arm at the side.[12]

The nerve gap or defect has now been made up by maneuvers that are physiologic and compatible with good nerve regeneration and without dependence on excessive joint flexion to provide approximation.

2. *Flexion. Joint flexion* will diminish tension on the suture line for protective purposes and will also provide end-to-end epineurial anastomosis, after which the inherent elasticity of the nerve can be slowly and gently stretched during a prolonged protective postoperative period (3 months). *Wrist flexion* will allow the distal segment to be advanced proximally 1 cm. *Elbow flexion* will allow the proximal fragment to be advanced distally 1 cm. *Adduction* of the abducted arm to the side of the body will allow the proximal segment to be advanced distally 1 cm.

This information has been documented numerous times during the course of our experience with peripheral nerve injuries. It is reliable and compatible with a good result. The 10% to 20% inherent elasticity of nerves is considered when these figures are used as guidelines in view of the 1 to 2 mm a day stretch potential of a peripheral nerve, provided that tethering points are eliminated.

Nerve gaps per se are not made up by primarily flexing joints but rather by mobilization of proximal and distal segments, transferal of the nerves so that they run in a straight line, release of tethering points, and use of joint flexion to relieve tension on the sutured nerve so that fine suture material can be used, along with gradual elongation of the nerve during a 3-month period after repair so that the inherent elasticity provides elongation of the nerve rather than harmful stretch of the suture line and the existing nerve fibers. Recognition of the concept of inherent elasticity and the ways of using it are essential to the success of this method.[12]

Shortening of the forearm or humerus has diminished the nerve defect by 6 cm in the humerus and 4 cm in the forearm. This technique is valuable in the management of triple nerve injuries in the forearm with tissue loss, an isolated radial nerve injury associated with an open fracture, and loss of several centimeters of radial nerve. Also, in the attempt to reapproximate several branches of the brachial plexus after an injury involving several trunks or cords, the alternative may be 10 sural nerve grafts measuring 10 cm in length or a decrease of the nerve gap by shortening the humerus 5 cm and thereby shortening the length of the graft and in certain situations providing end-to-end anastomosis.[12]

Fig. 23-6 is the intraoperative appearance of a 34-year-old male who had a close-range .30-.30 rifle injury to the axilla. The attending surgeons inserted a 12 cm vein graft to replace the damaged axillary artery. This clotted within 8 hours and necessitated a second and later a third operative procedure. The muscles of the forearm and hand were intermittently ischemic for 12 to 14 hours at a time and permanent partial loss of function occurred in many muscle fibers. Several muscle specimens removed from the forearm and from the first dorsal interosseous muscle at the time of the delayed nerve repair showed irreversible muscle death in over 50% of the muscle fibers observed.

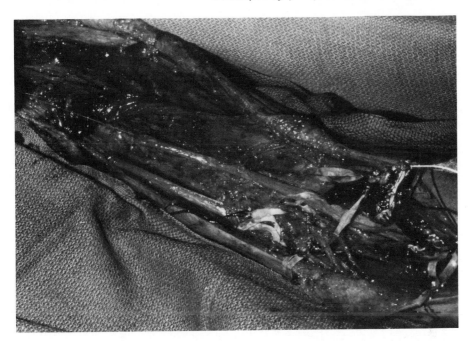

Fig. 23-6. This is the left arm during an operative procedure for management of a 34-year-old male who received a close range .30-.30 bullet wound that required a vein graft to replace the axillary artery and exploration of the axilla to repair median, ulnar, radial, and musculocutaneous nerves. Irreparable ischemia had affected over 50% of the forearm muscles and intrinsic muscles of the hand. The incision extends from the infraclavicular region to the wrist so that all nerves could be mobilized, each nerve could be redirected in a straight line from axilla to forearm, and fasciotomy of all forearm and arm muscles could be performed. The axilla is on the left, the elbow and distal nerve segments are on the right, and rubber tapes are around the individual nerves. The ulnar nerve has been transferred to the front of the medial condyle, and the median nerve has been transferred anterior to the pronator quadratus.

The actual loss of neural tissue was significant. After dissection of the distal segments of the brachial plexus, isolation of the vein graft, and mobilization of the proximal and distal segments of the median, ulnar, radial, and musculo-cutaneous nerves, the measurable defect in the peripheral nerves after mobilization and after cutting back proximal and distal segments but without application of traction to the nerve ends was 8 cm of median nerve, 7 cm of ulnar nerve, and 7 cm of radial nerve. With the arm at the side, the elbow flexed, and the wrist flexed, the remaining interval with minimal traction applied was 4 to 5 cm. The alternatives were three sural nerve grafts to each nerve with an average length of 7 cm for each segment or a total of about 63 cm of sural nerve. Muscle viability was compromised at least 50%, and nerve grafting in this situation was time consuming and unreliable.[12]

The second consideration was shortening of the humerus and insertion of a 4-hole inboard compression plate after removal of 5 cm of bone. This aspect

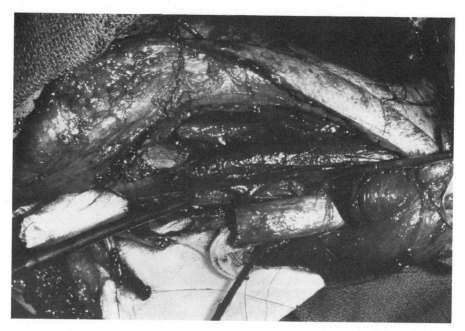

Fig. 23-7. Defect of about 7 cm was present in the median, ulnar, and radial nerves. In order to shorten the gap, a segment of the humeral shaft 5 cm long was removed from the midsection. After this was done, the proximal segment of the radial nerve was transposed from posterior to the humerus to a position anterior and medial to the humerus. The same realignment was done with the distal segment of the radial nerve, and when the elbow was flexed and the arm was placed at the side, the nerve ends could be brought together without tension. The white sponge is proximal, a bone hook is in the medullary canal over the proximal humeral shaft, the bone segment to be removed is in the center of the wound, and the long distal nerve segments have been mobilized for matching to the proximal nerves.

of the procedure required five additional minutes to expose the humerus and 20 minutes to apply the plate with the fixation screws. Fig. 23-7 shows the segment of humerus removed. After shortening of the humerus, the nerve gaps were reduced to 3 cm. This allowed relatively easy end-to-end anastomosis when the arm was adducted and when the elbow and wrist were flexed. After the nerves were sutured, the tension on the suture lines was minimal and the epineurial approximation using 7-0 nylon was sufficient to hold the nerve ends together without risk. Fig. 23-8 shows the appearance of the extremity after it was shortened. This patient has now been observed for 2 years. The musculo-cutaneous nerve has reinnervated the biceps and brachialis, the radial nerve shows 20% function in the brachioradialis and wrist extensors, the median demonstrates 20% function in the flexores digitorum profundi, and the ulnar nerve shows 30% action in the flexor carpi ulnaris and flexores digitorum profundi of the ring and little fingers. No intrinsic muscles are present and

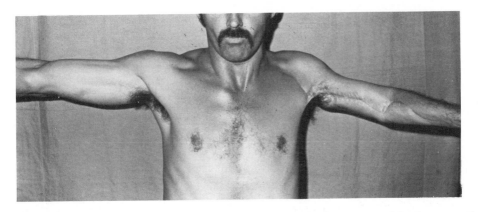

Fig. 23-8. Patient's extremity 2 years after the vein graft, shortening of the humerus 5 cm, and epineurial suture of the median, ulnar, and radial nerves. Sensory regeneration is in keeping with the advancing percussion test, which progressed at about 40 mm a month. Motor recovery was slower but has been progressing satisfactorily. The biceps muscle through the musculocutaneous has recovered to about 70% of normal. The forearm flexors and extensors are about 15% of normal. Muscle regeneration in the forearm and hand will be limited because of initial prolonged vascular insufficiency. I have used this technique since 1947. The motor and sensory recovery justify continued use of this concept of humeral shortening for epineurial suture without nerve graft or occasionally with nerve graft.

none are expected to recover because of the irreversible changes noted in muscle tissue attributable to the ischemia.

Sensory regeneration occurred at the rate of approximately 1 mm a day. At 24 months, the patient can recognize light touch, heat, cold, and pressure. Sweating is not present and two-point discrimination is greater than 20 mm in all digits. Fixed contractures of the finger flexors exist because of the fibrosis of muscles, and although splinting has been persistent and well tolerated by the patient, the fibrotic muscle tissue does not stretch easily. There are enough active motor fibers, however, to provide minimal function.

Several patients who have had humeral shortening have been observed for up to 20 years. Muscle action has not been compromised by the short humerus. There has been no functional or cosmetic problem related to the shortened extremity. I believe that this procedure should be considered in every instance where nerve tissue damage occurs at a high level in the arm or axilla so that end-to-end anastomosis can be accomplished in certain instances and shorter nerve grafts used in others.

Shortening of both bones of the forearm should always be considered when two or three nerve injuries have occurred and where neural tissue has been lost. Forearm bone shortening has been done in patients who have had damage to the dorsal and volar muscle mass and who have fixed flexion contractures of the fingers with little chance of improvement by tendon lengthening and tendon transfer. Alternatives such as vascular pedicle transfer of the gracilis muscle have been considered but shortening of both bones of the forearm, each 4 cm, has allowed end-to-end nerve repair, has diminished a contracture of musculotendinous units, and has made nerve grafting unnecessary.[12]

NERVE GRAFTING

Seddon and Brooks were moderately enthusiastic about nerve grafting around 1950. Instrumentation and suture material were inadequate to provide a consistently good result. Millesi reinitiated investigation with nerve grafting, and his technique has resulted in improvement of nerve regeneration by him and a few other investigators. The results, however, are not consistently dependable. Experimental work with nerve grafting is limited and inconclusive and the clinical assessment of the results has not been uniformly defined. Many factors affect the result of nerve grafting, and they are as follows:

1. Adequate passage of time is needed for regeneration. Three to 5 years must pass before a result is determined, even if the graft is done at the wrist or in the hand.
2. Full-thickness skin coverage is necessary, although subcutaneous tunneling has been described with questionable results.
3. The nerve graft and the proximal and distal segments of the nerve being grafted must have adequate vascular supply.
4. Stretch on the suture lines must be avoided.
5. Placement of the graft requires adequate magnification, small instrumentation, and small suture. The technique must be atraumatic. Alignment of the graft to corresponding fascicles is difficult or impossible, particularly if the gap is long.
6. The mechanism of revascularization is important.
7. Axon plasm must be stimulated by an intact anterior horn cell and must pass across both suture lines. Histologic studies have shown that the distal suture line causes more difficulty than does the proximal suture line. Thus, once the axons pass through the proximal junction, there may be difficulty in overcoming the distal junction. The concept that the distal suture line must be sectioned and redone has not been well documented. Detailed histologic examination of six patients who have had sural nerve grafts to the median and ulnar nerves show no evidence of axon regeneration through the grafts or the proximal or distal suture lines after 1 year.
8. In regard to the age of the patient, younger patients do show better clinical results than do older individuals.
9. The anatomic location of the nerve graft, that is, in the finger or at the wrist, the forearm, the arm, or the supraclavicular level, affects the results.

10. Nerve grafts show varying results as to motor recovery of a mild degree with no sensory recovery, or sensory improvement of a mild degree with no motor recovery. This is probably dependent on the congruity of the nerve graft with the proximal segment and the configurational alignment.

11. The complex rotational configuration prevents anatomic matching of the proximal and distal ends with the nerve graft.[26]

12. Anomalous motor and sensory innervation patterns, if present, do result in improved function that was not attributable to the nerve repair or the nerve graft.

Sensory recovery after nerve injury varies according to the kind of injury that has occurred. Overlap from adjacent sensory nerves does occur either because of ingrowth from peripheral nonmyelinated nerve fibers that have been injured but remain intact adjacent to the area of injury, or by peripheral sprouting of the injured nerve. For example, an abdominal flap placed on the foot will after 2 years acquire sufficient sensory endings to allow the patient to recognize sharp, dull, heat, and cold. Two-point discrimination is over 30 mm.

Since 1950 approximately 30 patients have had sural nerve or medial antebrachial cutaneous nerve grafts at Duke University Medical Center. Short segment grafts in the fingers or at the wrist for restoration of protective sensation have been reasonably successful. The patients have regained recognition of heat, cold, sharp, and dull, but two-point discrimination has been greater than 30 mm. Several nerve grafts were done to both median and ulnar nerves in the forearm in order to make up large nerve deficits that persisted even after immobilization and shortening. Minimal overall success resulted, and no motor recovery in the hand was observed and only moderate sensory recovery. The most satisfactory sensory grafts have been those done for pain associated with the superficial radial nerve. Patients who have had a 4 to 5 cm graft to satisfy the superficial radial nerve previously fibrosed or resected have had reasonably good results with partial pain relief about a year after insertion of the graft.

One patient with a 6 cm ulnar nerve gap was managed by three segments of sural nerve between the proximal and distal ends of the ulnar nerve. About 15 months later this patient showed 10% recovery of the hypothenar muscles, protective sensation with two-point discrimination greater than 30 mm along the course of the ulnar nerve, and no pain but significant cold intolerance. She continues to improve slowly but the result here will be rated as poor based on sensory regeneration and motor strength and functional recovery. Another patient with a high 3 cm radial nerve defect was grafted with 3 sural segments and after 2 years regained half of the normal strength in the wrist and finger extension muscles. *My experience at this time suggests that nerve grafting should be held in abeyance as a last resort rather than as the first choice.*

REFERENCES

1. Bora, W.: Repair of 7 cm nerve gap by mobilization and direct suture. Personal communication; course on peripheral nerves of the upper extremity, Durham, N.C., Sept. 14-16, 1978.
2. Cabaud, H. E., Rodkey, W. G., and McCarroll, H. R., Jr.: Experimental study—epineurial versus fascicular suture of lacerated nerves. Personal communication, Letterman Army Research Center, San Francisco, Calif., 1977.
3. Cameron, E. A., and French, E. B.: Saint Anthony's fire rekindled: gangrene due to therapeutic dose of ergotamine, Br. Med. J. **2:**28-30, 1960.
4. Clippinger, F. W., Goldner, J. L., and Roberts, J. M.: Use of the electromyograph in evaluating upper-extremity peripheral nerve lesions, J. Bone Joint Surg. **44-A:**1047-1060, 1962.
5. Gelberman, R. H., Urbaniak, J. R., Bright, D. S., and Levin, L. S.: Digital sensibility following replantation, J. Hand Surg. 3(4):313-319, July 1978.
6. Goldner, J. L.: Function of the hand following peripheral nerve injuries, American Academy of Orthopaedic Surgery instructional course lecture, Vol. X, 1953.
7. Goldner, J. L.: Peripheral nerve mapping, motor fibers, Durham, N.C., 1958-1978. Unpublished.
8. Goldner, J. L.: Anomalous innervation patterns of the hand and upper extremities, J. Bone Joint Surg. **48-A:**604, 1969.
9. Goldner, J. L., and Eguro, H.: Distribution of superficial radial nerve in 50 normal patients—observation, variations, pattern of sensation in the index and thumb. Durham, N.C. Unpublished data, 1971.
10. Goldner, J. L.: Sensory mapping of peripheral nerves in conjunction with geographic repair of lacerated nerves under local anesthesia, 1968-1974. Unpublished data.
11. Goldner, J. L., and Bright, D. S.: The effect of extremity blood flow on pain and cold tolerance. In Omer, G., and Spinner, M., editors: Management of peripheral nerve problems, Philadelphia, 1979, W. B. Saunders, Co.
12. Goldner, J. L.: Peripheral nerve gaps—alternates of treatment. Presented at Conference on peripheral nerves of the upper extremity, Duke University Medical Center and American Society for Surgery of the Hand, Durham, N.C., Sept. 14-16, 1978.
13. Goldner, J. L.: Volkmann's ischaemic contracture. In Flynn, J. E., editor: Hand surgery, ed. 2, Baltimore, 1975, The Williams & Wilkins Co.
14. Hakstian, R. W.: Funicular orientation by direct stimulation, J. Bone Joint Surg. **50-A:**1178-1186, 1968.
15. Kline, D.: Evoked action potentials as an aid to peripheral nerve repair. Personal communication; Conference on peripheral nerves of the upper extremity, Duke University Medical Center and American Society for Surgery of the Hand, Durham, N.C., Sept. 14-16, 1978.
16. Lyons, W. R., and Woodhall, B.: Atlas of peripheral nerve injuries, Philadelphia, 1949, W. B. Saunders Co.
17. Millesi, H.: The interfascicular nerve-grafting of the median and ulnar nerves, J. Bone Joint Surg. **54-A:**727-750, 1972.
18. Mitchell, S. W.: Injuries of the nerves and their consequences, Philadelphia, 1872, J. B. Lippincott Co.
19. Narakas, A.: Brachial plexus injuries—operative treatment. Conference on peripheral nerves of the upper extremity, Duke University Medical Center and American Society for Surgery of the Hand, Durham, N.C., Sept. 14-16, 1978.
20. Nashold, B. S., Goldner, J. L., Bright, D. S., Mullen, J., and Meyer, P.: Topography

of sensory and motor fasciculi in human median and sciatic nerves determined by electrical stimulation. Presented at American Association of Neurological Surgeons, annual meeting, Toronto, April 24-28, 1968.

21. Omer, G.: Personal communication. Conference on peripheral nerves of the upper extremity, Duke University Medical Center and American Society for Surgery of the Hand, Durham, N.C., Sept. 14-16, 1978.
22. Seddon, H. J.: The use of autogenous grafts for the repair of large gaps in peripheral nerves, Br. J. Surg. **35:**151-167, 1947.
23. Seddon, H. J.: Nerve grafting, J. Bone Joint Surg. **45-B:**447-461, August 1963.
24. Smith, J. W.: Factors influencing nerve repair. I. Blood supply to peripheral nerves, Arch. Surg. **93:**335-341, 1966.
25. Spinner, M.: Injuries to the major branches of peripheral nerves of the forearm, ed. 2, Philadelphia, 1978, W. B. Saunders Co.
26. Sunderland, S.: Observations on the treatment of traumatic injuries of peripheral nerves, Br. J. Surg. **35:**36-42, July 1947.
27. Sunderland, S.: Nerves and nerve injury, Baltimore, 1968, The Williams & Wilkins Co.
28. Tarlov, I. M.: Plasma clot suture of peripheral nerves and nerve roots, Springfield, Ill., 1950, Charles C Thomas, Publisher.
29. Woodhall, B., and Lyons, W. R.: Peripheral nerve injuries: the results of "early nerve suture." A preliminary report, Surgery **19:**757-789, 1946.
30. Woodhall, B., and Beebe, G. W.: Peripheral nerve regeneration. VA Medical Monograph, 26 June 1956, Superintendent of Documents, U.S. Government Printing Office, Washington, 25, D.C.

GENERAL DISCUSSION

Dr. Goldner: When does the budding start? Jack, do you want to talk about that?

Dr. Tupper: Microscopically it starts about 14 days to 21 days and each axon buds, depending on who you read, as many as 50 to 500 buds. According to the theory the bud that finds its way into the correct sheath distally is the one that hypertrophies; the others die off. There is a lot of buddings; that's the basis behind Drucker's theory that you get your best regeneration at 14 to 21 days.

Dr. Goldner: We had a panel at the American Society for Surgery of the Hand about 4 or 5 years ago, and we had a physiologist who had tissue cultures showing nerve budding. In some instances, depending on the animal, it occurs at 3 days and in others at 5 days. I don't know when the human budding begins, but it is relatively soon.

Question: Would there be any benefit to surrounding nerve anastomoses or neurolyses with Gelfoam or fat graft? Does anybody use these?

Dr. Goldner: I wrote an article in 1953 on tendon repair and we did some nerve repairs also with Gelfoam. We did find that Gelfoam was beneficial in preventing external fibrosis but not in improving internal regeneration. I still use Surgicel, and when I finish a nerve I wrap a piece of Surgicel around it. I feel better when I do it. I cover the suture line so I can't see it. It turns dark when it bleeds. When I have gone back to do a tendon repair at 4 to 6 weeks, for whatever the reason is, I believe the nerve peels off a little bit better.

Both Dr. Bright and Dr. Urbaniak have also used silicone just to piece under the nerve prior to doing a permanent repair. If you are doing a secondary excision or doing some bone or tendon work, and you're not ready to do the nerve repair, you may mobilize things by putting a piece of silicone under it. When you come back in a few weeks, that nerve just falls right out and it doesn't adhere to surrounding tissue. Don, do you want to comment on this?

Dr. Bright: We may use the silicone just on one side now and the Gelfoam as you mentioned.

Dr. Goldner: On what stimulator do you use the so-called special tips for nerve or fascicular recordings of evoked action potentials?

Dr. Bright: We use the Grass stimulator. They have several models. We use their medium model with the Grass isolation unit. The stimulator tips come from Avery Company. They produce small probes that are shielded all the way down to the tips. They must have special care if they are going to work. The neurophysiologist uses glass tips; they blow their own. Jack, do you have any comment about the electrode tips?

Dr. Tupper: The physiologists have voltage clamps. They are very small, and they can actually invade the single cell with tips that are available.

Dr. Goldner: Green or blue marking solution may help in identifying the fascicles. If the tourniquet is up and you cut the nerve, if you'll paint a little green over it, you may see the perineurium better. The bundles of similar sizes and shapes may then be matched a little easier than when you are just looking at a yellow surface that doesn't have any bleeding on it.

Dr. Goldner: Dr. Tupper, in replantations, if bone is not shortened and vein grafts are required, are primary nerve grafts done at this sitting?

Dr. Tupper: No, they are too much work.

Dr. Tupper: Dr. Goldner, you mentioned in your talk that you used magnification in clubfoot surgery.

Dr. Goldner: Yes, you have to see the posterior tibial nerve, the branch to the calcaneous, the posterior tibial vessel and branches, the various layers of the deltoid ligaments, and so on. If you have about a 3-power magnification and use the small Beaver blade and small instruments, you do a much less traumatic job than if you don't use any magnification.

Your associate may be only 30 years old and sees better; if you've got your glasses on and he doesn't have any on, then you will see better. We have rules here when we are doing small or precise surgery; for example, the person who puts the tourniquet on is the one who gets to do the case. Now that makes them get there ahead of you. Secondly, if they don't have their loupes, there is a question of whether they get to operate. This kind of keeps them on their toes.

Index